Treatment of Movement Disorders

Editor

JOSEPH JANKOVIC

NEUROLOGIC CLINICS

www.neurologic.theclinics.com

Consulting Editor
RANDOLPH W. EVANS

May 2020 • Volume 38 • Number 2

ELSEVIER

1600 John F. Kennedy Boulevard • Suite 1800 • Philadelphia, Pennsylvania, 19103-2899

http://www.theclinics.com

NEUROLOGIC CLINICS Volume 38, Number 2
May 2020 ISSN 0733-8619, ISBN-13: 978-0-323-70991-0

Editor: Stacy Eastman
Developmental Editor: Donald Mumford

Neurologic Clinics (ISSN 0733-8619) is published quarterly by Elsevier Inc., 360 Park Avenue South, New York, NY 10010–1710. Months of issue are February, May, August, and November. Periodicals postage paid at New York, NY, and additional mailing offices. Subscription prices are $326.00 per year for US individuals, $696.00 per year for US institutions, $100.00 per year for US students, $408.00 per year for Canadian individuals, $843.00 per year for Canadian institutions, $427.00 per year for international individuals, $843.00 per year for international institutions, $210.00 for foreign students/residents, and $100.00 for Canadian students/residents. To receive student/resident rate, orders must be accompanied by name of affiliated institution, date of term, and the *signature* of program/residency coordinator on institution letterhead. Orders will be billed at individual rate until proof of status is received. Foreign air speed delivery is included in all *Clinics* subscription prices. All prices are subject to change without notice. **POSTMASTER:** Send address changes to *Neurologic Clinics*, Elsevier Health Sciences Division, Subscription Customer Service, 3251 Riverport Lane, Maryland Heights, MO 63043. **Customer Service: Telephone: 1-800-654-2452 (U.S. and Canada); 314-447-8871 (outside U.S. and Canada). Fax: 314-447-8029. E-mail: journalscustomerservice-usa@elsevier.com (for print support); journalsonlinesupport-usa@elsevier.com (for online support).**

Reprints. For copies of 100 or more of articles in this publication, please contact the Commercial Reprints Department, Elsevier Inc., 360 Park Avenue South, New York, New York, 10010-1710; Tel.: +1-212-633-3874; Fax: +1-212-633-3820, and E-mail: reprints@elsevier.com.

Neurologic Clinics is also published in Spanish by Nueva Editorial Interamericana S.A., Mexico City, Mexico.

Neurologic Clinics is covered in *Current Contents/Clinical Medicine, MEDLINE/PubMed (Index Medicus), EMBASE/Excerpta Medica, and PsycINFO, and ISI/BIOMED.*

Contributors

CONSULTING EDITOR

RANDOLPH W. EVANS, MD
Clinical Professor, Department of Neurology, Baylor College of Medicine, Houston, Texas, USA

EDITOR

JOSEPH JANKOVIC, MD
Professor of Neurology, Distinguished Chair in Movement Disorders, Director, Parkinson's Disease Center and Movement Disorders Clinic, Department of Neurology, Baylor College of Medicine, Baylor St. Luke's Medical Center at the McNair Campus, Houston, Texas, USA

AUTHORS

HASSAAN H. BASHIR, MD
Fellow, Department of Neurology, Baylor College of Medicine, Parkinson's Disease Center and Movement Disorders Clinic, Houston, Texas, USA

KAILASH P. BHATIA, FRCP, MD
Professor, Department of Clinical and Movement Neurosciences, Queen Square Institute of Neurology, University College London, London, United Kingdom

JEFF M. BRONSTEIN, MD, PhD
Professor, Fred Silton Family Chair in Movement Disorders, Department of Neurology, David Geffen School of Medicine at UCLA, Los Angeles, California, USA

ERIC M. CHIN, MD
Fellow in Neurodevelopmental Disabilities, Department of Neurology and Developmental Medicine, Kennedy Krieger Institute, Baltimore, Maryland, USA

ANDREW FEIGIN, MD
Professor, Department of Neurology, NYU Langone Health, Marlene and Paolo Fresco Institute for Parkinson's and Movement Disorders, New York, New York, USA

JENNIFER G. GOLDMAN, MD, MS
Section Chief, Parkinson's Disease and Movement Disorders, Shirley Ryan AbilityLab, Professor, Departments of Physical Medicine and Rehabilitation and Neurology, Northwestern University Feinberg School of Medicine, Chicago, Illinois, USA

CARLOS MANUEL GUERRA, MD, MSc
Head of PRISMA Advanced Center for Parkinson, Movement Disorders and Dementia, San Luis Potosi, Professor of Cognition and Behavior, Faculty of Psychology, Autonomous University of San Luis Potosi, San Luis Potosi, Mexico

HILARY E. GWYNN, MD
Assistant, Department of Neurology and Developmental Medicine, Kennedy Krieger Institute, Baltimore, Maryland, USA

ALEXANDER H. HOON Jr, MD, MPH
Director, Phelps Center for Cerebral Palsy and Neurodevelopmental Medicine, Associate Professor, Department of Neurology and Developmental Medicine, Kennedy Krieger Institute, Baltimore, Maryland, USA

JOSEPH JANKOVIC, MD
Professor of Neurology, Distinguished Chair in Movement Disorders, Director, Parkinson's Disease Center and Movement Disorders Clinic, Department of Neurology, Baylor College of Medicine, Baylor St. Luke's Medical Center at the McNair Campus, Houston, Texas, USA

JOOHI JIMENEZ-SHAHED, MD
Medical Director, Movement Disorders Neuromodulation and Brain Circuit Therapeutics, Associate Professor, Neurology and Neurosurgery, Icahn School of Medicine at Mount Sinai, New York, New York, USA

H.A. JINNAH, MD, PhD
Professor, Departments of Neurology, and Human Genetics, Emory University School of Medicine, Atlanta, Georgia, USA

SHENG-HAN KUO, MD
Division of Movement Disorders, Assistant Professor, Department of Neurology, Columbia University Irving Medical Center, New York, New York, USA

KIMBERLY TSU KWEI, MD, PhD
Fellow, Division of Movement Disorders, Department of Neurology, Columbia University Irving Medical Center, New York, New York, USA

KATHRIN LAFAVER, MD
Associate Professor, Department of Neurology, Northwestern University Feinberg School of Medicine, Chicago, Illinois, USA

ANNA LATORRE, MD, PhD
Department of Clinical and Movement Neurosciences, Queen Square Institute of Neurology, University College London, London, United Kingdom

PHILIPP MAHLKNECHT, MD, PhD
Department of Neurology, Medical University Innsbruck, Innsbruck, Austria

KYLE T. MITCHELL, MD
Duke University Movement Disorders Center, Durham, North Carolina, USA

CAITLIN MULLIGAN, MD
Assistant Clinical Professor, Department of Neurosciences, University of California, San Diego, La Jolla, California, USA

WILLIAM GEORGE ONDO, MD
Director, Movement Disorders-Methodist Neurological Center, Professor of Neurology, Weill Cornell Medical School, Houston, Texas, USA

JILL L. OSTREM, MD
UCSF Movement Disorders and Neuromodulation Center, San Francisco, California, USA

WERNER POEWE, MD
Department of Neurology, Medical University Innsbruck, Innsbruck, Austria

SHENANDOAH ROBINSON, MD
Professor, Department of Neurosurgery, Johns Hopkins University School of Medicine, Baltimore, Maryland, USA

CHRISTINE M. STAHL, MD
Clinical Assistant Professor, Department of Neurology, NYU Langone Health, Marlene and Paolo Fresco Institute for Parkinson's and Movement Disorders, New York, New York, USA

ARJUN TARAKAD, MD
Assistant Professor, Department of Neurology, Parkinson's Disease Center and Movement Disorders Clinic, Baylor College of Medicine, Houston, Texas, USA

Contents

This article reviews scales that have been developed for, validated in, and/ or frequently used across multiple movement disorders with a focus on assessment of motor and nonmotor symptoms of Parkinson disease. Rating scales used in other disease states include those for essential tremor, dystonia (generalized dystonia, cervical dystonia, and blepharospasm), Tourette syndrome, Huntington disease, tardive dyskinesia, Wilson disease, ataxia, and functional movement disorders. Key features of each scale as well as cited criticisms and limitations of each scale are also discussed. Lastly, the article briefly discusses the emerging role of digital assessment tools (both wearable devices and digital interface applications).

The cardinal motor features of Parkinson disease (PD) are driven by striatal dopamine deficiency. Pharmacologic dopamine substitution is the mainstay of drug treatment of PD. Levodopa is still the most efficacious drug to treat PD motor symptoms. MAO-B inhibitors and dopamine agonists are useful options. The main limitation of levodopa is the development of motor response fluctuations and drug-induced dyskinesias. Adjunct MAO-B and COMT inhibitors as well as dopamine agonists and continuous infusions of levodopa intestinal gel or subcutaneous apomorphine are efficacious in reducing motor fluctuations and amantadine is the only drug with established efficacy in reducing dyskinesias.

Parkinson disease (PD) is well recognized by its motor features of bradykinesia, tremor, rigidity, and gait and balance difficulties. However, PD is also characterized by a myriad of nonmotor symptoms, which may occur even before motor symptoms, early in the course of disease, and throughout the advancing disease. These nonmotor symptoms span multiple different systems, invoke multiple different neurotransmitters, and require multiple strategies for treatment including pharmacologic and nonpharmacologic interventions and, often, multiple different disciplines. This article discusses symptoms, assessments, and therapeutics for the nonmotor symptoms of PD including those affecting mood, cognition, behavior, sleep, autonomic function, and sensory systems.

Kyle T. Mitchell and Jill L. Ostrem

Surgery in Parkinson disease is effective for a select group of patients when optimal medical management is not sufficient. Functional neurosurgery can be used as either a salvage therapy in patients with disabling symptoms or to maintain quality of life and independence before progression to severe disability in high-functioning patients. With recent technological advancements in imaging and targeting as well as novel neuromodulation paradigms, there are numerous options for targeted brain lesions and deep brain stimulation. Surgical decision making and postoperative management in Parkinson disease therefore often requires a multidisciplinary team effort with neurology, neurosurgery, neuropsychology, and psychiatry.

William George Ondo

Established medications that improve tremor include beta-adrenergic antagonists, primidone, topiramate, and ethanol. Less consistent efficacy is reported with many other medications, usually antiepileptic drugs. A number of investigational medications, including T-type calcium channel blockers and allosteric gamma-aminobutyric acid-A modulators, are being developed for tremor. Deep brain stimulation techniques continues to be refined and focused ultrasound thalamotomy now offers an incisionless surgical option. Finally a number of peripheral electrical and mechanical devices are under development for tremor.

H.A. Jinnah

The dystonias are a large and heterogenous group of disorders characterized by excessive muscle contractions leading to abnormal postures and/or repetitive movements. Their clinical manifestations vary widely, and there are many potential causes. Despite the heterogeneity, helpful treatments are available for the vast majority of patients. Symptom-based therapies include oral medications, botulinum toxins, and surgical interventions. For some subtypes of dystonia, specific mechanism-based treatments are available. Advances in understanding the biological basis for many types of dystonia have led to numerous recent clinical trials, so additional treatments are likely to become available in the very near future.

Joohi Jimenez-Shahed

Tourette syndrome is a complex neuropsychiatric disorder with a wide phenotypic spectrum, including tics and psychiatric comorbidities, such as obsessive-compulsive disorder and attention-deficit disorder. Often considered a neurodevelopmental disorder, it is most prevalent during childhood and treatment strategies can vary according to degree of severity and patient-specific symptom manifestations. This review focuses on established and emerging management options for tics, including behavioral interventions and nonpharmacologic therapies, medication management, and promising surgical approaches.

Huntington disease, a neurodegenerative disease characterized by progressive motor, behavioral, and cognitive decline, is caused by a CAG trinucleotide repeat expansion in the huntingtin gene on chromosome 4. Current treatments target symptom management because there are no disease-modifying therapies at this time. Investigation of RNA-based and DNA-based treatment strategies are emerging and hold promise of possible future disease-modifying therapy.

Tardive dyskinesia (TD) is an iatrogenic condition that encompasses a wide phenomenological spectrum of movement disorders caused by exposure to dopamine receptor blocking agents (DRBAs). TD may cause troublesome or disabling symptoms that impair quality of life. Due to frequent, often inappropriate, use of DRBAs, TD prevalence rates among patients exposed to DRBAs continue to be high. The judicious use of DRBAs is key to the prevention of TD, reduction of disease burden, and achieving lasting remission. Dopamine-depleting vesicular monoamine transporter type 2 inhibitors are considered the treatment of choice of TD.

Cerebral palsy is the most common cause of childhood motor disability, affecting 2 to 3/1000 children worldwide. Clinical abnormalities in tone, posture, and movement are the result of brain dysgenesis or injury early in life, and impairment varies in type, distribution, and in severity. The underlying brain disorder may also lead to other associated neurologic and systemic impairments. Variability in functional impairments, which can change during development, necessitates an individualized treatment plan. Treatment options are primarily symptomatic and directed toward optimizing independence, function, and/or ease of care—while limiting side effects. New promising disease-preventing and modifying treatments are emerging.

Wilson's disease is one of the few preventable movement disorders in which there are therapies that modify disease progression. This disease is caused by copper overload caused by reduced copper excretion secondary to genetic mutations in the ATP7B gene. Copper overload can lead to a variety of clinical presentations, including neurologic symptoms, liver failure, and/or psychiatric manifestations. There is often a delay in diagnosis of Wilson disease, and awareness of the diagnosis and management is important because of the treatable nature of this condition. This article reviews the clinical presentation, epidemiology, genetics, pathophysiology, diagnosis, and management of Wilson disease.

Paroxysmal dyskinesia (PxD) is a heterogeneous group of syndromes characterized by attacks of abnormal movements (dystonic, choreic, ballistic), triggered by detectable factors, without loss of consciousness. According to the precipitating factors, they are classified as paroxysmal kinesigenic dyskinesia (PKD), paroxysmal non-kinesigenic dyskinesia (PNKD), and paroxysmal exercise-induced dystonia (PED); mostly due to a genetic defect in the PRRT, PNKD (MR-1) and SLC2A1 gene respectively. PxD treatment is based on the combination of non-pharmacological and pharmacological approaches. While PKD has an exquisite response to antiepileptic drugs, in PNKD and PED the symptoms can be controlled by avoiding precipitating factors. Pharmacological and other non-pharmacological treatments are also available for PNKD and PED. In PxD refractory to conventional treatment, surgery might be a treatment option. In PRRT2-PKD and MR-1-PNKD treatment might not be needed with advancing age.

Cerebellar ataxia can be caused by a variety of disorders, including degenerative processes, autoimmune and paraneoplastic illness as well as by gene mutations inherited in autosomal dominant, autosomal recessive, or X-linked fashions. In this review, we highlight the treatments for cerebellar ataxia in a systematic way, to provide guidance for clinicians who treat patients with cerebellar ataxia. In addition, we review therapies currently under development for ataxia, which we feel is currently one of the most exciting fields in neurology.

Functional movement disorders (FMD) are commonly seen in neurologic practice and frequent sources of disability. Patients may present with tremor, weakness, dystonia, jerking movements, abnormal gait and speech, often combining several movement phenomenologies. Associated symptoms include chronic pain, depression, and anxiety. Treatment of FMD begins with an explanation of the diagnosis and needs to be tailored to patients' symptoms and comorbidities. There may be benefit from multidisciplinary treatment, including physical, occupational, and speech therapy, as well as psychotherapeutic interventions, especially cognitive behavioral therapy. The role for neuromodulation such as transmagnetic stimulation in FMD treatment requires further research.

NEUROLOGIC CLINICS

RELATED SERIES

Neuroimaging Clinics
Psychiatric Clinics
Child and Adolescent Psychiatric Clinics

THE CLINICS ARE AVAILABLE ONLINE!
Access your subscription at:
www.theclinics.com

Preface

Treatment of Movement Disorders

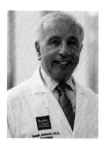

Joseph Jankovic, MD
Editor

Movement disorders are a group of neurologic conditions characterized phenomeno-logically by slowness and paucity of movement (hypokinetic disorders) or abnormal excessive involuntary movements (hyperkinesias). The hypokinetic movement disorders are exemplified by Parkinson disease and other parkinsonian disorders. Hyperkinetic movement disorders include tremors, dystonia, tics, chorea, athetosis, ballism, stereotypy, and akathisia. Ataxia, gait disorders, and spasticity are also often included among movement disorders. While the basal ganglia and their connections have been implicated in the pathophysiology of most of the movement disorders, some are caused by altered peripheral input as exemplified by hemifacial spasm and other peripherally induced movement disorders. A subset of movement disorders with varied phenomenology is caused by psychological factors, hence referred to in the past as "psychogenic" movement disorder in contrast to "organic" movement disorders. More recently adopted terminology, however, favors the term "functional" as this is less stigmatizing than "psychogenic," although many patients with this group of disorders perceive themselves as "dysfunctional."

Once considered primarily a diagnostic subspecialty of neurology, relying chiefly on phenomenology in making the diagnosis, movement disorders have evolved into one of the most therapeutically oriented areas of neurology. This transformation is largely due to better understanding of the pathogenesis and pathophysiology of movement disorders, advances in neuropharmacology and neurosurgical therapies, and improvements in designs of clinical trials that have led to the generation of evidence-based data on the efficacy and safety or therapeutic interventions. It is important to point out, however, that although physicians generally aspire to apply evidence-based medicine in clinical practice, this is not always possible. There are many reasons for this discrepancy, including the fact that most patients for whom we prescribe medications would not qualify for the original studies that led to their approval by the Food and Drug Administration, because they would not satisfy the inclusion-exclusion criteria due to

Neurol Clin 38 (2020) xiii–xiv
https://doi.org/10.1016/j.ncl.2020.03.001
0733-8619/20/© 2020 Published by Elsevier Inc.

demographic characteristics, comorbidities, concomitant medications, and other reasons.

In planning this special issue, I carefully considered and eventually selected what I consider are the most important current topics and invited the best experts to provide comprehensive, balanced, and authoritative reviews. I am pleased that I was able to assemble the most outstanding and renowned experts in the field. The authors were encouraged to provide the most up-to-date reviews and submit as many figures, treatment algorithms, and tables as possible to enhance the clinical and scientific value of each article. In addition, the authors were instructed to highlight the most important aspects in "Key Points."

This comprehensive issue, which includes 14 different topics, should be of interest not only to neurologists who are asked to evaluate and treat patients with Parkinson disease and other movement disorders but also to other clinicians, physiatrists, neurosurgeons, clinical investigators, as well as basic neuroscientists.

One of the many reasons why all invited authors accepted the challenge to provide the comprehensive and well-balanced reviews is that *Neurologic Clinics* is a well-established and prestigious brand of scientific and clinical publication. Furthermore, a unique feature of *Neurologic Clinics* is that the issues are not only viewed as books but also as collections of articles, cited in PubMed.

I wish to thank all the authors for their scholarly and timely contributions. I also wish to thank the editorial staff of Elsevier, particularly Donald Mumford, Senior Developmental Editor, for their professionalism and hard work. I also thank my colleague, friend, and tennis partner, Randolph Evans, MD, the consulting editor, who inspired this issue. Finally, I wish to express my deep appreciation to my wife, Cathy, for her support throughout this project and over the many decades of our shared lives.

Joseph Jankovic, MD
Professor of Neurology, Distinguished Chair in Movement Disorders, Director
Parkinson's Disease Center and Movement Disorders Clinic
Department of Neurology
Baylor College of Medicine
Baylor St. Luke's Medical Center at the McNair Campus
7200 Cambridge, 9th Floor, Suite 9A
Houston, TX 77030-4202, USA

E-mail address:
josephj@bcm.edu

Website:
http://www.jankovic.org

Clinical Rating Scales and Quantitative Assessments of Movement Disorders

Arjun Tarakad, MD

KEYWORDS

- Rating scales • Parkinson disease • Essential tremor • Dystonia
- Huntington disease • Wearables

KEY POINTS

- Rating scales are crucial for objective and standardized assessment of disease state, which is of particular importance when testing interventions in clinical trials.
- A vast number of rating scales are used across disease states as well as those developed for evaluation within specific diseases.
- Appropriate clinimetric testing for reliability, validity, and sensitivity to change are crucial when selecting appropriate scales to use in a given disease state.
- Digital assessment tools are a fast developing segment of objective assessments although standardization and validation against clinical assessments remain limiting factors in their use.

INTRODUCTION

When discussing disease states both in clinical and research contexts, objective quantification of symptoms is important to assess disease severity, progression, and response to treatment. The use of rating scales helps standardize examination findings and allows for comparison of a disease state across patients evaluated by different clinicians and sites. Within the specialty of movement disorders, clinical examination and phenomenology are of greater importance, given the general lack of physiologic, radiographic, serologic, or other biomarkers for most disease states. Clinical rating scales are of particular value in such cases. Successful rating scales require good reliability and reproducibility between raters, demonstrable validity in the disease state that they are monitoring, and sensitivity to change when tracking disease progression or disease interventions. Because of the extremely large number of rating scales developed and used across movement disorders, this review focuses on those scales most frequently used for and validated in the diseases discussed with

Department of Neurology, Parkinson's Disease Center and Movement Disorders Clinic, Baylor College of Medicine, 7200 Cambridge Street Suite 9A, Houston, TX 77030, USA
E-mail address: tarakad@bcm.edu

Neurol Clin 38 (2020) 231–254
https://doi.org/10.1016/j.ncl.2019.12.001
0733-8619/20/© 2020 Elsevier Inc. All rights reserved.

neurologic.theclinics.com

a focus on Parkinson disease (PD) as detailed in **Table 1** and other common movement disorders **(Table 2)**.

SCALES IN PARKINSON DISEASE

PD presents numerous challenges when developing rating scales due to its heterogeneous presentation, variable progression, and wide constellation of potential symptoms.

Comprehensive and Motor Scales

Several comprehensive scales have been developed, with the Unified Parkinson's Disease Rating Scale (UPDRS) and the revised version, the Movement Disorders Society Unified Parkinson's Disease Rating Scale (MDS-UPDRS), being best known and most widely used.[1,2] The UPDRS has 4 main sections with both physician- and patient-derived parts: part I for mentation, behavior, and mood; part II for activities of daily living; part III for motor symptoms; and part IV for complications. Overall scores and parts II and III subscores have demonstrated good interrater reliability, with defined minimal clinically important difference (MCID) in scores when assessing disease state, although assessment of specific items (speech and facial immobility) as well as part IV testing may be less reliable.[3–5] Other criticisms for this scale have included ambiguous text anchors and instructions, as well as limitations in assessment of nonmotor symptoms.[6] The MDS-UPDRS was developed in the early 2000s to address limitations with the original UPDRS, with the final version being released after supported clinimetric testing in 2008.[2] Significant changes included more clearly defined anchors, with all items being rated on a 0 to 4 scale and a greater focus on milder impairment and disability scores.[7] The MDS-UPDRS showed high correlations with the UPDRS in clinimetric testing,[2] also has defined MCID values, and has validated versions across other languages.[8–13]

Because of the lengthy administration time needed for the UPDRS and MDS-UPDRS, more recently, the Parkinson's Disease Composite Scale (PDCS) was used as a tool for more rapid evaluation that takes into account motor and nonmotor symptoms as well as treatment complications in PD.[14] It has been validated against the MDS-UPDRS, although consistency in some sections has been drawn into question.[14,15]

The Unified Dyskinesia Rating Scale (UDysRS) is a 4-part scale developed specifically to comprehensively rate dyskinesias in PD. Part I and II cover patient reported "On" and "Off" dyskinesia-associated disability. Part III is clinician-rated dyskinesia severity across 7 body regions and is based off the Abnormal Involuntary Movement Scale (AIMS) discussed in the tardive dyskinesia section of this article. Part IV is an objective disability rating based on the clinician-rated segment.[16] The scale has shown good reliability, stability across different "On" and "Off" states, defined MCID values for parts I and II, and has been translated into several other languages.[16–21]

The Parkinson's Disease Quality of Life Questionnaire has both a 39-question (PDQ-39) and a shorter 8-question (PDQ-8) version with questions across domains of mobility, emotional well-being, stigma, social support, cognition, communication, and bodily discomfort.[22] It has shown strong correlation with MDS-UPDRS parts I and II and has been widely translated and validated in multiple countries.[23–29]

The Hoehn and Yahr scale (HY), is a widely used scale in PD, which stratifies disability and impairment across 5 stages.[30] Strengths of this scale include its quick, simple, and reproducible rating, whereas criticisms include the lack of distinction between disability and impairments and focus on postural stability without sufficiently capturing other motor impairments.[31]

Table 1
Selected commonly used rating scales in Parkinson disease

	Scale	Details and Scoring
Comprehensive Scales	Unified Parkinson's Disease Rating Scale (UPDRS)	Four-part scale covering mood, activities of daily living, motor symptoms, and complications. Part I: 0–16; Part II: 0–52; Part III: 0–108; Part IV: 0–23 Total score: 0–199
	Movement Disorder Society Unified Parkinson's Disease Rating Scale (MDS-UPDRS)	Four-part scale covering nonmotor aspects experiences, motor experiences, motor symptoms, and complications. Part I: 0–52; Part II: 0–52; Part III: 0–132; Part IV: 0–24 Total: 0–260
Psychiatric Scales	Beck's Depression Inventory II (BDI-II)	21 items rated on a 0–3 scale. Total score: 0–63
	Hospital Anxiety and Depression Scale (HADS)	14 items (7 anxiety and 7 depression) rated on a 0–3 scale. Depression total score: 0–21 Anxiety total score: 0–21
	Parkinson's Anxiety Scale (PAS)	12 items across 3 sections rated on a 0–4 scale. Persistent anxiety: 0–20; episodic anxiety: 0–16; avoidance behavior: 0–12 Total score: 0–48
	Questionnaire for Impulsive-Compulsive Disorders in Parkinson's Disease (QUIP)	5 questions (yes/no) across 4 domains Total score: 0–5 for each domain
Autonomic Scales	Scales for Outcomes In Parkinson's Disease Autonomic Scale (SCOPA-AUT)	23 items rated on 0–3 scale Total score: 0–69
	Non-Motor Symptom Assessment Scale for Parkinson's Disease (NMSS)	30 questions across 9 domains scored as product of severity (rated 0–3) and frequency (rated 1–4) Total score: 0–360

(continued on next page)

Table 1
(continued)

	Scale	Details and Scoring
Cognitive Scales	Montreal Cognitive Assessment (MoCA)	30 point scale across 8 sections Total score: 0–30
	Parkinson's Disease-Cognitive Rating Scale (PD-CRS)	9-item scale with individual item scoring as well as fronto-subcortical and posterior-cortical scoring. Fronto-subcortical score: 0–104 Posterior-cortical score: 0–30 Total score: 0–134
Sleep	Epworth Sleepiness Scale (ESS)	8 items rated on a 0–3 scale Total score: 0–24
	Parkinson's disease Sleep Scale 2 (PDSS-2)	15 questions rated on a 0–4 scale Total score: 0–60

Table 2
Selected commonly used rating scales in other movement disorders

	Scale	Details and Scoring
Essential Tremor	Fahn-Tolosa-Marin Tremor Rating Scale (FTM-TRS)	21 items rated on a 0–4 point scale. Total score: 0–84
	Tremor Research Group Essential Tremor Rating Scale (TETRAS)	21 items (9 performance and 12 activities of daily living items) rated on a 0–4 point scale. Performance score: 0–36; activities of daily living score: 0–48 Total score: 0–84
Dystonia	Burke Fahn Marsden Dystonia Rating Scale (BFMDRS)	9 body areas rated as product of provoking factor (0–4 points), severity factor (0–4 points), and weighting for given region (0.5 or 1 point). Total score: 0–120
	Unified Dystonia Rating Scale (UDRS)	14 body areas with ratings for severity (0–4 points) and duration (0–4 points) for a maximum of 8 points per region. Total score: 0–112
	Toronto Western Spasmodic Torticollis Rating Scale (TWSTRS)	19 items rated across 3 subscales. Severity subscale: 0–35; disability subscale: 0–30; pain subscale: 0–20 Total score: 0–85
Tourette Syndrome	Yale Global Tic Severity Scale (YGTSS)	Motor and phonic tic severity separately rated across 5 items on a scale of 0–5. Impairment rated on a scale of 0–50 (with 10 point increments). Motor tic severity: 0–25; phonic tic severity: 0–25; total tic severity (motor + phonic): 0–50 Total score (total tic severity + impairment): 0–100
Huntington Disease	Unified Huntington's Disease Rating Scale (UHDRS)	4 components (motor function, cognition, behavior, and functional abilities). Motor assessment contains 15 items rated on 0–4 point scale. UHDRS total motor score: 0–60
Tardive Dyskinesia	Abnormal Involuntary Movement Scale (AIMS)	14 items (first 7 items rating movements in body regions on a 0–4 scale) Total AIMS score (first 7 items): 0–28
Wilson Disease	Unified Wilson's Disease Rating Scale (UWDRS)	34 items across 3 parts with items 2–30 being rated on a 0–4 point scale. Items 31–34 rated as yes (1) or no (0). Part 1 (level of consciousness) score: 0–3; Part 2 (patient/family reported items) score: 0–40; Part 3 (neurologic examination) score: 0–142

(continued on next page)

Table 2
(continued)

Scale		Details and Scoring
Ataxia	International Cooperative Ataxia Rating Scale (ICARS)	19 items rated across 4 domains. Postural and gait disturbances subscale: 0–34 Limb ataxia subscale: 0–52; dysarthria subscale: 0–8; occulomotor subscale: 0–6 Total score: 0–100
	Scale for the Assessment and Rating of Ataxia (SARA)	8 items rated on severity (ranging from 0–4 to 0–8 point scales). Mean score calculated when both sides assessed. Total score: 0–40
Functional Movement Disorders	Simplified Functional Movement Disorders Rating Scale (S-FMDRS)	9 items rated on a scale of 0–3 for both severity and duration. Total score: 0–54

Psychiatric Scales

Mood disturbances are a well-recognized feature of PD. Numerous scales have been used in assessing depression in PD with the Beck Depression Inventory II (BDI-II) scale, a self-rating multiple choice questionnaire in which the patient rates how they have been feeling during the past 2 weeks, being one of the most widely used, with demonstrated validity in PD.[32,33] The Geriatric Depression Scale (GDS) is a self-reported scale with both 30-question (GDS-30) and 15-question (GDS-15) versions that have been validated in PD,[32,34,35] although more recently it has been suggested that this scale may not adequately distinguish depression from apathy, fatigue, or anxiety in patients with PD.[36]

Other depression scales include the Hamilton Depression Scale (Ham-D), a clinician-rated screening scale that is one of the most widely used depression scales in general and has been validated in several PD studies but has not demonstrated factorial validity,[32,37] and the Montgomery-Asberg Depression Rating Scale (MADRS), which was initially developed to better assess changes in depression brought on by treatment as compared with the Ham-D.[38] The MADRS consists of a 10 questions each rated on a 0 to 6 point scale and has been validated in patients with PD.[35,39] One criticism of the Ham-D and MADRS has been the screening of somatic symptoms, which are generally less accurate when assessing depression in patients with PD due to overlap with other features of the disease.[40] The Hospital Anxiety and Depression Scale (HADS) is a scale aimed at screening mood disorders and distinguishing depression from anxiety. The scale's use has been supported and validated in PD.[32,35,41,42] A potential positive of this scale in PD relative to other scales discussed here is the absence of scoring cognitive and somatic symptoms, which may overlap with other features in patients with PD. However, it has also been suggested that some questions on this scale such as "feeling tense" or "feeling slowed down" do not adequately distinguish from somatic symptoms in patients with PD and that the scale cannot sufficiently discriminate between anxiety and depression in patients with PD.[43]

Hamilton Anxiety Rating Scale (HARS) is a 14-item clinician rated scale that is one of the more broadly evaluated and validated scales for anxiety in PD.[41,42,44,45] A criticism has been that it may focus specifically on generalized anxiety symptoms.[46] The Beck's Anxiety Inventory (BAI) has been widely used and validated outside of PD but has not been validated in PD populations.[42] Criticisms of this scale include the inclusion of somatic symptoms that may be endorsed by patients with PD due to other aspects of disease[43] and its focus primarily on panic symptoms.[46] The Parkinson's Anxiety Scale is a newer 12-item scale covering 3 domains (persisting anxiety, episodic anxiety, and avoidance behavior) developed specifically for use in the PD with items derived both from the HARS and BAI. The scale can be quickly administered and has been validated in PD populations.[47,48] The Geriatric Anxiety Inventory may have additional applicability, given PD's typical presentation later in life[49] and has shown the best balance of sensitivity and specificity (86% and 88%, respectively) when compared with other anxiety scales in PD.[48]

Several scales have been developed to examine impulsive and compulsive behavior in PD. The Questionnaire for Impulsive-Compulsive Disorders in Parkinson's Disease (QUIP) is a brief self-assessment screening questionnaire that looks for impulse control disorders in the categories of gambling, sex, buying, and eating.[50] It has been widely used and validated, with criticisms including limited sensitivity for punding, walkabout, and compulsive medication use, as well as not inquiring into sweet food preference.[50,51] Related to the QUIP is the QUIP-RS, a patient-reported clinician-rated scale designed to measure severity of impulse control disorders.[52] Criticisms include limits in assessing dopamine dysregulation syndrome.[51]

The Scales for Outcomes in Parkinson's disease (SCOPA) research project has led to the development of a group of scales intended to cover all relevant areas within PD.[53–58] The SCOPA Psychiatric Complications (SCOPA-PC) is a 7-item clinician-rated questionnaire with assessments of both psychotic and compulsive behavior.[54] Limitations from the impulsive and compulsive behavior standpoint include combining shopping and gambling together as compulsive behavior and not including compulsive eating or medication use.[51]

Autonomic Scales

The SCOPA autonomic scale (SCOPA-AUT) is intended to screen for autonomic dysfunction and impairment. The scale consists of 26 questions covering gastrointestinal, urinary, cardiovascular, thermoregulatory, and sexual dysfunction.[58] Although the scale has been criticized for being long, it has been independently validated on multiple occasions.[59,60] The Non-Motor Symptom Assessment Scale for Parkinson's Disease (NMSS) is a 30-item scale covering cardiovascular, sleep/fatigue, mood/cognition, perceptual problems, attention/memory, gastrointestinal, urinary, sexual function, and other domains.[61,62] The scale has shown good correlation with the SCOPA-AUT.[62]

Cognitive

The Montreal Cognitive Assessment (MoCA) is a 30-point scale that covers multiple cognitive domains including spatiotemporal orientation, sustained attention, visuospatial function, executive function, verbal memory, language, naming, and abstract thinking. It has been widely used and validated within PD populations.[63–65] Strengths include the multiple available versions of the test and short administration time (typically about 10 minutes), whereas criticisms include different cutoffs for illiterate patients and possible limitations in detecting change within a patient.[66,67] The Mattis Dementia Rating Scale second edition (DRS-2) assesses attention, initiation/perseveration, construction, conceptualization, and memory. It is considered suitable across most levels of cognitive impairment and most types of dementia. Criticisms include potential ceiling effects and an absence of alternate versions of the scale.[66] The SCOPA Cognitive (SCOPA-COG) scale is a 10-item scale designed to be specific and sensitive to detecting cognitive deficits in PD.[68] It has demonstrated good validity and reliability leading to its recommendation as a screening tool,[66] although the limited assessments on its sensitivity to change have been unfavorable.[67] The Parkinson's Disease-Cognitive Rating Scale was developed to fully cover cognitive deficits associated with PD including both cortical and subcortical deficits.[69] The scale has been validated for patients with PD in multiple studies, is sensitive to change, and shows high sensitivity and specificity for detection of PD dementia,[69–71] as well as some utility in patients with nondemented PD and those with mild cognitive impairment.[72]

Sleep

The Epworth Sleepiness Scale (ESS) is an 8-item self-assessment designed to assess excessive daytime sleepiness.[73] It has been widely used and validated in patients with PD,[74] although it is limited in scope to daytime sleepiness and may not be accurate in picking up associated sleep disorders.[74,75] The Pittsburgh Sleep Quality Index is a 19-question self-rated questionnaire that has been used within the PD population and validated within the general and specific patient populations but has drawn criticism due to being weighted toward sleep habits over sleep disturbances or daytime somnolence.[74] The Parkinson's Disease Sleep Scale (PDSS) is a 15-item scale designed to assess various aspects of sleep in PD, including insomnia, rapid eye movement sleep behavior disorder nocturia, overnight motor symptoms, and daytime somnolence.[76] This scale has demonstrated clinical utility, correlating with both the ESS and HY,[77] but has limitations in its design as a screen for nocturnal disturbance rather than for screening or diagnosis of specific sleep disorders and may be difficult for patients with PD to use.[74] A revised version of the scale, the PDSS-2, was developed to be easier for patients with PD to complete and cover additional sleep disturbances such as symptoms of restless legs syndrome.[78]

Fatigue and pain

The Parkinson Fatigue Scale is a self-reported 16-item scale developed to measure severity of fatigue and its impact on daily function.[79] It is available in both a polytomous version (rating items from 1 "strongly disagree" to 5 "strongly agree) and a dichotomous version (rating items as 0 or 1), with validation studies favoring the former.[80–82] The Fatigue Severity Scale is a 9-item scale that has been widely used and validated in patients with PD and without PD in assessing severity of fatigue.[81,83,84] It has been praised for being short and easy to use, making it suitable for screening.[81] The Multidimensional Fatigue Inventory is a 20-item self-report scale.[85] It has been widely used and validated in patients with PD as a measure of fatigue severity,[81,86] although its length (10–20 minutes to administer) make it less practical for screening.[81] The King's Parkinson's Disease Pain Scale is a rater-interview–based scale consisting of 14 items across 7 domains (musculoskeletal pain, chronic pain, fluctuation-related pain, nocturnal pain, orofacial pain, discoloration/edema, and radicular pain).[87] The scale has been validated, and a self-administered patient questionnaire version (the King's Parkinson's Disease Pain Questionnaire) has also been developed.[87,88]

SCALES IN ESSENTIAL TREMOR

The Fahn-Tolosa-Marin Tremor Rating Scale (FTM-TRS) is a widely used scale that was developed to assess rest, postural, and action tremor. The scale is divided into several parts: direct clinician assessment of position and severity of tremor, clinician assessment of tremor with specific tasks, a patient questionnaire of functional disability from tremor, and overall disability from tremor rated by the patient and clinician.[89] Criticisms of the scale include limited interrater reliability, limitations in assessing more severe essential tremor (ET) leading to a ceiling effect, and ambiguity of anchors when rating severity.[89–92] It is also worth noting that although this scale is widely used in ET, it was not specifically developed to assess tremor in ET but rather tremor in general.

The Tremor Research Group Essential Tremor Rating Assessment Scale was developed to overcome limitations of other tremor rating scales in ET (namely the FTM-TRS). It is divided into performance (clinician rated) and activities of daily living (patient rated) sections.[90] Strengths of the scale include no need for additional equipment (test only requires a pen and paper), clear anchors for clinician rated segments, inclusion of assessment of wing-beating tremor, good intra- and interrater reliability, and sensitivity to change.[90,91,93] Limitations of the scale include only assessing tremor (as opposed to other motor or nonmotor aspects of ET).

Other scales used in ET include the Bain and Findley Clinical Tremor Rating Scale (BF-TRS), which was initially developed for assessing tremor in upper limbs in patients with ET and dystonic tremor. It has both a clinician-rated segment and a patient self-administered questionnaire to assess activities of daily living.[94] It has been widely used and does not require any additional equipment, including a pen or paper, but only assesses upper extremity tremor, and has been criticized for using subjective anchors in rating, which can hurt reliability.[92] The Glass Scale is a simple 1-question scale to assess upper extremity tremor in ET involving asking one question: "Over the last week, when you were sitting down at the table, how did you drink water from a glass?" with 4 answer choices to rate severity. The scale has been validated and shown to be reliable, albeit limited in scope.[95]

The Quality of life Essential Tremor Questionnaire is a 30-item scale covering 5 domains: physical, psychosocial, communication, hobbies/leisure, and work/finance. The scale has demonstrated reliability and validity in patients with ET across multiple studies[96–99] and may be used in conjunction with scales listed earlier, which focus primarily on tremor and motor impairments from this. Lastly, the Essential Tremor Embarrassment Assessment is a 14-item self-assessment scale that has been validated to measure embarrassment in patients with ET.[100]

SCALES IN DYSTONIA

Dystonia can vary in presentation from focal to generalized, and different scales have been developed depending on areas of involvement.

Generalized Dystonia

The Burke Fahn Marsden Dystonia Rating Scale (BFMDRS) evaluates 9 body areas including the eyes, mouth, speech and swallowing, neck, trunk, and right and left arm and leg. It rates both severity and provoking factor on a scale of 0 to 4 and takes the product of these 2 scores multiplied by a weighting factor (0.5 for eyes, mouth, and neck and 1.0 for others) with a maximum score of 120.[101] The BFMDRS has been validated and has shown good interrater reliability, and sensitivity to change.[101–103] Criticisms include variable definition of body areas, variable score distribution, and subjectivity in patient-rated speech and swallowing components.[103,104] The Unified Dystonia Rating Scale was developed to address limitations of the BFMDRS and includes ratings for 14 body areas, including the upper face, lower face, jaw and tongue, larynx, neck, trunk, and right and left proximal and distal arm/hand and leg/foot. It rates both severity and duration in each section on a scale of 0 to 4 with a maximal total score of 112.[103] The scale has been validated and has shown good inter- and intrarater reliability and sensitivity to change.[102,103]

Cervical Dystonia

The Toronto Western Spasmodic Torticollis Rating Scale (TWSTRS) is a 3-component scale covering symptom severity, disability, and pain with scores ranging from 0 to 85. The scale has been validated and has shown good intra- and interrater reliability.[104] Criticisms of the scale include its complexity, unclear definition of midline for assessing range of motion, and lack of separate scoring for dystonic tremor.[104] The Cervical Dystonia Impact Scale (CDIP-58) is a patient-rated questionnaire consisting of 58 questions divided into domains of head and neck symptoms, pain and discomfort, upper limb activities, walking, sleep, annoyance, mood, and psychosocial functioning.[105] The scale has been validated, has shown good reliability, and has defined MCID with treatment.[104–106] The Comprehensive Cervical Dystonia Rating Scale was developed by revising the TWSTRS to a second version (TWSTRS-2) addressing several criticisms including adding rating for head tremor and eliminating the variable scaling of items.[107,108] It also includes a newly developed psychiatric scale specific to cervical dystonia (TWSTRS-PSYCH) and an unmodified version of the CDIP-58 to assess quality of life.[108]

Blepharospasm

The Blepharospasm Disability Index (BSDI) is a patient-rated scale that measures impairment of specific activities of daily living caused by blepharospasm.[104] It has shown good intrarater reliability and sensitivity to change.[109,110] Criticisms include its focus on disability related to sight rather than specifically measuring dystonic motor abnormalities and less sensitivity to mild changes.[104,111] The Jankovic Rating Scale is a 2-item clinician-rated scale to rate the severity and frequency of blepharospasm, which has shown correlation with the BSDI as well as validity and reliability.[110,112]

SCALES IN TOURETTE SYNDROME

The paroxysmal and heterogeneous nature of tics, including the ability of patients to suppress their tics, present challenges when attempting to objectively quantify severity of Tourette syndrome (TS). Scales largely rely on patient reporting of symptoms, whether this is through the form of a self-administered questionnaire or clinician guided. Although obsessive compulsive disorder and attention deficit disorder are frequently comorbid with TS,[113] scales assessing these conditions are not unique to the TS population and beyond the scope of this article.

The Yale Global Tic Severity Scale (YGTSS) is a semistructured clinician-rated scale that assesses the characteristics of motor and phonic tics over the previous week on dimensions of number, frequency, intensity, complexity, and interference, as well as a separate impairment rating (based on interpersonal, academic, and occupational interference).[114] It has been widely validated and has shown good consistency and reliability and sensitivity to change with defined MCID when determining treatment response.[114–117]It has also been praised for its comprehensive nature and sensitivity to change.[118] The primary criticisms of this scale are training required for administration and the long duration to administer the test (about 20 minutes).[118]

The Tourette Syndrome Clinical Global Impression scale is a 7-point clinician-rated scale that assesses overall severity (ranging from "normal" to "extremely severe").[119] It has been validated against other scales including the YGTSS and shows good interrater reliability, although its short duration is also its weakness because it does not capture details or subdivide TS symptoms such as the YGTSS.[118–120] The Shapiro Tourette Syndrome Severity Scale is a clinician-rated scale that evaluates tic severity and interference through 5 items. The scale has shown good intra- and interrater reliability and validity, with primary criticism being that it does not assess frequency, distribution, complexity, or time frame of tics.[118,121] The Gilles de la Tourette Syndrome Quality of Life is a 27-item self-assessment measuring psychological, physical, obsessive-compulsive, and cognitive impact of TS. It has demonstrated validity and reliability.[122,123]

SCALES IN HUNTINGTON DISEASE

Huntington disease (HD) can present with a wide constellation of motor, cognitive, and psychiatric symptoms much as PD, and as such, a comprehensive rating scale, the Unified Huntington's disease Rating Scale (UHDRS), has been developed. The UHDRS assesses motor function, cognitive function, behavioral abnormalities, and functional capacity in HD.[124] The motor section of the scale uses standardized ratings of oculomotor function, dysarthria, chorea, dystonia, gait, and postural stability. This was updated in 1999 with the removal of dysarthria.[125] The total motor score of the UHDRS (UHDRS-TMS) has been validated, shows good reliability and sensitivity to change, and is widely used in the assessment of motor symptoms of HD,[124–126] with strengths being the comprehensive nature in assessing motor symptoms and the short administration time (about 5 minutes).[125] Further shortened versions including subscales assessing specific motor features have also been developed.[125,127] Criticisms include floor and ceiling effects in premanifest patients and patients with advanced HD, respectively.[128] Cognitive assessment within the UHDRS is by phonetic verbal fluency, symbol digit modalities test, and the Stroop interference test.[124] These 3 tests cover multiple cognitive domains including visual attention, working memory, symbolic encoding, psychomotor speed, cognitive flexibility, response inhibition, selective attention, language, and executive functioning. The cognitive subscale has been validated and has shown good reliability, although it has had mixed results on sensitivity to detecting change.[124,129–133] Criticisms include a small number of tests being inadequate in sufficiently capturing all relevant cognitive domains.[129] The behavioral assessment of the UHDRS measures frequency and severity of symptoms related to effect, thought content, and coping styles, covering domains of irritability/aggression, apathy, depression, obsessive-compulsive behaviors, and psychosis. Items are rated on a 5-point scale covering the previous month.[124] The behavior subscale has shown good reliability, although more mixed results on validity of individual components.[124,134–137]

The UHDRS For Advanced Patients (UHDRS-FAP) was developed to better assess patients with advanced HD due to ceiling effects exhibited by the UHDRS.[128] It retains the motor function, cognition, and behavior sections of the original UHDRS but replaces the functional capacity assessment with a somatic domain section. The motor section assesses 13 areas including gait, dysphagia, capacity of feeding, toileting, clothing, cerebellar or pyramidal impairment, the presence of synkinesia, and tendon retractions.[128] The motor score within the UHDRS-FAP may better distinguish between patients with severe HD when directly compared with the UHDRS-TMS and shows greater sensitivity to change in patients with advanced HD.[138,139] The cognitive section of the UHDRS-FAP includes pointing tasks, simple commands, temporal orientation questions, praxis evaluations, automatic series, daily activity participation rating, and categorical and functional matching tasks including the Stroop task as in the original UHDRS.[128] The cognitive section has shown good validity and reliability, as well as sensitivity to change.[128,139] The behavior section of the UHDRS-FAP converts the 4-point scale used for behavior assessment in the UHDRS into binary (yes/no) answers about apparent sadness, anxiety, apathy, irritability, aggressiveness, agitation, obsession, and delirium. This was done to simplify testing in patients with advanced HD with more limited communication abilities; however, neither the UHDRS-FAP nor the original UHDRS behavioral components seem sensitive to detecting change in patients with advanced HD.[128] The somatic section of the UHDRS-FAP assesses 9 items including digestion, continence, pressure ulcers, hyperhidrosis, hypersalivation, and hypersomnia.

The MoCA (discussed earlier in context of PD) has also been used and validated in HD across several stages of disease[140–142] and has been identified as suitable in assessing severity of cognitive dysfunction in HD (with some caveats).[129] Several previously discussed behavior rating scales including the BDI and HADS have also been applied and validated in HD.[134]

SCALES IN TARDIVE DYSKINESIA

The Abnormal Involuntary Movement Scale (AIMS) is a 12-item scale measuring the severity of abnormal movements across 7 regions (the face, lips, jaw, tongue, upper extremities, lower extremities, and trunk) as well as clinical judgment of severity, patient awareness, incapacitation due to movements, and dental status. This scale was later revised to include 2 additional items of edentulousness and disappearance of abnormal movements during sleep.[143,144] Although the original scale lacked detailed instructions leading to high interrater variability, these have since been developed.[144–146] A criticism of the use of the AIMS is that although assessments may often include a total AIMS score (the sum of scores across body regions in the first 7 items of the scale),[147,148] a total score was not included in the scale's original development.[144] This has more recently been revisited to define clinically relevant changes within the AIMS scale.[149] The Simpson Dyskinesia Scale consists of 4 sections, including facial symptoms (14 items), neck and trunk movements (6 items), extremities (12 items), and whole body (2 items), each scored on a scale of 1 to 6.[150] The scale has demonstrated good reliability and validity, although it is notably long and more complex than the AIMS with abbreviated and modified versions of the scale also available.[150,151] The extrapyramidal symptom rating scale was assessed to develop 4 drug-induced movement disorders — parkinsonism, akathisia, dystonia, and TD — with the TD segment being broken into orofacial, and trunk/limb dyskinesia. The scale has shown good interrater reliability and correlates well with AIMS scores.[152,153]

SCALES IN WILSON DISEASE

The Unified Wilson's Disease Rating Scale (UWDRS) divides neurologic manifestations into dystonia, ataxic, and parkinsonian components across 27 items consisting of 9 patient questionnaire items and 18 clinician-rated segments (on a scale of 0–4 ranging from no symptoms to "worst characteristic possible").[154] A shortened version of the UWDRS termed the minimal UWDRS consists only of the first 9 (patient questionnaire) items and has shown good correlation with the UWDRS total score,[155] whereas the UWDRS total score has shown good reliability and validity when assessing patients with Wilson disease.[155,156] The Global Assessment Scale for Wilson's Disease (GAS for WD) consists of 2 "tiers" with Tier 1 covering global disability and Tier 2 being the neurologic assessment. The Tier 2 subscale consists of 13 items including Wilson facies, scholastic performance, depression, psychosis, dystonia, tremor, chorea, parkinsonism, speech, swallowing, salivation, posture and gait, and Kayser Fleischer rings with items rated from 0 to 4. In addition, there is a 14th item marking the presence or absence of uncommon features (emotional lability, seizures over preceding month, myoclonus, stereotypy, tics, pyramidal signs, and eye movement abnormalities) with a maximum of 4 points derived from this item. The GAS for WD has been shown good interrater reliability, validity, and sensitivity to change.[157] The neurologic subscale of the UWDRS and the Tier 2 subscale of the GAS for WD have shown to correlate well with each other.[155]

SCALES IN ATAXIA

The International Cooperative Ataxia Rating Scale (ICARS) is a 19-item scale that consists of 4 subscales assessing posture and gait, kinetic functions, speech disorders, and oculomotor disorders.[158] The scale has demonstrated good reliability, although it has been criticized for potentially redundant and contradictory scoring and its length (more than 20 minutes to administer).[159–161] The Scale for the Assessment and Rating of Ataxia (SARA) is an 8-item scale that assesses gait, stance, sitting, speech disturbance, finger chase, nose-finger test, fast alternating hand movements, and heel-shin slide (with limb kinetic functions being rated independently for both sides and the mean of these values being used in final score calculation).[162] The scale has shown high interrater reliability and validity.[161,162] A distinguishing feature from the ICARS is a lack of an oculomotor assessment. Both ICARS and SARA correlate well with each other but have shown limitations in discriminating ataxia when present in conjunction with additional movement disorders.[163]

SCALES IN FUNCTIONAL (PSYCHOGENIC) MOVEMENT DISORDERS

The psychogenic movement disorder rating scale (PMDRS) rates 10 phenomena (rest tremor, action tremor, dystonia, chorea, bradykinesia, myoclonus, tics, athetosis, ballism, and cerebellar incoordination) across 14 body regions as well as 2 additional functions (gait and speech). Each phenomenon is initially rated as present or absent, with those present being graded in severity and duration from 0 to 4 for each body region. Global severity and incapacitation is also rated from 0 to 4 for each phenomenon. The scale has shown good reliability, validity, and sensitivity to change.[164] Because of the large number of items in the scale, a simplified version, the simplified functional movement disorders rating scale, was developed. In this scale, the phenomenology of abnormal movements was removed in favor of presence or absence of any abnormal movement in a particular body region. The number of body regions was also reduced from 14 to 9 with symptom severity and duration being rated from 0 to 3. The resulting scale showed good correlation with PMDRS scores as well as reliability and sensitivity to change.[165]

DIGITAL ASSESSMENT TOOLS

A more recent and fast developing area within the assessment of movement disorders is the use of computer-assisted technologies in quantifying disease characteristics. These technologies largely fall into 2 general categories of wearable devices and digital interfaces or "apps." Most wearable devices currently used derive data from a combination of gyroscopes and accelerometers to determine patient position and movement, although the use of additional sensors such as surface electromyography and optical sensors have also been explored, as have sensors to assess nonmotor components of disease, such as heart rate.[166] Digital interfaces meanwhile refer to interaction between the patient and a program (such as a finger-tapping test)[167] that may or may not be used in conjunction with passive sensor monitoring.

The appeal for such technologies is obvious in the realm of research, as it has the potential to remove variability seen between raters. They also would diminish the need of an experienced clinician in assessments (allowing for more frequent or continuous monitoring as well as broadening the scale of potential research subjects). Although many of these devices/technologies have been validated against clinical scales, there has been a lack of validation to patient-centered scales, and a lack of standardization across different tools and devices, making assessments of individual tools challenging.[168]

DISCLOSURE

The author has nothing to disclose.

REFERENCES

1. Fahn S, Marsden CD, Calne DB, et al. Recent developments in Parkinson's disease, vol. 2. Florham Park (NJ): Macmillan Healthc Inf; 1987.
2. Goetz CG, Tilley BC, Shaftman SR, et al. Movement disorder society-sponsored revision of the Unified Parkinson's Disease Rating Scale (MDS-UPDRS): Scale presentation and clinimetric testing results. MovDisord 2008;23(15):2129–70.

3. Siderowf A, McDermott M, Kieburtz K, et al. Test-retest reliability of the Unified Parkinson's Disease Rating Scale in patients with early Parkinson's disease: Results from a multicenter clinical trial. MovDisord 2002;17(4):758–63.

4. Richards M, Marder K, Cote L, et al. Interrater reliability of the unified Parkinson's disease rating scale motor examination. MovDisord 1994;9(1):89–91.

5. Hauser RA, Gordon MF, Mizuno Y, et al. Minimal clinically important difference in Parkinson's disease as assessed in pivotal trials of pramipexole extended release. Parkinsons Dis 2014;2014:1–8.

6. Movement Disorder Society Task Force on Rating Scales for Parkinson's Disease. The Unified Parkinson's Disease Rating Scale (UPDRS): Status and recommendations. MovDisord 2003;18(7):738–50.

7. Goetz CG, Fahn S, Martinez-Martin P, et al. Movement Disorder Society-sponsored revision of the Unified Parkinson's Disease Rating Scale (MDS-UPDRS): Process, format, and clinimetric testing plan. MovDisord 2007; 22(1):41–7.

8. Martinez-Martin P, Rodriguez-Blazquez C, Alvarez-Sanchez M, et al. Expanded and independent validation of the Movement Disorder Society–Unified Parkinson's Disease Rating Scale (MDS-UPDRS). J Neurol 2013;260(1):228–36.

9. Kashihara K, Kondo T, Mizuno Y, et al. Official Japanese Version of the International Parkinson and Movement Disorder Society-Unified Parkinson's Disease Rating Scale: Validation Against the Original English Version. MovDisordClinPract 2014;1(3):200–12.

10. Zitser J, Peretz C, Ber David A, et al. Validation of the Hebrew version of the Movement Disorder Society—Unified Parkinson's Disease Rating Scale. ParkinsonismRelatDisord 2017;45:7–12.

11. Akbostanci MC, Bayram E, Yilmaz V, et al. Turkish Standardization of Movement Disorders Society Unified Parkinson's Disease Rating Scale and Unified Dyskinesia Rating Scale. MovDisordClinPract 2018;5(1):54–9.

12. Goetz CG, Stebbins GT, Wang L, et al. IPMDS-sponsored scale translation program: process, format, and clinimetric testing plan for the MDS-UPDRS and UDysRS. MovDisordClinPract 2014;1(2):97–101.

13. Horváth K, Aschermann Z, Ács P, et al. Minimal clinically important difference on the Motor Examination part of MDS-UPDRS. ParkinsonismRelatDisord 2015; 21(12):1421–6.

14. Stocchi F, Radicati FG, Chaudhuri KR, et al. The Parkinson's Disease Composite Scale: results of the first validation study. Eur J Neurol 2018;25(3):503–11.

15. Martinez-Martin P, Radicati FG, Rodriguez Blazquez C, et al. Extensive validation study of the Parkinson's Disease Composite Scale. Eur J Neurol 2019; 26(10):1281–8.

16. Goetz CG, Nutt JG, Stebbins GT. The Unified Dyskinesia Rating Scale: Presentation and clinimetric profile. MovDisord 2008;23(16):2398–403.

17. Goetz CG, Stebbins GT, Theeuwes A, et al. Temporal stability of the Unified Dyskinesia Rating Scale. MovDisord 2011;26(14):2556–9.

18. Colosimo C, Martínez-Martín P, Fabbrini G, et al. Task force report on scales to assess dyskinesia in Parkinson's disease: Critique and recommendations. MovDisord 2010;25(9):1131–42.

19. Cubo E, Goetz CG, Stebbins GT, et al. Independent Spanish Validation of the Unified Dyskinesia Rating Scale. MovDisordClinPract 2014;1(3):213–8.

20. Skorvanek M, Minar M, Grofik M, et al. Validation of the Official Slovak Version of the Unified Dyskinesia Rating Scale (UDysRS). Parkinsons Dis 2015;2015:1–7.

21. Makkos A, Kovács M, Pintér D, et al. Minimal clinically important difference for the historic parts of the Unified Dyskinesia Rating Scale. ParkinsonismRelatDisord 2019;58:79–82.
22. Peto V, Jenkinson C, Fitzpatrick R. PDQ-39: a review of the development, validation and application of a Parkinson's disease quality of life questionnaire and its associated measures. J Neurol 1998;245(S1):S10–4.
23. Bushnell DM, Martin ML. Quality of life and Parkinson's disease: translation and validation of the US Parkinson's Disease Questionnaire (PDQ-39). QualLife Res 1999;8(4):345–50.
24. Kohmoto J, Ohbu S, Nagaoka M, et al. Validation of the Japanese version of the Parkinson's Disease Questionnaire. RinshoShinkeigaku 2003;43(3):71–6 [in Japanese].
25. Ma H-I, Hwang W-J, Chen-Sea M-J. Reliability and validity testing of a Chinese-translated version of the 39-item Parkinson's Disease Questionnaire (PDQ-39). QualLife Res 2005;14(2):565–9.
26. Galeoto G, Colalelli F, Massai P, et al. Quality of life in Parkinson's disease: Italian validation of the Parkinson's Disease Questionnaire (PDQ-39-IT). Neurol Sci 2018;39(11):1903–9.
27. Jesus-Ribeiro J, Vieira E, Ferreira P, et al. Reliability and Validity of 39-Item Parkinson's Disease Questionnaire and Parkinson's Disease Quality of Life Questionnaire. Acta Med Port 2017;30(5):395.
28. Suratos CTR, Saranza GRM, Sumalapao DEP, et al. Quality of life and Parkinson's disease: Philippine translation and validation of the Parkinson's disease questionnaire. J ClinNeurosci 2018;54:156–60.
29. Skorvanek M, Martinez-Martin P, Kovacs N, et al. Relationship between the MDS-UPDRS and quality of life: a large multicenter study of 3206 patients. ParkinsonismRelatDisord 2018;52:83–9.
30. Hoehn MM, Yahr MD. Parkinsonism: onset, progression and mortality. Neurology 1967;17(5):427–42.
31. Goetz CG, Poewe W, Rascol O, et al. Movement disorder society task force report on the hoehn and yahr staging scale: status and recommendations. MovDisord 2004;19(9):1020–8.
32. Torbey E, Pachana NA, Dissanayaka NNW. Depression rating scales in Parkinson's disease: A critical review updating recent literature. J AffectDisord 2015; 184:216–24.
33. Visser M, Leentjens AFG, Marinus J, et al. Reliability and validity of the Beck depression inventory in patients with Parkinson's disease. MovDisord 2006; 21(5):668–72.
34. Schrag A, Barone P, Brown RG, et al. Depression rating scales in Parkinson's disease: Critique and recommendations. MovDisord 2007;22(8):1077–92.
35. Goodarzi Z, Mrklas KJ, Roberts DJ, et al. Detecting depression in Parkinson disease: A systematic review and meta-analysis. Neurology 2016;87(4):426–37.
36. Lopez FV, Split M, Filoteo JV, et al. Does the Geriatric Depression Scale measure depression in Parkinson's disease? Int J GeriatrPsychiatry 2018;33(12): 1662–70.
37. Broen MPG, Moonen AJH, Kuijf ML, et al. Factor analysis of thehamilton depression rating scale in Parkinson's disease. ParkinsonismRelatDisord 2015;21(2): 142–6.
38. Montgomery SA, Åsberg M. A new depression scale designed to be sensitive to change. Br J Psychiatry 1979;134(4):382–9.

39. Ketharanathan T, Hanwella R, Weerasundera R, et al. Diagnostic validity and factor analysis of montgomery-asberg depression rating scale in parkinson disease population. J GeriatrPsychiatry Neurol 2016;29(3):115–9.
40. Leentjens AFG, Marinus J, Van Hilten JJ, et al. The contribution of somatic symptoms to the diagnosis of depressive disorder in Parkinson's Disease. J NeuropsychiatryClinNeurosci 2003;15(1):74–7.
41. Mondolo F, Jahanshahi M, Granà A, et al. Evaluation of anxiety in Parkinson's disease with some commonly used rating scales. Neurol Sci 2007;28(5):270–5.
42. Leentjens AFG, Dujardin K, Marsh L, et al. Anxiety rating scales in Parkinson's disease: A validation study of the Hamilton anxiety rating scale, the Beck anxiety inventory, and the hospital anxiety and depression scale. MovDisord 2011; 26(3):407–15.
43. Leentjens AFG, Dujardin K, Marsh L, et al. Anxiety rating scales in Parkinson's disease: critique and recommendations. MovDisord 2008;23(14):2015–25.
44. Kummer A, Cardoso F, Teixeira AL. Generalized anxiety disorder and the Hamilton Anxiety Rating Scale in Parkinson's disease. ArqNeuropsiquiatr 2010;68(4): 495–501.
45. Stefanova E, Ziropadja L, Petrović M, et al. Screening for anxiety symptoms in Parkinson Disease. J GeriatrPsychiatry Neurol 2013;26(1):34–40.
46. Martinez-Martin P, Rojo-Abuin JM, Dujardin K, et al. Designing a new scale to measure anxiety symptoms in Parkinson's disease: item selection based on canonical correlation analysis. Eur J Neurol 2013;20(8):1198–203.
47. Leentjens AFG, Dujardin K, Pontone GM, et al. The Parkinson Anxiety Scale (PAS): Development and validation of a new anxiety scale. MovDisord 2014; 29(8):1035–43.
48. Dissanayaka NNW, Torbey E, Pachana NA. Anxiety rating scales in Parkinson's disease: a critical review updating recent literature. IntPsychogeriatr 2015; 27(11):1777–84.
49. Mele B, Holroyd-Leduc J, Smith EE, et al. Detecting anxiety in individuals with Parkinson disease: A systematic review. Neurology 2018;90(1):e39–47.
50. Weintraub D, Hoops S, Shea JA, et al. Validation of the questionnaire for impulsive-compulsive disorders in Parkinson's disease. MovDisord 2009; 24(10):1461–7.
51. Evans AH, Okai D, Weintraub D, et al. Scales to assess impulsive and compulsive behaviors in Parkinson's disease: Critique and recommendations. MovDisord 2019;34(6):791–8.
52. Weintraub D, Mamikonyan E, Papay K, et al. Questionnaire for impulsive-compulsive disorders in Parkinson's Disease–rating scale. MovDisord 2012; 27(2):242.
53. Marinus J, Visser M, Martínez-Martín P, et al. A short psychosocial questionnaire for patients with Parkinson's disease: the SCOPA-PS. J ClinEpidemiol 2003; 56(1):61–7.
54. Visser M, Verbaan D, van Rooden SM, et al. Assessment of psychiatric complications in Parkinson's disease: The SCOPA-PC. MovDisord 2007;22(15):2221–8.
55. Martínez-Martín P, Benito-León J, Burguera JA, et al. The SCOPA–motor scale for assessment of Parkinson's disease is a consistent and valid measure. J ClinEpidemiol 2005;58(7):674–9.
56. Verbaan D, Marinus J, Visser M, et al. Cognitive impairment in Parkinson's disease. J NeurolNeurosurgPsychiatry 2007;78(11):1182–7.
57. Marinus J, Visser M, van Hilten JJ, et al. Assessment of sleep and sleepiness in Parkinson Disease. Sleep 2003;26(8):1049–54.

58. Visser M, Marinus J, Stiggelbout AM, et al. Assessment of autonomic dysfunction in Parkinson's disease: The SCOPA-AUT. MovDisord 2004;19(11):1306–12.

59. Rodriguez-Blazquez C, Forjaz MJ, Frades-Payo B, et al, Longitudinal Parkinson's Disease Patient Study, Estudio Longitudinal de Pacients con Enfermedad da Parkinson Group. Independent validation of the scales for outcomes in Parkinson's disease-autonomic (SCOPA-AUT). Eur J Neurol 2010;17(2):194–201.

60. Forjaz MJ, Ayala A, Rodriguez-Blazquez C, et al, Longitudinal Parkinson's Disease Patient Study, Estudio longitudinal de pacientes con enferedad de Parkinson- ELEP Group. Assessing autonomic symptoms of Parkinson's disease with the SCOPA-AUT: a new perspective from Rasch analysis. Eur J Neurol 2010; 17(2):273–9.

61. Chaudhuri KR, Martinez-Martin P, Brown RG, et al. The metric properties of a novel non-motor symptoms scale for Parkinson's disease: Results from an international pilot study. MovDisord 2007;22(13):1901–11.

62. Martinez-Martin P, Rodriguez-Blazquez C, Abe K, et al. International study on the psychometric attributes of the Non-Motor Symptoms Scale in Parkinson disease. Neurology 2009;73(19):1584–91.

63. Gill DJ, Freshman A, Blender JA, et al. The montreal cognitive assessment as a screening tool for cognitive impairment in Parkinson's disease. MovDisord 2008; 23(7):1043–6.

64. Nie K, Zhang Y, Wang L, et al. A pilot study of psychometric properties of the Beijing version of Montreal Cognitive Assessment in patients with idiopathic Parkinson's disease in China. J ClinNeurosci 2012;19(11):1497–500.

65. Ozdilek B, Kenangil G. Validation of the Turkish version of the montreal cognitive assessment scale (MoCA-TR) in patients With Parkinson's Disease. ClinNeuropsychol 2014;28(2):333–43.

66. Skorvanek M, Goldman JG, Jahanshahi M, et al. Global scales for cognitive screening in Parkinson's disease: Critique and recommendations. MovDisord 2018;33(2):208–18.

67. Faust-Socher A, Duff-Canning S, Grabovsky A, et al. Responsiveness to Change of the Montreal Cognitive Assessment, Mini-Mental State Examination, and SCOPA-Cog in Non-Demented Patients with Parkinson's Disease. DementGeriatrCognDisord 2019;47(4-6):1–11.

68. Marinus J, Visser M, Verwey NA, et al. Assessment of cognition in Parkinson's disease. Neurology 2003;61(9):1222–8.

69. Pagonabarraga J, Kulisevsky J, Llebaria G, et al. Parkinson's disease-cognitive rating scale: a new cognitive scale specific for Parkinson's disease. MovDisord 2008;23(7):998–1005.

70. Serrano-Dueñas M, Serrano M, Villena D, et al. Validation of the Parkinson's Disease-cognitive rating scale applying the movement disorder society task force criteria for dementia associated with Parkinson's Disease. MovDisordClinPract 2017;4(1):51–7.

71. Martínez-Martín P, Prieto-Jurczynska C, Frades-Payo B. Psychometric attributes of the Parkinson's Disease-Cognitive Rating Scale. An independent validation study. Rev Neurol 2009;49(8):393–8 [in Spanish].

72. Fernández de Bobadilla R, Pagonabarraga J, Martínez-Horta S, et al. Parkinson's disease-cognitive rating scale: Psychometrics for mild cognitive impairment. MovDisord 2013;28(10):1376–83.

73. Johns MW. A new method for measuring daytime sleepiness: the epworth sleepiness scale. Sleep 1991;14(6):540–5.

74. Högl B, Arnulf I, Comella C, et al. Scales to assess sleep impairment in Parkinson's disease: Critique and recommendations. MovDisord 2010;25(16): 2704–16.

75. Nishiyama T, Mizuno T, Kojima M, et al. Criterion validity of the Pittsburgh Sleep Quality Index and Epworth Sleepiness Scale for the diagnosis of sleep disorders. Sleep Med 2014;15(4):422–9.

76. Chaudhuri KR, Pal S, DiMarco A, et al. The Parkinson's disease sleep scale: a new instrument for assessing sleep and nocturnal disability in Parkinson's disease. J NeurolNeurosurgPsychiatry 2002;73(6):629–35.

77. Tse W, Liu Y, Barthlen GM, et al. Clinical usefulness of the Parkinson's disease sleep scale. ParkinsonismRelatDisord 2005;11(5):317–21.

78. Trenkwalder C, Kohnen R, Högl B, et al. Parkinson's disease sleep scale-validation of the revised version PDSS-2. MovDisord 2011;26(4):644–52.

79. Brown RG, Dittner A, Findley L, et al. The Parkinson fatigue scale. ParkinsonismRelatDisord 2005;11(1):49–55.

80. Nilsson MH, Bladh S, Hagell P. Fatigue in Parkinson's disease: measurement properties of a generic and a condition-specific rating scale. J PainSymptomManage 2013;46(5):737–46.

81. Friedman JH, Alves G, Hagell P, et al. Fatigue rating scales critique and recommendations by the Movement Disorders Society task force on rating scales for Parkinson's disease. MovDisord 2010;25(7):805–22.

82. Martinez-Martin P, Wetmore JB, Arbelo JM, et al. Validation study of the Parkinson's Fatigue Scale in advanced Parkinson's disease. PatientRelatOutcome Meas 2019;10:141–52.

83. Krupp LB, LaRocca NG, Muir-Nash J, et al. The fatigue severity scale. Arch Neurol 1989;46(10):1121.

84. Hagell P, Höglund A, Reimer J, et al. Measuring fatigue in Parkinson's disease: a psychometric study of two brief generic fatigue questionnaires. J PainSymptomManage 2006;32(5):420–32.

85. Smets EM, Garssen B, Bonke B, et al. The Multidimensional Fatigue Inventory (MFI) psychometric qualities of an instrument to assess fatigue. J Psychosom Res 1995;39(3):315–25.

86. Elbers RG, van Wegen EEH, Verhoef J, et al. Reliability and structural validity of the Multidimensional Fatigue Inventory (MFI) in patients with idiopathic Parkinson's disease. ParkinsonismRelatDisord 2012;18(5):532–6.

87. Chaudhuri KR, Rizos A, Trenkwalder C, et al. King's Parkinson's disease pain scale, the first scale for pain in PD: An international validation. MovDisord 2015;30(12):1623–31.

88. Martinez-Martin P, Rizos AM, Wetmore J, et al. First comprehensive tool for screening pain in Parkinson's disease: the King's Parkinson's Disease Pain Questionnaire. Eur J Neurol 2018;25(10):1255–61.

89. Stacy MA, Elble RJ, Ondo WG, et al, TRS study group. Assessment of interrater and intrarater reliability of the Fahn-Tolosa-Marin Tremor Rating Scale in essential tremor. MovDisord 2007;22(6):833–8.

90. Elble R, Comella C, Fahn S, et al. Reliability of a new scale for essential tremor. MovDisord 2012;27(12):1567–9.

91. Ondo W, Hashem V, LeWitt PA, et al. Comparison of the Fahn-Tolosa-Marin clinical rating scale and the essential tremor rating assessment scale. MovDisordClinPract 2018;5(1):60–5.

92. Elble R, Bain P, JoãoForjaz M, et al. Task force report: Scales for screening and evaluating tremor: Critique and recommendations. MovDisord 2013;28(13): 1793–800.

93. Voller B, Lines E, McCrossin G, et al. Alcohol challenge and sensitivity to change of the essential tremor rating assessment scale. MovDisord 2014;29(4):555–8.

94. Bain PG, Findley LJ, Atchison P, et al. Assessing tremor severity. J NeurolNeurosurgPsychiatry 1993;56(8):868–73.

95. Gironell A, Martínez-Corral M, Pagonabarraga J, et al. The Glass scale: A simple tool to determine severity in essential tremor. ParkinsonismRelatDisord 2010; 16(6):412–4.

96. Tröster AI, Pahwa R, Fields JA, et al. Quality of life in Essential Tremor Questionnaire (QUEST): Development and initial validation. ParkinsonismRelatDisord 2005;11(6):367–73.

97. Martínez-Martín P, Jiménez-Jiménez FJ, CarrozaGarcía E, et al. Most of the Quality of Life in Essential Tremor Questionnaire (QUEST) psychometric properties resulted in satisfactory values. J ClinEpidemiol 2010;63(7):767–73.

98. Kovács M, Makkos A, Janszky J, et al. Independent validation of the Quality of Life in Essential Tremor Questionnaire (QUEST). IdeggyogySz 2017;70(5–6): 193–202.

99. Güler S, Turan FN. Turkish version quality of life in essential tremor questionnaire (quest): validity and reliability study. IdeggyogySz 2015;68(9–10):310–7.

100. Traub RE, Gerbin M, Mullaney MM, et al. Development of an essential tremor embarrassment assessment. ParkinsonismRelatDisord 2010;16(10):661–5.

101. Burke RE, Fahn S, Marsden CD, et al. Validity and reliability of a rating scale for the primary torsion dystonias. Neurology 1985;35(1):73–7.

102. Susatia F, Malaty IA, Foote KD, et al. An evaluation of rating scales utilized for deep brain stimulation for dystonia. J Neurol 2010;257(1):44–58.

103. Comella CL, Leurgans S, Wuu J, et al, Dystonia Study Group. Rating scales for dystonia: A multicenter assessment. MovDisord 2003;18(3):303–12.

104. Albanese A, Sorbo F Del, Comella C, et al. Dystonia rating scales: Critique and recommendations. MovDisord 2013;28(7):874–83.

105. Cano SJ, Warner TT, Linacre JM, et al. Capturing the true burden of dystonia on patients: the Cervical Dystonia Impact Profile (CDIP-58). Neurology 2004;63(9): 1629–33.

106. Espay AJ, Trosch R, Suarez G, et al. Minimal clinically important change in the Toronto Western Spasmodic Torticollis Rating Scale. ParkinsonismRelatDisord 2018;52:94–7.

107. Comella C, Perlmutter J, Jinnah H, et al. Reliability of the severity subscale of the revised toronto spasmodic torticollis rating scale (TWSTRS-2) (S15.001). Neurology 2015;84(14 Supplement):S15.001.

108. Comella CL, Perlmutter JS, Jinnah HA, et al. Clinimetric testing of the comprehensive cervical dystonia rating scale. MovDisord 2016;31(4):563–9.

109. Jankovic J, Comella C, Hanschmann A, et al. Efficacy and safety of incobotulinumtoxinA (NT 201, Xeomin) in the treatment of blepharospasm-a randomized trial. MovDisord 2011;26(8):1521–8.

110. Jankovic J, Kenney C, Grafe S, et al. Relationship between various clinical outcome assessments in patients with blepharospasm. MovDisord 2009;24(3): 407–13.

111. Wabbels B, Jost WH, Roggenkämper P. Difficulties with differentiating botulinum toxin treatment effects in essential blepharospasm. J NeuralTransm 2011; 118(6):925–43.

112. Jankovic J, Orman J. Botulinum A toxin for cranial-cervical dystonia: A double-blind, placebo-controlled study. Neurology 1987;37(4):616.
113. Roth J. The colorful spectrum of Tourette syndrome and its medical, surgical and behavioral therapies. ParkinsonismRelatDisord 2018;46:S75–9.
114. Leckman JF, Riddle MA, Hardin MT, et al. The Yale Global Tic Severity Scale: initial testing of a clinician-rated scale of tic severity. J Am Acad Child Adolesc-Psychiatry 1989;28(4):566–73.
115. Storch EA, Murphy TK, Geffken GR, et al. Reliability and validity of the Yale Global Tic Severity Scale. Psychol Assess 2005;17(4):486–91.
116. McGuire JF, Piacentini J, Storch EA, et al. A multicenter examination and strategic revisions of the Yale Global Tic Severity Scale. Neurology 2018;90(19): e1711–9.
117. Storch EA, De Nadai AS, Lewin AB, et al. Defining treatment response in pediatric tic disorders: a signal detection analysis of the Yale Global Tic Severity Scale. J Child AdolescPsychopharmacol 2011;21(6):621–7.
118. Martino D, Pringsheim TM, Cavanna AE, et al. Systematic review of severity scales and screening instruments for tics: critique and recommendations. Mov-Disord 2017;32(3):467–73.
119. Cohen DJ, Bruun RD, Leckman JF, editors. Tourette's syndrome and tic disorders: clinical understanding and treatment. Oxford (England): John Wiley & Sons; 1988.
120. Walkup JT, Rosenberg LA, Brown J, et al. The validity of instruments measuring tic severity in Tourette's syndrome. J Am Acad Child AdolescPsychiatry 1992; 31(3):472–7.
121. Shapiro AK, Shapiro ES, Young JG, et al. In: Gilles de la Tourette syndrome. 2nd edition; 1988. p. xxiv, 558-xxiv, 558.
122. Cavanna AE, Schrag A, Morley D, et al. The Gilles de la Tourette Syndrome-quality of life scale (GTS-QOL): development and validation. Neurology 2008; 71(18):1410–6.
123. Cavanna AE, Luoni C, Selvini C, et al. The Gilles de la Tourette Syndrome-quality of life scale for children and adolescents (C&A-GTS-QOL): development and validation of the Italian version. Behav Neurol 2013;27(1):95–103.
124. Unified Huntington's Disease Rating Scale: reliability and consistency. Huntington Study Group. MovDisord 1996;11(2):136–42.
125. Mestre TA, Forjaz MJ, Mahlknecht P, et al. Rating scales for motor symptoms and signs in huntington's disease: critique and recommendations. MovDisord-ClinPract 2018;5(2):111–7.
126. Siesling S, van Vugt JPP, Zwinderman KAH, et al. Unified Huntington's disease rating scale: a follow up. MovDisord 1998;13(6):915–9.
127. Siesling S, Zwinderman AH, van Vugt JP, et al. A shortened version of the motor section of the Unified Huntington's disease rating scale. MovDisord 1997;12(2): 229–34.
128. Youssov K, Dolbeau G, Maison P, et al. The unified huntington's disease rating scale for advanced patients: validation and follow-up study. MovDisord 2013; 28(14):1995–2001.
129. Mestre TA, Bachoud-Lévi A-C, Marinus J, et al. Rating scales for cognition in Huntington's disease: critique and recommendations. MovDisord 2018;33(2): 187–95.
130. Busse M, Quinn L, Debono K, et al. A randomized feasibility study of a 12-week community-based exercise program for people with Huntington's disease. J NeurolPhysTher 2013;37(4):149–58.

131. Piira A, van Walsem MR, Mikalsen G, et al. Effects of a one year intensive multi-disciplinary rehabilitation program for patients with Huntington's Disease: a prospective intervention study. PLoSCurr 2013;5.

132. HORIZON Investigators of the Huntington Study Group and European Huntington's Disease Network. A randomized, double-blind, placebo-controlled study of latrepirdine in patients with mild to moderate Huntington disease. JAMA Neurol 2013;70(1):25–33.

133. Ravina B, Romer M, Constantinescu R, et al. The relationship between CAG repeat length and clinical progression in Huntington's disease. MovDisord 2008;23(9):1223–7.

134. Mestre TA, van Duijn E, Davis AM, et al. Rating scales for behavioral symptoms in Huntington's disease: critique and recommendations. MovDisord 2016; 31(10):1466–78.

135. Rickards H, Souza J De, Crooks J, et al. Discriminant analysis of beck depression inventory and hamilton rating scale for depression in Huntington's disease. J NeuropsychiatryClinNeurosci 2011;23(4):399–402.

136. Rickards H, De Souza J, van Walsem M, et al. Factor analysis of behavioural symptoms in Huntington's disease. J NeurolNeurosurgPsychiatry 2011;82(4):411–2.

137. van Duijn E, Reedeker N, Giltay EJ, et al. Course of irritability, depression and apathy in Huntington'sdisease in relation to motor symptoms during a two-year follow-up period. Neurodegener Dis 2013;13(1):9–16.

138. Winder JY, Achterberg WP, Marinus J, et al. Assessment scales for patients with advanced Huntington's disease: comparison of the UHDRS and UHDRS-FAP. MovDisordClinPract 2018;5(5):527–33.

139. Winder JY, Achterberg WP, Gardiner SL, et al. Longitudinal assessment of the Unified Huntington's Disease Rating Scale (UHDRS) and UHDRS–For Advanced Patients (UHDRS-FAP) in patients with late stage Huntington's disease. Eur J Neurol 2019;26(5):780–5.

140. Videnovic A, Bernard B, Fan W, et al. The Montreal Cognitive Assessment as a screening tool for cognitive dysfunction in Huntington's disease. MovDisord 2010;25(3):401–4.

141. Gluhm S, Goldstein J, Brown D, et al. Usefulness of the Montreal Cognitive Assessment (MoCA) in Huntington's disease. MovDisord 2013;28(12):1744–7.

142. Bezdicek O, Majerova V, Novak M, et al. Validity of the montreal cognitive assessment in the detection of cognitive dysfunction in Huntington's Disease. ApplNeuropsycholAdult 2013;20(1):33–40.

143. Abnormal Involuntary Movement Scale (117-AIMS). In: Guy W, editor. ECDEU assessment manual for psychopharmacology: revised.; Rockville (MD): 1976.

144. Kane JM, Correll CU, Nierenberg AA, et al, Tardive Dyskinesia Assessment Working Group. Revisiting the abnormal involuntary movement scale. J ClinPsychiatry 2018;79(3) [pii:17cs11959].

145. Munetz MR, Benjamin S. How to examine patients using the abnormal involuntary movement scale. Psychiatr Serv 1988;39(11):1172–7.

146. Lane RD, Glazer WM, Hansen TE, et al. Assessment of tardive dyskinesia using the Abnormal Involuntary Movement Scale. J NervMent Dis 1985;173(6):353–7.

147. Anderson KE, Stamler D, Davis MD, et al. Deutetrabenazine for treatment of involuntary movements in patients with tardive dyskinesia (AIM-TD): a double-blind, randomised, placebo-controlled, phase 3 trial. Lancet Psychiatry 2017; 4(8):595–604.

148. Müller T. Valbenazine for the treatment of tardive dyskinesia. Expert Rev Neurother 2017;17(12):1135–44.
149. Stacy M, Sajatovic M, Kane JM, et al. Abnormal involuntary movement scale in tardive dyskinesia: Minimal clinically important difference. MovDisord 2019; 34(8):1203–9.
150. Simpson GM, Lee JH, Zoubok B, et al. A rating scale for tardive dyskinesia. Psychopharmacology (Berl) 1979;64(2):171–9.
151. Woerner MG, Correll CU, Alvir JMJ, et al. Incidence of tardive dyskinesia with risperidone or olanzapine in the elderly: results from a 2-year, prospective study in antipsychotic-naïve patients. Neuropsychopharmacology 2011;36(8): 1738–46.
152. Chouinard G, Margolese HC. Manual for the extrapyramidal symptom rating scale (ESRS). Schizophr Res 2005;76(2–3):247–65.
153. Gharabawi GM, Bossie CA, Lasser RA, et al. Abnormal Involuntary Movement Scale (AIMS) and Extrapyramidal Symptom Rating Scale (ESRS): cross-scale comparison in assessing tardive dyskinesia. Schizophr Res 2005;77(2–3): 119–28.
154. Członkowska A, Tarnacka B, Möller JC, et al. Unified Wilson's Disease Rating Scale - a proposal for the neurological scoring of Wilson's disease patients. NeurolNeurochir Pol 2007;41(1):1–12.
155. Volpert HM, Pfeiffenberger J, Gröner JB, et al. Comparative assessment of clinical rating scales in Wilson's disease. BMC Neurol 2017;17(1):140.
156. Leinweber B, Möller JC, Scherag A, et al. Evaluation of the Unified Wilson's Disease Rating Scale (UWDRS) in German patients with treated Wilson's disease. MovDisord 2008;23(1):54–62.
157. Aggarwal A, Aggarwal N, Nagral A, et al. A novel global assessment scale for Wilson's Disease (GAS for WD). MovDisord 2009;24(4):509–18.
158. Trouillas P, Takayanagi T, Hallett M, et al. International cooperative ataxia rating scale for pharmacological assessment of the cerebellar syndrome. The Ataxia Neuropharmacology Committee of the World Federation of Neurology. J Neurol Sci 1997;145(2):205–11.
159. Storey E, Tuck K, Hester R, et al. Inter-rater reliability of the international cooperative ataxia rating scale (ICARS). MovDisord 2004;19(2):190–2.
160. Schmitz-Hübsch T, Tezenas du Montcel S, Baliko L, et al. Reliability and validity of the International Cooperative Ataxia Rating Scale: A study in 156 spinocerebellar ataxia patients. MovDisord 2006;21(5):699–704.
161. Salcı Y, Fil A, Keklicek H, et al. Validity and reliability of the international cooperative ataxia rating scale (ICARS) and the scale for the assessment and rating of ataxia (SARA) in multiple sclerosis patients with ataxia. MultSclerRelatDisord 2017;18:135–40.
162. Schmitz-Hubsch T, du Montcel ST, Baliko L, et al. Scale for the assessment and rating of ataxia: Development of a new clinical scale. Neurology 2006;66(11): 1717–20.
163. Brandsma R, Lawerman TF, Kuiper MJ, et al. Reliability and discriminant validity of ataxia rating scales in early onset ataxia. Dev Med Child Neurol 2017;59(4): 427–32.
164. Hinson VK, Cubo E, Comella CL, et al. Rating scale for psychogenic movement disorders: scale development and clinimetric testing. MovDisord 2005;20(12): 1592–7.

165. Nielsen G, Ricciardi L, Meppelink AM, et al. A simplified version of the psychogenic movement disorders rating scale: the simplified functional movement disorders rating scale (S-FMDRS). MovDisordClinPract 2017;4(5):710–6.
166. Jalloul N. Wearable sensors for the monitoring of movement disorders. Biomed J 2018;41(4):249–53.
167. Lee CY, Kang SJ, Hong S-K, et al. A validation study of a smartphone-based finger tapping application for quantitative assessment of bradykinesia in Parkinson's Disease. PLoS One 2016;11(7):e0158852. Lebedev MA, ed.
168. Merola A, Sturchio A, Hacker S, et al. Technology-based assessment of motor and nonmotor phenomena in Parkinson disease. Expert Rev Neurother 2018; 18(11):825–45.

Pharmacologic Treatment of Motor Symptoms Associated with Parkinson Disease

Werner Poewe, MD*, Philipp Mahlknecht, MD, PhD

KEYWORDS

- Parkinson disease (PD) • Treatment • Dopamine • Dyskinesia • Motor fluctuations
- Recommendation • Guideline
- Movement disorders society (MDS) evidence-based medicine (EBM) review update

KEY POINTS

- Although there is still no neuroprotective therapy for PD, a large number of drugs are available to improve motor symptoms, making it the best treatable of all neurodegenerative diseases.
- Although levodopa remains the gold standard for PD therapy, enzyme inhibitors to enhance central dopamine activity and dopamine agonists have been a cornerstone in medical management for decades.
- The medical armamentarium is continuing to expand, particularly beyond the dopaminergic arena to drugs that stimulate or inhibit nondopaminergic receptors involved in multiple basal ganglia synaptic transmission pathways.
- The present review gives an overview of the current state of the art in medical management of PD in accordance with recommendations of the MDS EBM review update (Fox and colleagues 2018).

INTRODUCTION

Parkinson disease (PD) is the second most common neurodegenerative disorder with an estimated 6 million people affected worldwide.[1] PD prevalence has increased by 74% between 1990 and 2016 and prevalence figures are expected to further increase by 2- to 3-fold until 2030. The disease is clinically defined by the presence of cardinal motor features, including bradykinesia, rigidity, and a characteristic asymmetric 5-Hz resting tremor of the distal extremities.[2] Bradykinesia is the anchor symptom defining a parkinsonian syndrome and is associated with reduced speed and amplitude of movement, the latter typically showing a decrement with repetitive motor sequences.

Department of Neurology, Medical University Innsbruck, Anichstrasse 35, Innsbruck 6020, Austria
* Corrresponding author.
E-mail address: WERNER.POEWE@I-MED.AC.AT

Neurol Clin 38 (2020) 255–267
https://doi.org/10.1016/j.ncl.2019.12.002
0733-8619/20/© 2020 Elsevier Inc. All rights reserved.

Bradykinesia impacts on multiple activities of daily living, including gait with slowness and reduced step length, finger dexterity with problems in handwriting and use of utensils, and voice with hoarseness and low volume speech.

Although there is currently no cure or intervention that can slow the progression of PD, recent insights into the molecular pathways involved in PD pathogenesis have revealed multiple novel targets for pharmacologic interventions that could modify the progression of PD. Most prominent among those are approaches that directly or indirectly target a-syn proteostasis, including small-molecule chaperones, enhancers of glucocerebrosidase, inhibitors of LRRK2, and anti-a-syn immunotherapies designed to prevent cell-to-cell transmission of pathogenic a-syn assemblies.[3–6]

These approaches will not be further reviewed here. Instead, we aim to review the large and growing number of drugs that have been shown to significantly improve the motor symptoms associated with PD, making it the best treatable of all neurodegenerative diseases.

CLASSES OF ANTIPARKINSONIAN DRUGS

The first successful pharmacologic therapy for the motor symptoms of PD using belladonna extracts was based on serendipity (see later discussion) and effects were mainly on tremor and rigidity. The breakthrough in the medical management of PD occurred when striatal dopamine deficiency was discovered to be the key defect in central neurotransmission responsible for the cardinal motor features of the disease. This opened the door for pharmacologic dopamine substitution as the mainstay of current drug therapies to treat the motor symptoms of PD.

Dopaminergic Drugs

Since the introduction of levodopa as an approach to restore striatal dopamine transmission multiple refinements of this basic strategy have evolved, including the use of enzyme inhibitors to improve brain delivery of levodopa or enhance central dopamine activity and the development of direct acting dopamine receptor agonists (**Fig. 1**).

Levodopa
Levodopa is the aromatic amino acid precursor of dopamine, which, unlike dopamine, is able to cross the blood-brain barrier and, on action of central aromatic amino acid decarboxylase (AADC), is converted to dopamine. This process occurs in remaining nigrostriatal projection neurons presumably involving presynaptic storage and release of the neurotransmitter but likely also ectopically in serotonergic neurons potentially leading to unregulated synaptic dopamine release in the striatum.[7]

The dramatic efficacy of levodopa in alleviating the motor symptoms of PD was first shown in the 1960s and multiple randomized controlled trials have since established the efficacy of the drug in controlling the motor symptoms in early PD.[8,9] Until now no drug—with the possible exception of the dopamine agonist apomorphine—has been found to equal levodopa's symptomatic effect size.

Oral levodopa formulations are marketed as combinations with non-brain penetrant inhibitors of AADC (carbidopa or benserazide) to enhance central bioavailability and reduce peripheral dopaminergic side effects, particularly nausea. The short half-life of standard oral levodopa of around 90 minutes requires multiple daily doses and intestinal absorption occurs mainly in the duodenum and proximal jejunum making systemic drug delivery vulnerable to delayed gastric emptying or competition for jejunal absorption by dietary amino acids. Taken together these peripheral pharmacokinetic factors give rise to fluctuating levodopa plasma levels that are the main reason for the development of motor response fluctuations with chronic therapy.

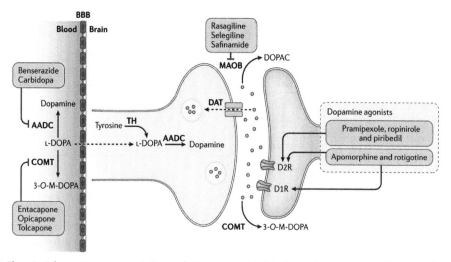

Fig. 1. Schematic representation of the nigrostriatal dopamine synapse showing the site and mode of action of dopaminergic drugs to treat the motor symptoms of PD. AADC, aromatic amino acid decarboxylase; BBB, blood-brain barrier; COMT, catechol-o-methyl-transferase; DOPAC, dioxy phenylacetate; MAO-B, monoamine-oxidase B; TH, tyrosine-hydroxylase. (*From* Poewe W, Seppi K, Tanner CM, et al. Parkinson disease. *Nat Rev Dis Prim.* 2017;3:1-21; with permission.)

Different orally active extended-release formulations of levodopa have been developed to provide more continuous drug delivery and are licensed to treat motor fluctuations in many countries (Madopar CR, Sinemet CR, Rytary) and several novel approaches are in clinical development. In addition a levodopa/carbidopa intestinal gel formulation is available for continuous intestinal delivery via percutaneous endoscopic gastrostomy tubes for patients with motor complications that are refractory to oral therapies (see section on Treatment of Levodopa-induced motor complications below).

Levodopa formulations with rapid onset of effect are useful for patients needing "rescue" from OFF periods (see later discussion) and a dispersible formulation of levodopa/benserazide is available in the European Union; an inhalable powder formulation for intrapulmonary delivery has been recently approved in the United States (Inbrija).[10,11]

Dopamine agonists

Dopamine agonists (DAs) are a class of drugs that exert their antiparkinsonian efficacy via direct stimulation of striatal dopamine receptors with preferential affinity to the D2-receptor subfamily. The first member of this class, introduced in the 1970s, was the ergoline compound bromocriptine,[12] and several other ergoline DAs followed. They were largely superseded by newer nonergoline compounds (**Table 1**) following reports of retroperitoneal, pleural, and cardiovalvular fibrosis induced by the ergot compounds bromocriptine, pergolide, and cabergoline—very likely related to their activity at 5-HT2B serotonergic receptors expressed on fibroblasts of these tissues.[13,14]

DAs are the most extensively studied class of antiparkinsonian drugs in terms of randomized controlled trials, with 29 such trials involving more than 5000 patients published by 2009.[15] Their efficacy to improve the motor symptoms of PD as early

Table 1			
Pharmacologic profile of (nonergot) dopamine agonists			
Drug	**DA-Receptor-Affinity**	**Half-Life (h)**	**Elimination Route**
Piribedil	D2	12	Hepatic/renal
Pramipexol[a]	D2	8–12	Renal
Ropinirol[a]	D2	6	Renal
Rotigotine (transdermal patch with 24 h delivery)	D2>D1	5–7	Renal
Apomorphine (s.c.)	D2>D1	0.5	

[a] Prolonged-/extended-release forms available.

monotherapy or adjunct to levodopa is firmly established as is their efficacy in reducing motor fluctuations.[8]

There is also solid evidence to show that effects sizes in reducing motor symptoms are smaller with DAs and that the risk to induce dyskinesias in early monotherapy is substantially smaller compared with levodopa.[15] The major limiting side effects of DAs are daytime somnolence and impulse control disorders—both common and with potentially catastrophic consequences, such as falling asleep at the wheel or the breakdown of social and professional relations due to impulse dyscontrol.[16]

Enzyme inhibitors

Blocking the metabolism of central dopamine via inhibition of monoamine-oxidase (MAO) was suggested already in the very early days of levodopa treatment as a strategy to enhance efficacy. It had to be abandoned because the then available nonselective MAO inhibitors were associated with the risk of inducing hypertensive crisis after ingestion of tyramine-rich food ("cheese effect") due to central serotonergic overactivity. The development of selective inhibitors of the B-type of the enzyme, which mainly metabolizes dopamine, paved the way of MAO inhibition into clinical practice in PD. Current MAO-B inhibitors include the irreversible enzyme blockers selegiline and rasagiline, and safinamide, which is a reversible inhibitor with additional indirect glutamatergic activity.[17] Their antiparkinsonian effect size is smaller than that of levodopa or DAs.

With combined levodopa/decarboxylase inhibitor therapy the peripheral metabolism of levodopa is shifted toward o-methylation via the enzyme catechol-o-methyl-transferase (COMT). COMT inhibitors prolong the half-life and bioavailability of levodopa thereby extending the duration of effect of individual doses. The nitrocatechol compounds entacapone, tolcapone, and opicapone have all been shown to be effective in reducing OFF-time when added to levodopa in patients with motor response fluctuations.[8]

Nondopaminergic Drugs

The first successful use of pharmacologic agents to treat the motor symptoms of PD dates back to the 1860s when Ordenstein, working under Charcot at the Salpetriere Hospital in Paris, observed beneficial effects of plant extracts from *Hyoscyamus niger*, which contained belladonna alkaloids, such as atropine and hyoscyamine—substances that were much later shown to have anticholinergic properties leading to the introduction of synthetic anticholinergics into PD therapy in the 1930s. Anticholinergics still have some limited use in modern anti-PD therapy, particularly to control PD tremor. Because of their potential to induce or worsen cognitive dysfunction they should not be used in patients older than 65 years or those with cognitive impairment.

If anticholinergics are not effective in the treatment of PD tremor or are difficult to tolerate because of adverse effects, botulinum toxin injections into the hand and arm muscles may provide effective control of the tremor for about 3 to 4 months, after which time the treatment must be repeated.[18]

Similar to the first use of anticholinergics the antiparkinsonian efficacy of an N-methyl-d-aspartate (NMDA) receptor antagonist was discovered by serendipity and before its mechanism of action was known.[19] Although modestly effective, amantadine today is rarely used as initial monotherapy of PD but is the only currently available drug with proven efficacy to reduce levodopa-induced dyskinesias (LID) (see section on Treatment of levodopa-induced motor complications below).

The past 2 decades have seen an expanding understanding of multiple nondopaminergic receptors and pathways that directly or indirectly modify the basal ganglia cortical motor circuits, offering a multitude of potential targets for nondopaminergic drugs to treat the motor symptoms of PD.[20] Despite numerous clinical trials only very few agents have eventually been approved for PD therapy. These include the adenosine A2-antagonist istradefylline and the combined sodium and calcium channel blocker with additional MAO-B-inhibitory activity zonisamide, which are both marketed in Japan (istradefylline recently also in the United States) as adjunctive therapies in levodopa-treated patients with response fluctuations.[8,21,22]

EARLY MONOTHERAPY

There is a large and consistent body of evidence from randomized controlled clinical trials for the efficacy of levodopa, DAs, or MAO-B inhibitors as initial monotherapies to treat the motor symptoms in early PD (**Table 2**).[8] Despite decades of dopaminergic drug development and numerous clinical trials, levodopa still remains the drug with the greatest effect size and is thus regarded as the gold standard of symptomatic efficacy in the pharmacologic management of PD motor symptoms. The short half-life of levodopa standard formulations require at least 3 daily doses with many authors recommending 4 times daily dosing at around 4-hourly intervals to reduce fluctuations in plasma levels during the waking day. Although doses as low as 3 times 50 mg have shown efficacy over placebo, clinically meaningful and sustained responses are usually observed from a daily dose threshold of 300 mg onward.[23,24] The most important limitation to initiating treatment with levodopa in early PD is the potential to induce motor complications, which—depending on age, disease duration, and dose—affects a large proportion of patients after more than 3 years of sustained therapy[25] (see later discussion). Several randomized controlled trials have shown that early monotherapy with DAs carries a significantly reduced risk for the development of dyskinesias compared with monotherapy with levodopa over up to 5 years.[8,26] This has led to the recommendation of starting therapy with levodopa-sparing strategies (DAs or MAO-B inhibitors) with later adjunct of levodopa when required to maintain adequate symptomatic control.[27] These trial results and practice recommendations were unfortunately misinterpreted by patients and doctors alike, giving rise to the phenomenon of "levodopa-phobia" where the drug was withheld despite a need for better symptomatic control.[28] As recently shown in a large pragmatic trial involving more than 1600 subjects with early PD global symptom control as assessed by the mobility domain score of the PDQ-39 was consistently better with levodopa compared with treatment with DAs or MAO-B inhibitors (the PD-Med trial). Almost all patients started on a levodopa-sparing drug (DA or MAO-B inhibitor) eventually required additional levodopa and there were no major differences in the incidence of dyskinesias after extended follow-up

Table 2
Treatments for symptomatic monotherapy and as adjunct to levodopa in early stable disease (based on movement disorders society evidence-based medicine review update)

Class	Drug	Commonly Used Dose Range	Recommendations According to MDS EBM Review Update[a]
(Nonergot) dopamine agonists	Pramipexole (ER)	0.26–3.15 mg (base)	Efficacious Clinically useful
	Ropinirole (PR)	2–24 mg	Efficacious Clinically useful
	Rotigotine	2–8 mg	Efficacious Clinically useful
	Piribedil	150–300 mg	Efficacious Clinically useful
Levodopa/ peripheral decarboxylase inhibitor	Standard formulation	300–1000 mg	Efficacious Clinically useful
	Controlled release	100–200 mg (nocte)	Efficacious Clinically useful
MAO-B inhibitors	Rasagiline	1 mg	Efficacious Clinically useful
	Selegeline	5–10 mg	Efficacious Clinically useful
Others	Anticholinergics	Dose range depends on type of drug	Likely efficacious Clinically useful
	Amantadine	100–300 mg	Likely efficacious Possibly useful

Abbreviations: COMT, catechol-o-methyl-transferase; ER, extended release; LID, levodopa-induced dyskinesias; MAO-B, Monoamine-oxidase B; MF, motor fluctuations; PR, prolonged release.
[a] Recommendations are given for (1) efficacy conclusions and (2) implications for clinical practice according to the movement disorders society (MDS) evidence-based medicine (EBM) review update 2018.[8] Only drugs with the designation *(likely) efficacious* and *(possibly) clinically useful* are listed.

over 7 years—despite earlier development of this complication in the levodopa group.[29]

Nevertheless, initiating treatment with an MAO-B inhibitor is a viable option for patients with early disease and mild symptoms: in the placebo-controlled phase of the ADAGIO trial about 90% of subjects randomized to rasagiline did not need additional drugs over the first 9 months.[30] Similarly, the median time to need for levodopa in the DATATOP trial was 24 months in patients receiving selegiline versus 15 months in those not receiving selegeline,[31] and in the PD-MED trial less than 20% of patients allocated to MAO-B inhibitor therapy with selegiline or rasagiline were discontinued because of lack of efficacy.[29] The symptomatic effect size of DAs is generally perceived greater than that of MAO-B inhibitors, although the PD-Med trial did not support this notion, but on the contrary showed slightly greater benefit on the PDQ39 outcome in the MAO-B inhibitor arm.

In many national guidelines worldwide DAs are still recommended as an initial monotherapy option particularly for patients with increased risk to develop drug-induced dyskinesias with levodopa, mainly those with disease onset before the age of 60 to 70 years.[27] Although this approach has the advantage of delaying the development of dyskinesias and the convenience of enabling once-daily dosing with extended-release or transdermal patch formulations, it cannot prevent motor complications in the long term due to the need for adjunct levodopa. In addition, these benefits of DAs come with a price of poorer symptomatic control and increased risks for daytime somnolence, hallucinosis, leg edema, and impulse control disorders when compared with levodopa. In a recent prospective follow-up study of patients treated with DAs the cumulative incidence of impulse control disorders was 46% over 5 years.[32]

Nondopaminergic drugs, such as anticholinergics or amantadine, still have a limited role as alternatives to dopaminergic therapies as early monotherapies in certain patient populations. For example, young patients with tremor as a chief complaint may derive sufficient benefit from anticholinergics for some time, and amantadine monotherapy can provide satisfactory motor control in those with early and mild disease, before dopamine replacement becomes necessary.

In summary, levodopa remains the most effective drug to treat the motor symptoms in PD and should be used freely whenever required to achieve adequate control and satisfactory quality of life. Initiating treatment with levodopa-sparing strategies may be a preferred option in early mild disease (MAO-B inhibitors) or in subjects with young-onset PD and high risk for LID. Counseling patients about the different risk-benefit profiles of levodopa versus DAs is mandatory and should ideally include partners or caregivers, who should also be aware of the risks of excessive sleepiness and impulse control disorders with dopamine agonists.[16] **Table 3** provides a summary of the benefit-risk profiles of the main classes of dopaminergic drugs used to treat the motor symptoms of PD.

ADJUNCT THERAPIES IN STABLE DISEASE

Several of the drugs discussed above also have established efficacy to enhance motor control in patients already on levodopa. Their use as adjunct therapy may be a preferred strategy to avoid or delay further increases in the total levodopa dose or dose frequency. Evidence from controlled clinical trials has shown this type of efficacy for all of the commonly used DAs as well as for the 2 MAO-B inhibitors selegiline and rasagiline (See **Table 2**).[8] The combined MAO-B and glutamate release inhibitor zonisamide has shown similar efficacy but is currently licensed in Japan only.[22] The COMT inhibitor tolcapone has also been studied in a trial in patients on stable levodopa without motor fluctuations, where it led to improved motor control, but the drug is licensed only to treat patients with motor fluctuations (see later discussion).

Table 3
Benefit/risk profile of dopaminergic Parkinson disease therapies

	MAO-B Inhibitors	Dopamine Agonists	Levodopa
Benefit			
Symptomatic effect size	+	++	+++
Risks			
Peripheral dopaminergic AEs (nausea, hypotension)	−/+	+	+
EDS	−/+	++	+
Leg edema	−	+	−
Psychosis	−/+	++	+
Impulse control disorders	−/+	+++	−/+
Motor complications	−	−	+++

−, negligible; +, low; ++, moderate; +++, marked (for AEs >10% risk).
Abbreviations: AE, adverse events; EDS, excessive daytime somnolence.

TREATMENT OF LEVODOPA-INDUCED MOTOR COMPLICATIONS

Most patients treated with levodopa will develop motor complications comprising response oscillations and LID,[2] as well as levodopa-resistant axial motor symptoms, including freezing of gait, dysarthria, and dysphagia.

The most common types of motor response oscillations are wearing off, and other phenomena include delayed-on or no-on as well as early-morning akinesia. These are generally considered to be among the most troublesome symptoms by advanced PD patients. Dyskinesias can be related to on-off cycle with on-period chorea, biphasic dyskinesias, and, often painful, off-period dystonia. Severe and disabling dyskinesias are less frequent but are troublesome for patients and require medical attention, whereas milder forms of dyskinesias are more frequent, but rarely troublesome and do not require treatment if other components of motor function are adequately maintained. Levodopa-induced motor complications have been found to develop in 20% to 50% of patients after only 2 to 5 years ($\sim$10% per year) after introduction of levodopa.[33,34] Pathophysiological mechanisms include peripheral pharmacokinetic factors, such as short half-life of levodopa, erratic gastrointestinal absorption due to delayed gastric emptying and/or intestinal absorption failure, as well as central pharmacodynamic mechanisms and molecular alterations at presynaptic and postsynaptic dopaminergic and serotonergic transmission sites.[35] Risk factors for the development of levodopa-related motor complications are cumulative levodopa dose, daily levodopa doses of $\geq$ 400 mg (and/or >4 mg/kg), longer PD duration at the time of starting levodopa, female sex, low body weight, and early onset of PD, especially heritable young-onset autosomal recessive PD (parkin, PINK1, and DJ-1).[34,36]

In line with the above-mentioned risk factors for levodopa-induced motor complications, there has been a belief that holding levodopa therapy back until required in later PD, especially before the age of 70 years, will delay the onset of these side effects, substantiated by open label studies.[29,37] On the other side, the introduction of levodopa in patients with longer disease duration and/or in high doses has been shown to result in a shortened period of good effect before motor complications begin, thus suggesting that PD duration is the crucial factor with regard to development of response oscillations and LID.[38,39] Therefore, the current common approach is to introduce levodopa as soon as needed to maintain good symptom control and quality of life.

As soon as response oscillations and LID have started, the principle of their pharmacologic management is to provide more continuous and reliable dopaminergic drug delivery—either simply by increasing the dosage of dopaminergic medication, dividing the levodopa dosage into smaller but more frequent doses (levodopa dose fractionation), or by modifying the peripheral pharmacokinetics of levodopa (**Table 4**). Although extended levodopa formulations have existed for a long time and have mainly been used for reversal of nighttime and early-morning OFF-periods, a novel levodopa formulation has recently been approved in the United States; IPX-066 (Rytary) consists of microspheres of different sizes that deliver levodopa at different rates providing a more prolonged clinical response translating into increases of daily "on" duration by approximately 3 h compared with immediate release levodopa and 1.5 h compared with levodopa/entacapone.[40,41]

Adding transdermal (rotigotine) or extended-release (pramipexole, ropinirole) DAs can help alleviating motor fluctuations. Prolonging the synaptic availability of dopamine by use of COMT inhibitors (entacapone, tolcapone, or opicapone) or centrally active MAO-B inhibitors (selegeline, rasagiline, or safinamide) is another established strategy. Continuous drug delivery via pump devices is available for subgroups of patients with late-stage PD using levodopa/carbidopa (Duodopa pump) via a

Table 4
Efficacious treatments for motor fluctuations and/or levodopa-induced dyskinesias (based on movement disorders society evidence-based medicine review update)

Class	Drug	Commonly Used Daily Dose Range	Effects on	Recommendations According to MDS EBM Review Update[a]
(Nonergot) Dopamine agonists	Pramipexole (ER)	0.26–3.15 mg (base)	MF	Efficacious Clinically useful
	Ropinirole (PR)	2–24 mg	MF	Efficacious Clinically useful
	Rotigotine	2–8 mg	MF	Efficacious Clinically useful
	Apomorphine s.c.	3–30 mg (intermittent) 16–72 mg (continuous)	MF	Efficacious Clinically useful[b]
Levodopa/ peripheral decarboxylase inhibitor	Standard formulation	400–1000 mg	MF	Efficacious Clinically useful
	Extended release	855–2205 mg	MF	Efficacious Clinically useful
	Intestinal infusion	600–1800 mg	MF	Efficacious Clinically useful[b]
	Levodopa inhaled powder	1–2 42 mg capsules (up to 5 times a day)	MF	Not yet reviewed by MDS EBM committee
COMT inhibitors	Entacapone	600–1600 mg	MF	Efficacious Clinically useful
	Tolcapone	300–600 mg	MF	Efficacious Possibly useful[b]
	Opicapone	50 mg	MF	Efficacious Clinically useful
MAO-B inhibitors	Rasagiline	1 mg	MF	Efficacious Clinically useful
	Safinamide	50–100 mg	MF	Efficacious Clinically useful
Others	Amantadine	100–300 mg	LID	Efficacious Clinically useful
	Istradefylline	20–40 mg	MF	Likely efficacious Possibly clinically useful

Abbreviations: COMT, catechol-o-methyl-transferase; ER, extended release; LID, levodopa-induced dyskinesias; MAO-B, monoamine-oxidase B; MF, motor fluctuations; PR, prolonged release.
[a] Recommendations are given for (1) efficacy conclusions and (2) implications for clinical practice according to movement disorders society (MDS) evidence-based medicine (EBM) review update 2018.[8] Only drugs with the designation (likely) efficacious and (possibly) clinically useful are listed.
[b] Acceptable risk profile with specialized monitoring.

percutaneous duodenal tube or the dopamine agonist apomorphine via subcutaneous infusion. Continuous drug delivery may also alleviate LID and, potentially, help to avoid long-term evolution of motor fluctuations and LIDs in patients with early-stage PD, but this concept still needs to be tested. If strategies of modified drug delivery fail and wearing off and sudden offs persists, "rescue" therapies are available with dispersible formulation of levodopa, inhalable powder formulation of levodopa for intrapulmonary delivery recently approved in the United States (Inbrija),[10,11] and subcutaneous application of the dopamine agonist apomorphine (APO-go Pen). The only currently available effective drug to treat LID remains the noncompetitive NMDA receptor antagonist amantadine. Amantadine is now available in the United States as an extended-release formulation (ADS-5102 or Gocovri), administered as a nighttime 68.5- or 137-mg capsule, for the treatment of LID and motor fluctuations.[42]

The medical armamentarium has recently expanded beyond the dopaminergic arena to drugs that stimulate or inhibit nondopaminergic receptors involved in multiple basal ganglia synaptic transmission pathways.

Adenosine A2a receptors are selectively localized to the cell bodies and terminals of the indirect striatal output pathway involved in development of motor fluctuations. From the many developed adenosine A2A receptor antagonists, istradefylline is the only one that has undergone positive testing in large clinical trials and has so far been licensed in Japan[21] and has been recently approved by the US Drug and Food Administration (Nourianz) to treat OFF-time. The drug also shows promise in the treatment of freezing of gait, postural abnormalities, and cognitive dysfunction.[21] Zonisamide, another nondopaminergic drug acting at GABA and glutamatergic synapses and usually used as an antiepileptic agent, has been found to reduce "wearing offs" and has also been approved as a treatment of motor fluctuations in Japan.[22] The above-mentioned MAO-B inhibitor safinamide has also an antiglutamatergic mode of action and is therefore believed to reduce dyskinesias in addition to increasing ON-time.

Although not a medical treatment, deep brain stimulation of the subthalamic nucleus and globus pallidus internus should be mentioned at this stage, as it has been proven as a highly efficacious treatment of both motor fluctuations and levodopa-induced dyskinesias (LIDs)[8] (see Kyle T. Mitchell and Jill L. Ostrem's article, "Surgical Treatment of Parkinson's Disease," in this issue of Neurologic Clinics).

TREATMENT OF LEVODOPA-RESISTANT MOTOR COMPLICATIONS

In addition to levodopa-induced motor complications, motor disability in advancing PD is driven by the emergence of often poorly levodopa-responsive disturbances of gait and balance, dysphagia, and dysarthria. After 15 to 20 years into the disease more than 80% of patients will have developed postural instability, freezing of gait, and recurrent falls, and more than half will suffer from dysphagia and choking.[43,44] Despite the high impact these symptoms have on mobility and quality of life in patients with advanced PD, there have only been few trials assessing the effect on medical treatments on these symptoms. The only drug that has been designated as likely efficacious and possibly useful by the MDS EBM task force in treating gait disorder in PD and potentially reducing falls is rivastigmine.[8,45] The mechanisms by which acetylcholine esterase inhibitors might exert such effects remain to be fully elucidated. Trials with other drugs from the same class of substances and with methylphenidate have provided less convincing results and they are not (yet) recommended for this indication.

DISCLOSURE

W. Poewe has received consultancy and lecture fees in relation to clinical drug programs for PD from AbbVie, AstraZeneca, BIAL, Biogen, Biohaven, Britannia, Grünenthal, Intec, Ipsen, Lundbeck, Novartis, Neuroderm, Orion Pharma, Oxford Biomedica, Prexton, Regenera, Roche, Sunovion, Sun Pharma, Takeda, Teva, UCB and Zambon. Royalties: Thieme, Wiley Blackwell, Oxford University Press and Cambridge University Press. P. Mahlknecht has received an educational grant from Medtronic.

REFERENCES

1. GBD 2016 Parkinson's Disease Collaborators. Global, regional, and national burden of Parkinson's disease, 1990–2016: a systematic analysis for the Global Burden of Disease Study 2016. Lancet Neurol 2018;17(11):939–53.
2. Poewe W, Seppi K, Tanner CM, et al. Parkinson disease. Nat Rev Dis Prim 2017; 3:1–21.
3. Jankovic J, Goodman I, Safirstein B, et al. Safety and tolerability of multiple ascending doses of PRX002/RG7935, an anti-α-synuclein monoclonal antibody, in patients with Parkinson disease: a randomized clinical trial. JAMA Neurol 2018;75(10):1206–14.
4. Jankovic J. Pathogenesis-targeted therapeutic strategies in Parkinson's disease. Mov Disord 2019;34(1):41–4.
5. Brys M, Fanning L, Hung S, et al. Randomized phase I clinical trial of anti-α-synuclein antibody BIIB054. Mov Disord 2019;34(8):1154–63.
6. Poewe W, Mahlknecht P, Jankovic J. Emerging therapies for Parkinson's disease. Curr Opin Neurol 2012;25(4):448–59.
7. Rylander D, Parent M, O'Sullivan SS, et al. Maladaptive plasticity of serotonin axon terminals in levodopa-induced dyskinesia. Ann Neurol 2010;68(5):619–28.
8. Fox SH, Katzenschlager R, Lim S-Y, et al. International Parkinson and Movement Disorder Society evidence-based medicine review: update on treatments for the motor symptoms of Parkinson's disease. Mov Disord 2018;33(8):1248–66.
9. LeWitt PA, Fahn S. Levodopa therapy for Parkinson disease: a look backward and forward. Neurology 2016;86(14 Suppl 1):S3–12.
10. LeWitt PA, Hauser RA, Pahwa R, et al. Safety and efficacy of CVT-301 (levodopa inhalation powder) on motor function during off periods in patients with Parkinson's disease: a randomised, double-blind, placebo-controlled phase 3 trial. Lancet Neurol 2019;18(2):145–54.
11. Gupta HV, Lyons KE, Pahwa R. Old drugs, new delivery systems in Parkinson's disease. Drugs Aging 2019. https://doi.org/10.1007/s40266-019-00682-9.
12. Calne DB, Teychenne PF, Leigh PN, et al. Treatment of parkinsonism with bromocriptine. Lancet 1974;2(7893):1355–6.
13. Antonini A, Poewe W. Fibrotic heart-valve reactions to dopamine-agonist treatment in Parkinson's disease. Lancet Neurol 2007;6(9):826–9.
14. Steiger M, Jost W, Grandas F, et al. Risk of valvular heart disease associated with the use of dopamine agonists in Parkinson's disease: a systematic review. J Neural Transm 2009;116(2):179–91.
15. Stowe RL, Ives NJ, Clarke C, et al. Dopamine agonist therapy in early Parkinson's disease. Cochrane Database Syst Rev 2008;(2):CD006564.
16. Voon V, Napier TC, Frank MJ, et al. Impulse control disorders and levodopa-induced dyskinesias in Parkinson's disease: an update. Lancet Neurol 2017; 16(3):238–50.
17. Huot P, Fox SH, Brotchie JM. Monoamine reuptake inhibitors in Parkinson's disease. Parkinsons Dis 2015;2015:609428.
18. Mittal SO, Lenka A, Jankovic J. Botulinum toxin for the treatment of tremor. Parkinsonism Relat Disord 2019;63:31–41.
19. Schwab RS, Poskanzer DC, England AC, et al. Amantadine in Parkinson's disease. Review of more than two years' experience. JAMA 1972;222(7):792–5.

20. Fox SH, Brotchie JM, Lang AE. Non-dopaminergic treatments in development for Parkinson's disease. Lancet Neurol 2008;7(10):927–38.
21. Torti M, Vacca L, Stocchi F. Istradefylline for the treatment of Parkinson's disease: is it a promising strategy? Expert Opin Pharmacother 2018;19(16):1821–8.
22. Matsunaga S, Kishi T, Iwata N. Combination therapy with zonisamide and antiparkinson drugs for Parkinson's disease: a meta-analysis. J Alzheimers Dis 2017; 56(4):1229–39.
23. Fahn S, Oakes D, Shoulson I, et al. Levodopa and the progression of Parkinson's disease. N Engl J Med 2004;351(24):2498–508.
24. Verschuur CVM, Suwijn SR, Boel JA, et al. Randomized delayed-start trial of levodopa in Parkinson's disease. N Engl J Med 2019;380(4):315–24.
25. Chaudhuri R, Poewe W, Brooks D. Motor and nonmotor complications of levodopa: phenomenology, risk factors, and imaging features. Mov Disord 2018; 33(6):909–19.
26. Goetz CG, Poewe W, Rascol O, et al. Evidence-based medical review update: pharmacological and surgical treatments of Parkinson's disease: 2001 to 2004. Mov Disord 2005;20(5):523–39.
27. Ferreira JJ, Katzenschlager R, Bloem BR, et al. Summary of the recommendations of the EFNS/MDS-ES review on therapeutic management of Parkinson's disease. Eur J Neurol 2013;20(1):5–15.
28. Espay AJ, Lang AE. Common myths in the use of levodopa in Parkinson disease: when clinical trials misinform clinical practice. JAMA Neurol 2017;74(6):633–4.
29. PD Med Collaborative Group, Gray R, Ives N, Rick C, et al. Long-term effectiveness of dopamine agonists and monoamine oxidase B inhibitors compared with levodopa as initial treatment for Parkinson's disease (PD MED): a large, open-label, pragmatic randomised trial. Lancet 2014;384(9949):1196–205.
30. Rascol O, Fitzer-Attas CJ, Hauser R, et al. A double-blind, delayed-start trial of rasagiline in Parkinson's disease (the ADAGIO study): prespecified and post-hoc analyses of the need for additional therapies, changes in UPDRS scores, and non-motor outcomes. Lancet Neurol 2011;10(5):415–23.
31. Parkinson Study Group. Effects of tocopherol and deprenyl on the progression of disability in early Parkinson's disease. N Engl J Med 1993;328(3):176–83.
32. Corvol J-C, Artaud F, Cormier-Dequaire F, et al. Longitudinal analysis of impulse control disorders in Parkinson disease. Neurology 2018;91(3):e189–201.
33. Ahlskog JE, Muenter MD. Frequency of levodopa-related dyskinesias and motor fluctuations as estimated from the cumulative literature. Mov Disord 2001;16(3): 448–58.
34. Aquino CC, Fox SH. Clinical spectrum of levodopa-induced complications. Mov Disord 2015;30(1):80–9.
35. Bastide MF, Meissner WG, Picconi B, et al. Pathophysiology of L-dopa-induced motor and non-motor complications in Parkinson's disease. Prog Neurobiol 2015;132:96–168.
36. Warren Olanow C, Kieburtz K, Rascol O, et al. Factors predictive of the development of levodopa-induced dyskinesia and wearing-off in Parkinson's disease. Mov Disord 2013;28(8):1064–71.
37. Hauser RA, Rascol O, Korczyn AD, et al. Ten-year follow-up of Parkinson's disease patients randomized to initial therapy with ropinirole or levodopa. Mov Disord 2007;22(16):2409–17.
38. Cilia R, Akpalu A, Sarfo FS, et al. The modern pre-levodopa era of Parkinson's disease: insights into motor complications from sub-Saharan Africa. Brain 2014;137(Pt 10):2731–42.

39. Katzenschlager R, Head J, Schrag A, et al. Fourteen-year final report of the randomized PDRG-UK trial comparing three initial treatments in PD. Neurology 2008; 71(7):474–80.

40. Pahwa R, Lyons KE, Hauser RA, et al. Randomized trial of IPX066, carbidopa/levodopa extended release, in early Parkinson's disease. Parkinsonism Relat Disord 2014;20(2):142–8.

41. Stocchi F, Hsu A, Khanna S, et al. Comparison of IPX066 with carbidopa-levodopa plus entacapone in advanced PD patients. Parkinsonism Relat Disord 2014;20(12):1335–40.

42. Pahwa R, Tanner CM, Hauser RA, et al. ADS-5102 (Amantadine) extended-release capsules for levodopa-induced dyskinesia in Parkinson disease (EASE LID Study): a randomized clinical trial. JAMA Neurol 2017;74(8):941–9.

43. Hely MA, Morris JGL, Reid WGJ, et al. Sydney multicenter study of Parkinson's disease: non-L-dopa-responsive problems dominate at 15 years. Mov Disord 2005;20(2):190–9.

44. Hely MA, Reid WGJ, Adena MA, et al. The Sydney Multicenter Study of Parkinson's disease: the inevitability of dementia at 20 years. Mov Disord 2008;23(6): 837–44.

45. Henderson EJ, Lord SR, Brodie MA, et al. Rivastigmine for gait stability in patients with Parkinson's disease (ReSPonD): a randomised, double-blind, placebo-controlled, phase 2 trial. Lancet Neurol 2016;15(3):249–58.

Treatment of Nonmotor Symptoms Associated with Parkinson Disease

Jennifer G. Goldman, MD, MS[a,b,*],
Carlos Manuel Guerra, MD, MSc[c,d]

KEYWORDS

- Anxiety • Apathy • Autonomic symptoms • Cognition • Dementia • Depression
- Psychosis • Sensory symptoms

KEY POINTS

- Parkinson disease (PD) is complicated by some element of nonmotor features in most cases, present as early as prodromal signs, to de novo and newly diagnosed PD, and into advanced disease.
- Many nonmotor features are intricately related to each other, such that mood, cognitive, behavioral, and sleep disorders may overlap in symptomatology and treatments.
- Nonmotor features such as mood disorders, cognitive impairment, psychosis, sleep dysfunction, and bladder, bowel, and blood pressure dysfunction can affect quality of life.
- Management of nonmotor symptoms in PD requires inquiry and evaluation regarding symptoms and a multidisciplinary approach with both pharmacologic and nonpharmacologic treatment strategies.

INTRODUCTION

Parkinson disease (PD) is well recognized as a complex neurodegenerative disorder with a myriad of motor and nonmotor symptoms.[1,2] Nonmotor symptoms can predate the classic motor signs (bradykinesia, tremor, rigidity, gait, and postural impairment) of PD.[3,4] Nonmotor symptoms may occur throughout all stages of PD, from prodromal, to early stages, to advanced disease, and can inform different PD subtypes with therapeutic and prognostic implications (**Table 1**).[5,6] The conceptualization of "nonmotor

[a] Parkinson's Disease and Movement Disorders, Shirley Ryan AbilityLab, 355 East Erie Street, Chicago, IL 60611, USA; [b] Departments of Physical Medicine and Rehabilitation and Neurology, Northwestern University Feinberg School of Medicine, Chicago, IL 60611, USA; [c] PRISMA Advanced Care Center for Parkinson's, movement disorders and Dementia, San Luis Potosi, México; [d] Facutly of Psychology, Autonomous University of San Luis Potosí Sierra de las Cascadas 117, Lomas 4a seccion San Luis Potosí 78216, México
* Corresponding author.
E-mail address: jgoldman02@sralab.org

Neurol Clin 38 (2020) 269–292
https://doi.org/10.1016/j.ncl.2019.12.003
0733-8619/20/© 2019 Elsevier Inc. All rights reserved.

PD" has expanded our understanding of disease pathophysiology, neurotransmitters beyond dopamine, clinical subtypes, and interdisciplinary treatment approaches (**Fig. 1**).[7–9] This article reviews therapeutic approaches for symptoms affecting mood, cognition, behavior, sleep, autonomic function, and sensory systems, drawing from evidence-based recommendations where appropriate (**Table 2**).[10]

MOOD DISORDERS

Depression and anxiety are common features in PD, with an estimated prevalence of 30% to 50% individually, with some reports of even higher frequencies.[11,12] Some mood symptoms may overlap with other PD symptoms (eg, reduced facial expression, slowness, changes in sleep and appetite), which can make diagnosis challenging. These mood symptoms are infrequently self-referred by patients themselves; the Global Parkinson's Disease Survey demonstrated that, although 50% were classified as depressed, only 1% of the population self-reported depression.[13] Thus, clinicians must implement a proactive and systematic search for mood disorders, as well as many other nonmotor symptoms discussed in this review.

There are no specific clinical features that differentiate mood disorders in PD patients from non-PD persons. Both depression and anxiety in PD may be subsyndromal and not fully meet DSM-5 (*Diagnostic and Statistical Manual of Mental Disorders*, 5th edition) criteria. Mood disorders negatively affect physical and cognitive performance in PD and are a major cause of caregiver burden and reduced health-related quality of life.[14,15]

Epidemiologic studies demonstrate that the presence of depression or anxiety increases the risk of PD.[16] Female sex, advanced PD, and cognitive impairment are the most consistently reported risk factors for the development of depression in PD. Genetic risk factors for depression and anxiety have not yet been clearly defined (eg, GBA associated with depression; SNA-Rep-1 with a protective role),[17,18] although variable genetic expression influences information-processing pathways in PD and may underlie depression and cognitive changes in some subtypes of PD.[19,20] In PD, depression and anxiety can occur together or separately, be episodic or chronic, and can relate to intrinsic neurobiological changes (eg, dopaminergic, serotonergic, noradrenergic, cholinergic systems) underlying PD and/or reactions or adjustments to PD and PD-related changes. Depression and anxiety can also occur as nonmotor fluctuations in 44% of PD patients, particularly as related to "off" periods and experienced as dysphoria, anxiety, and panic symptoms.[21,22] Depression may be more

Table 1		
Nonmotor symptoms across the PD spectrum		
Prodromal/Premotor	**Early**	**Moderate/Advanced**
• REM sleep behavior disorder • Hyposmia/anosmia • Depression • Anxiety • Constipation • Excessive sleepiness	• Depression • Anxiety • Mild cognitive impairment • Constipation • Bladder dysfunction • Fatigue	• Depression • Anxiety • Dementia • Constipation • Bladder dysfunction • Orthostatic hypotension • Psychosis • Impulse control disorders • Apathy • Fatigue • Sleep disturbances, excessive sleepiness

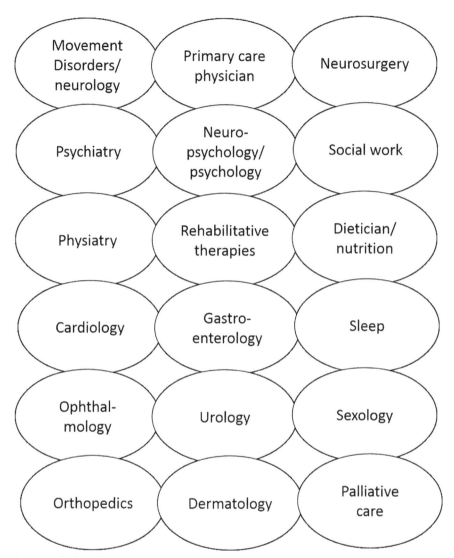

Fig. 1. Multidisciplinary approach to nonmotor symptoms in Parkinson disease: potential team members and specialists.

related to axial motor symptoms, whereas anxiety has been reported as more often present in patients with motor fluctuations and onset before 55 years.[23] Of interest, patients with PIGD (postural instability and gait difficulty) or rigid-predominant motor subtypes may be more prone to mood disorders.[24]

There is limited evidence to guide pharmacologic treatment of depression specifically in PD, and most evidence comes from some studies in PD as well as use of antidepressants and therapies in non-PD populations.[10] A systematic review reported statistically significant improvement of depression with selective serotonin reuptake inhibitors (SSRIs),[25] and a network meta-analysis concluded that SSRIs had "satisfying efficacy" for depression in PD, improved activities of daily living and motor function but had some adverse effects. The same study also reported that serotonin and

Table 2
Nonmotor features of Parkinson disease, interventions studied, and potential treatments

Nonmotor Category	Nonmotor Symptoms	Possible Treatments/Interventions Studied	Caveats and Other Information
Mood disorders	Depression	• Selective serotonin reuptake inhibitors • Selective serotonin norepinephrine inhibitors • Tricyclic antidepressants • MAO-B inhibitors • Dopamine agonists • Cognitive behavioral therapy • Transcranial magnetic stimulation • Electroconvulsive treatment • Physical exercise	• Serotonin syndrome • Tricyclics effects in elderly • Drug-drug interactions
	Anxiety	• Selective serotonin reuptake inhibitors • Selective serotonin norepinephrine inhibitors • Buspirone • Benzodiazepines • Cognitive behavioral therapy	• Benzodiazepine effects in elderly, balance, and/or cognitive problems
Cognitive disorders	Mild cognitive impairment	• Cholinesterase inhibitors • Rasagiline • Atomoxetine • Cognitive exercise/rehabilitation	• Trials with insufficient evidence of efficacy to date
	Dementia	• Cholinesterase inhibitors • Memantine	• Rivastigmine, FDA approved in USA • Monitor for bradycardia, hypotension, tremor, gastrointestinal symptoms with cholinesterase inhibitors

Behavioral issues	Psychosis	• Reduce or discontinue dopaminergic medication • Pimavanserin • Clozapine • Quetiapine	• Pimavanserin, FDA approved in USA • Blood count monitoring with clozapine • Monitor for sedation, hypotension with clozapine and quetiapine • Avoid dopamine-blocking antipsychotics
	Impulse control disorders	• Reduce or discontinue dopaminergic medication • Naltrexone • Cognitive behavioral therapy	• Monitor for dopamine agonist withdrawal syndrome
	Apathy	• Dopamine agonists • Rivastigmine • Antidepressants	• May be more noticeable by care partner
Sleep disorders	Insomnia	• Adjust dopaminergic regimen at nighttime • Eszopiclone • Melatonin • Antidepressants • Sleep hygiene	• Depends on etiology
	Sleep-related movement disorders	• Dopamine agonists • Gabapentin, pregabalin • Benzodiazepines • Iron supplementation, if indicated	• Differentiate between restless legs syndrome and periodic limb movements
	Sleep-disordered breathing REM sleep behavior disorder	• Continuous positive airway pressure • Melatonin • Benzodiazepines	• Monitor for safety in bedroom
	Excessive daytime sleepiness	• Modafinil • Caffeine • Continuous positive airway pressure	• Depends on etiology

(continued on next page)

Table 2
(continued)

Nonmotor Category	Nonmotor Symptoms	Possible Treatments/Interventions Studied	Caveats and Other Information
Autonomic dysfunction	Orthostatic hypotension	• Increased fluids, salt, caffeine, if appropriate • Compression stockings, abdominal binders, head of bed elevation • Fludrocortisone • Midodrine • Droxidopa • Pyridostigmine	• Monitor for supine hypertension
	Constipation	• Increased fluids, fiber, exercise • Lubiprostone • Probiotics and prebiotic fiber • Macrogol • Stool softeners • Osmotic laxatives	
	Bladder – irritative	• Solifenacin • Mirabegron • Trospium • Oxybutynin • Botulinum toxin injections	• Monitor for anticholinergic/central nervous system effects of medications
	Bladder – obstructive	• Evaluation for prostate issues • Catheterization	
	Sexual dysfunction	• Sildenafil • Counseling	
Fatigue	Fatigue	• Rasagiline • Methylphenidate • Modafinil • Acupuncture	• Methylphenidate in elderly or cardiac history

Sensory system dysfunction	Hyposmia/anosmia	• Increase flavoring/spices in food, make visually appealing	• Caution if unable to smell, eg, rotten food, smoke
	Vision	• Glasses, prisms • Artificial tears for dry eyes	• Depends on etiology • Consider vision specialists
	Pain	• Rotigotine • NSAIDs • Baclofen • Benzodiazepines • Gabapentin	• Depends on etiology • Monitor/minimize opioids
Musculoskeletal	Arthritic changes	• Physical and occupational therapy • Treat pain, if applicable	
	Postural changes (camptocormia, Pisa syndrome)	• Adjust dopaminergic medications • Benzodiazepines • Baclofen • Botulinum toxin injections • Physical therapy • Consider deep brain stimulation	
Skin	Seborrheic dermatitis	• Shampoos, lotions, creams	• Referral to dermatology
	Hyperhidrosis	• Adjust dopaminergic medications • Nonpharmacologic strategies • Botulinum toxin injections (eg, palms)	
	Melanoma risk		• Skin surveillance
Other	Sialorrhea	• Botulinum toxin injections • Glycopyrrolate • Ipratropium bromide spray	• Counsel regarding dental hygiene
	Dysphagia	• Adjustment to diet • Thickeners, if appropriate	• Referral to speech-language pathology for evaluation
	Weight loss	• Adjustments to diet • Assess eating, swallowing, calories, energy expenditure	• Referral to dietician/nutrition

norepinephrine reuptake inhibitors (SNRIs) are safe with high efficacy and good tolerance.[26] Although tricyclic antidepressants may demonstrate similar efficacy in depression compared with SSRIs, their side effects (eg, cardiac arrhythmias, orthostasis, confusion) limit their use especially in PD patients and older adults.[27] The dopamine agonists pramipexole and rotigotine have improved measures of depression when compared with placebo in PD.[28,29] Support for a relationship between dopamine pathways, dopamine agonists, and mood comes from the emergence of depression or apathy with dopaminergic agonist withdrawal or with rapid medication reduction after deep brain stimulation (DBS).[30] There is also evidence for nondopaminergic pathways in depression in early depressed patients with PD.[31] Although there remains a need for more randomized controlled trials, medication treatment of depression in PD encompasses SSRIs, SNRIs, tricyclic antidepressants (TCAs), and monoamine oxidase-B (MAO-B) inhibitors. Therapeutic strategies ideally should be individualized, potentially taking into account not only comorbidities but also phenotype and genotype.[32] Trials of medications for anxiety specifically in PD are lacking, with medications such as SSRIs and SNRIs, and sometimes buspirone, typically used.[10,33] Benzodiazepines are used judiciously, recognizing possible cognitive, balance, and sedative effects. If anxiety is related to nonmotor fluctuations or "off" periods, one may adjust dopaminergic medications, often in conjunction with anxiolytics.

Nonpharmacologic interventions are important strategies for mood disorders, and a multidisciplinary approach may have benefits beyond pharmacotherapy alone.[34] Cognitive behavioral therapy (CBT) improves depression with maintenance of control over 6 months of follow-up and with effects comparable with antidepressant medications for mild depression.[35,36] CBT can also lower anxiety and caregiver burden.[37] Successful delivery of CBT and psychotherapy has occurred using telecommunication technologies in pilot studies.[38,39] There is a growing literature of effects of physical exercise and activity on mood in PD. Transcranial magnetic stimulation and DBS demonstrate some evidence in PD depression, but requires further research. There is no strong supporting evidence for neuromodulation in anxiety at present.[40]

COGNITIVE DYSFUNCTION

Recognition of cognitive impairment in PD has grown with respect to phenotype, progression, biomarkers, and treatments in recent years.[41] Cognitive impairment may occur in 15% to 20% of de novo unmedicated PD patients, and mild cognitive impairment (PD-MCI) in about 25% (with reports up to 60%) after PD diagnosis.[42] The cumulative incidence for dementia increases to 75% to 90% over time, with 10% of patients manifesting dementia within 3 years of diagnosis, and increasing to 46% by 10 years and 83% by 20 years in longitudinal studies.[43] Cognitive decline and dementia contribute to decreased quality of life and increased risk of institutionalization, caregiver burden, and health-related costs.[44] Some studies suggest that cognitive decline may occur in some individuals at risk for developing PD, but this has not been well defined.[45]

Typical cognitive symptoms include a mixture of impaired executive function, attention, memory, and visuoperceptual skills. Language is less impaired compared with Alzheimer disease. In addition, 2 cognitive phenotypes have been proposed, "frontostriatal" or "posterior cortical," with differing progression and associated genotypes.[46]

Neuropsychological evaluation is an essential part of determining the characteristics and severity of cognitive impairment. The Movement Disorder Society (MDS) Rating Scales Review Committee published recommendations regarding global measures for cognitive screening in PD and proposing, with their methodology for

"Recommended" scales, the Montreal Cognitive Assessment, Mattis Dementia Rating Scale (2nd edition) and the Parkinson's Disease-Cognitive Rating Scale.[47] Assessments should measure premorbid cognitive levels and the impact of cognitive deficits on functional abilities. In addition, 89% of PD patients have at least one comorbid neuropsychiatric symptom, about 60% of which are clinically significant and may affect the evaluation.[48]

Mild cognitive impairment in PD (PD-MCI) is an evolving construct.[49] Diagnostic criteria have been proposed for PD-MCI, with both abbreviated and comprehensive assessments.[50] PD-MCI is heterogeneous, manifesting with different clinical presentations, often with multiple domains involved, and different rates of progression. Impaired semantic verbal fluency and visuospatial/visuoconstructive abilities may portend poorer prognosis.[51] PD dementia (PDD) is a syndrome representing a decline in more than one cognitive area (not necessarily memory), significant impact on everyday activities, and often associated with behavioral features (eg, apathy, depression, psychosis, excessive daytime sleepiness).[52] Older age, longer disease duration, worse motor function, comorbid neuropsychiatric features, rapid eye movement (REM) sleep behavior disorder, and cognitive impairment at baseline are risk factors for PDD.[53] Neuroimaging studies using different modalities (eg, structural MRI, functional MRI, nuclear medicine scans) demonstrate correlates of PD-MCI and PDD, with a range of cortical and subcortical atrophy patterns and disrupted corticostriatal connectivity.[54,55] Genetic mutations may contribute to PD cognitive impairment with stronger associations for synuclein duplications or triplications, GBA mutations, MAPT haplotypes H1/H1, and APOE e4 in some, in contrast to LRRK2 mutation carriers.[56]

The primary neural pathways contributing to cognitive dysfunction in PD include dopaminergic (frontostriatal, mesocortical), cholinergic (corticopetal), and noradrenergic systems, and form the basis of proposed treatments.[57] Rivastigmine is the only pharmacologic treatment with level A evidence and Food and Drug Administration (FDA) approval in the United States for PDD, whereas donepezil and galantamine have been considered "possibly useful" for PDD in MDS evidence-based medicine reviews.[10] Rivastigmine, rasagiline, and atomoxetine have been studied in randomized controlled trials for PD-MCI but did not provide significant benefit for primary cognitive outcomes. Management of cognitive impairment in PD should consider evaluation of PD and non-PD medications (eg, discontinuing anticholinergics or sedating medications), comorbid medical or neurologic issues, comorbid neuropsychiatric symptoms, and pharmacologic and nonpharmacologic interventions that address medication needs, safety, driving, and psychosocial impact. Physical activity and exercise improve cognition in PD, as may pairing cognitive tasks with exercise or cognitive exercises.[58,59]

BEHAVIORAL ISSUES

Psychosis in PD encompasses illusions, hallucinations, and delusions. Though not always the case, psychosis can be a frightening condition, especially for people with PD and caregivers. Psychosis has been associated with poor outcomes and increased caregiver burden.[60] Visual hallucinations are the most common sensory modality in PD, though auditory, tactile, and olfactory hallucinations can occur. Delusions most often have themes of paranoia or infidelity. Older age, cognitive impairment or dementia, and exposure to PD medications increase risk, although neither dosage, duration of administration, nor route of administration correlate with psychosis.[61] Minor hallucinations, however, can occur in 42% of untreated de novo PD patients, and long-term cumulative prevalence may be 60%.[62,63]

The etiology of PD psychosis is complex with potential contributions from neuro-chemical changes (eg, hypersensitivity of mesocorticolimbic D2/D3 receptors, seroto-ninergic/dopaminergic imbalances, and cholinergic deficits), sleep disturbances including REM sleep behavior disorder (RBD), cognitive impairment, and changes in the visual pathways from retina to visual association cortices.

Assessments for PD psychosis should begin with asking the patient about these phenomena. Several rating scales have been deemed "Recommended" by the MDS (eg, the Neuropsychiatric Inventory, Schedule for Assessment of Positive Symptoms [SAPS], Positive and Negative Syndrome Scale, Brief Psychiatric Rating Scale, and Clinical Global Impression Scale as secondary outcome).[64] New scales allow wider evaluation of symptoms, such as North-East Visual Hallucinations Interview (NEVH-I); the Scale for Assessment of Positive Symptoms adapted for PD (SAPS-PD), which focuses on the hallucinations and delusions items of the SAPS, was used in the pima-vanserin randomized controlled trial for PD psychosis.[65]

Treatment includes managing comorbid medical conditions and discontinuing or lowering doses of nonessential medications and, when able, dopaminergic medica-tions. When appropriate, antipsychotics with low dopamine antagonism or possibly cholinesterase inhibitors may be considered.[10,66] Typical or atypical antipsychotics with dopamine antagonism should be avoided. The selective 5-HT2A inverse agonist, pimavanserin, has been approved by the FDA in the United States for PD psychosis. Clozapine has demonstrated efficacy for PD psychosis without motor worsening in randomized clinical trials, but blood count monitoring for agranulocytosis is required. Quetiapine has been commonly used, despite the lack of evidence-based medicine in clinical trials.

Apathy, defined as loss of motivation and goal directed behavior, may occur in about 40% of PD patients. Apathy may have affective and cognitive components but can be independent from depression or cognitive impairment.[67] Symptoms such as executive deficits, verbal memory impairment, and bradyphrenia may occur. Apathy has been associated with decreased cingulate and inferior frontal gyri volumes on neuroimaging studies.[68] In the MDS review, the only "Recommended" scale was the 14-item Apathy Scale.[69] After DBS and withdrawal of dopamine medications, some PD patients may experience apathy. Levodopa and dopamine agonists, conversely, may improve motivation. Piribedil, a dopamine agonist, has been consid-ered as "possibly useful" in efficacy for apathy post–subthalamic nucleus (STN) DBS stimulation. In a randomized controlled trial, measures of apathy improved signifi-cantly in the rivastigmine group compared with placebo. Other considerations may include antidepressants, stimulants, cholinesterase inhibitors, or dopamine agonists, depending on the clinical symptomatology of apathy and associated depression, cognitive impairment, or DBS.[10,67]

Impulse control disorders (ICDs) are now recognized to occur in PD, with an asso-ciation with dopaminergic agonists and dopaminergic therapies. ICDs include repet-itive, often reward-associated, behaviors such as compulsive gambling or shopping, eating, sexual behaviors, dopamine dysregulation syndrome (compulsion for PD medication), and punding (repetitive non–goal-directed activity). These behaviors are more common in treated PD patients, but have been recognized in untreated pa-tients.[70,71] ICDs occur in 14% of PD patients, with one-third of them having more than one. The 5-year cumulative incidence is 46% and is greater in patients with dyski-nesia.[72,73] Besides dopamine agonist use, other associated medication features include higher levodopa doses and use of amantadine or MAO-B inhibitors.[74] Other risk factors include history of addiction (alcohol, gambling) in one's family, impulsive-ness, younger age, male sex, mood disorders, and early PD-onset age.[75] Cognitive dysfunction such as impaired executive function and set shifting or impulsive decision-making may occur in those with ICDs. These features may relate to altered striatal, cingulate, and orbitofrontal activation together with abnormal corticostriatal connectivity, enhanced during the "on" state.[76]

Instruments for detecting ICD include the Questionnaire for Impulsive-Compulsive Disorders in Parkinson Disease, the Questionnaire for Impulsive-Compulsive Disorders in Parkinson Disease-Rating Scale, and the Parkinson Impulse-Control Scale for the Severity Rating of Impulse-Control Behaviors in Parkinson Disease.[70] Patients should be counseled regarding ICDs, and routine surveillance should occur. ICD behaviors often disappear after discontinuing dopamine agonist or dopaminergic treatment, but one must be cautious to avoid dopamine agonist withdrawal syndrome, which can manifest as anxiety, panic attacks, dysphoria, dysautonomia, sleep disturbance, and cravings.[77,78] STN DBS may positively affect ICD behaviors, but there are some reports of worsened ICD after surgery, possibly secondary to high-dose medication.[79] Interventions such as naltrexone or CBT require further study.

SLEEP DISTURBANCES

Sleep disturbances are frequent across all stages of PD and represent a broad spectrum of symptomatology: disturbances of sleep (insomnia, sleep-related movement disorders, sleep-disordered breathing, parasomnias, RBD), disturbances of wakefulness (excessive daytime sleepiness), and circadian system dysfunction.[80] Sleep disturbances are associated with decreased quality of life in PD patients.[81] An estimated 40% to 98% of PD patients experience some form of sleep disturbances compared with 12% of the non-PD population.[82]

RBD is characterized by vivid dreams with involuntary vocalizations, jerks, and motor behaviors during REM sleep, usually associated with negative emotional content. This behavior is possible because of the loss of physiologic muscle atonia, and the involuntary movements may confer risk of injury to the patient and bed partner.[83] RBD is strongly associated with the development of a synucleinopathy over time (eg, PD, dementia with Lewy bodies, or multiple system atrophy), with 33.1% converting at 5 years and 90.4% at 14 years.[84]

Polysomnography (PSG)-confirmed RBD in PD occurs in about 39% to 46%, and in 25% of *de novo* patients.[85] RBD-PD patients are more likely to have an akinetic/rigid phenotype, more severe nonmotor and motor symptoms, increased falls, dyskinesias, hallucinations, and cognitive decline.[86] PSG is the gold standard for RBD diagnosis; screening questionnaires may be used but have relatively low specificity.[87–89]

Management includes education, ensuring a safe sleep environment, and avoiding medications that can aggravate RBD when possible (eg, SSRIs, SNRIs, or TCAs). Melatonin and clonazepam are pharmacologic strategies for treating RBD, alone or in combination, but caution regarding benzodiazepines, especially in older adults, is advised.[10] Rivastigmine may be helpful according to bed partners.[90]

Insomnia encompasses difficulties with sleep initiation, maintenance, and/or early-morning awakenings. It represents the most common sleep disorder in PD, affecting up to 80% of patients, with sleep fragmentation being the most frequent type of insomnia. Risk factors include advanced disease and female sex, along with inadequate sleep habits, REM sleep latency, and quality of sleep.[91] Besides PD-related degeneration in brain areas controlling sleep-wake homeostasis, motor and nonmotor symptoms also may result in fragmented sleep (eg, overnight tremors, rigidity and akinesia, painful dystonic spasms, nocturia, depression, anxiety, and hallucinations). Because insomnia in PD has many causes, a detailed medical and sleep history and examination is encouraged along with consideration for scales (eg, Parkinson

Disease Sleep Scale, second version and the Scale for Outcomes in PD-Sleep).[92,93] Optimizing nocturnal PD symptom management and counseling about sleep hygiene are advised. CBT may improve patient-reported sleep outcomes and physician-reported clinical global impression of change, and medications such as rotigotine may improve sleep efficiency while reducing sleep-onset latency and overnight awakenings. Antidepressants, eszopiclone, melatonin, and sodium oxybate have also been proposed as therapeutic strategies for insomnia, with weak evidence.[94–96]

Sleep-related movement disorders such as restless legs syndrome (RLS) and periodic limb movement disorder may occur in PD. The prevalence of RLS in PD is variable, but estimated in 21.6%. PD patients with RLS tend to have greater nonmotor symptoms such as depression, anxiety, dysautonomia, and low-weight malnutrition.[80] There is no evidence that RLS progresses to PD, although it frequently accompanies PD.[97] Treatment of RLS in PD includes dopamine agonists, gabapentin, pregabalin, and intravenous iron (if serum ferritin levels are low), and avoiding medications known to exacerbate RLS (eg, dopamine antagonists, antidepressants, anticholinergics, and antihistaminergics).[10] One should be mindful of augmentation as a complication; it may be preferable to start or switch treatment to pregabalin or gabapentin over dopamine agonists in these patients.[98]

Excessive daytime sleepiness (EDS) in PD ranges in prevalence from 20% to 60%, with 11.8% of de novo PD patients reporting EDS and increasing to 23.4% at 5 years.[99,100] EDS may represent an early, premotor manifestation of synuclein-related neurodegeneration.[101] PD patients with EDS are predominantly male, older, and have greater cognitive impairment, depression, autonomic dysfunction, RBD, motor and nonmotor symptoms.[102] The Epworth Sleepiness Scale is a self-reported instrument useful for diagnosis, but objective measures such the Multiple Sleep Latency Test may be useful. Informant corroboration may also be helpful.[103] Management includes identifying causes of EDS (eg, sedating medications, poor nighttime sleep), adjusting medications as appropriate, and counseling about driving safety. Good sleep-hygiene habits and regular physical exercise with adequate exposure to bright light should be encouraged.[104] Wakefulness-promoting drugs such as modafinil may be effective in treating EDS.[10] Caffeine use improved the clinical global impression of change in one study, but no changes were observed in the Epworth scale.[105]

Circadian dysfunction in PD such as with diurnal symptom fluctuation and seasonal variability of motor and nonmotor symptoms may reflect central pathophysiologic neurodegenerative processes and underlying sleep-wake disturbances in PD.[106,107] Pathologic effects of sleep and circadian alterations in PD may result in a "pathogenic feedback loop," with one feeding the other.[108] Circadian-based interventions (eg, light therapy), used in sleep medicine and psychiatry, demonstrate potential benefit for sleep-wake cycles, mood, and motor manifestations of PD.[109,110]

AUTONOMIC DYSFUNCTION

Autonomic dysfunction in PD, common in more advanced disease, is also recognized as an early disease marker with loss of postganglionic sympathetic skin nerve fibers and cardiac sympathetic/parasympathetic denervation.[111–113] About 71% of PD patients have at least one autonomic dysfunction manifestation, with mild symptoms worsening over time.[114] There is an independent progression between autonomic dysfunction and motor impairment, but it is highly associated with nonmotor symptoms, older age, male sex, poor levodopa response, and PIGD subtypes.

Cardiovascular symptoms may present at any phase of PD and do not correlate with dopaminergic deficit or motor fluctuations.[115] The Schellong test (lying-to-standing orthostatic test) is an effective screening tool for cardiovascular disturbances, and *meta*-iodobenzylguanidine scintigraphy is the best method of differential disease diagnostics.[116,117] Complaints of transient visual impairment, nausea, dizziness, and lightheadedness are present in half of PD patients, but orthostatic hypotension (OH) is the most frequent symptom.[118] OH can present simultaneously with or before motor symptoms and should be considered an intrinsic symptom of PD, with central (nigrostriatal and noradrenergic) and peripheral nervous system contributions. Dopaminergic treatment also can lower blood pressure. Management involves reviewing current medications and eliminating unnecessary drugs such as antihypertensives if no longer necessary. Nonpharmacologic strategies include elevating the head position during sleep, ensuring sufficient fluid intake (2–3 L/d) and/or sodium-enriched diet, using support stockings or abdominal binders, exercising, and eating smaller meals for patients with postprandial hypotension. Medications include fludrocortisone, which may be used with monitoring for lower extremity edema and congestive heart failure,[119] midodrine (or its metabolite, desglymidodrine), which increases vascular resistance while monitoring for nocturnal supine hypertension,[120] or droxidopa, a prodrug converted into norepinephrine, with longer duration of action and lesser nocturnal increase of blood pressure.[10,121] Pyridostigmine (an acetylcholinesterase inhibitor) reduces OH without supine hypertension, but its effect is modest. Other agents such as desmopressin, octreotide, methylphenidate, and yohimbine can be used for specific conditions.[122]

Urinary dysfunction occurs in 27% to 85% of PD patients, with urgency and nocturia as the most frequently reported nonmotor symptoms (56% versus 62%, respectively) using the Nonmotor Symptoms Questionnaire.[123] Detrusor hyperreflexia is the most frequent urinary problem in PD (in 45% to 100% of patients), but not all patients are always symptomatic. Urinary symptoms generally correlate with disease progression and may be divided in irritative (urgency, frequency, urge incontinence) or obstructive (hesitancy, reduced urinary stream, straining to urinate, incomplete emptying) categories. Anticholinergic drugs are the first options for irritative bladder symptoms, with the goal of avoiding older muscarinic drugs that can exacerbate cognitive dysfunction. Selective M3 receptor antagonists or β3-adrenergic receptor agonists may provide other options. In a small pilot study, solifenacin did not meet the primary outcome of change in mean number of micturitions per 24-hour period, although further study may be needed.[124] Botulinum toxin injections into the detrusor may provide benefit, and there may be improvement in lower urinary tract symptoms following STN DBS.[125,126] Obstructive bladder symptoms should raise suspicion of nonneurologic causes, such as prostatic hypertrophy or, possibly, detrusor underactivity. Anticholinergic medications may require discontinuation, and intermittent catheterization may be effective.

Gastrointestinal symptoms are common in PD, and the entire gastrointestinal tract may be dysfunctional, ranging in symptoms from salivary excess, dysphagia, gastroparesis, small intestine dysmotility, constipation, defecatory dysfunction, and weight loss.[127] Lewy bodies are present within the enteric nervous system, and it has been hypothesized that PD "begins in the gut," as suggested by α-synuclein abnormality found in the enteric nervous system and theories about the gut microbiome starting an inflammatory process that leads to neurodegeneration.[128,129] *Helicobacter pylori* infection also may interfere with PD medication absorption and affect motor fluctuations.[130]

Weight loss may occur in about 52% of PD patients, with malnutrition in 20%.[131] Weight loss may begin even in premotor stages, possibly because of increased energy expenditure and reduced energy intake, although this is not fully known. Low body weight and weight loss are associated with increased disease severity and dyskinesias, along with reduced quality of life, and may be influenced by various factors (eg, hormones, health fragility, medications, energy balance, decreased olfaction).[132] Early identification should urge dietary strategies against weight loss, and medication doses should be adjusted to body weight to lower the risk of dyskinesia.

Excessive salivation occurs in 90% of patients with advanced PD, 70% of all patients at all stages, and 40% on disease presentation. Oropharyngeal bradykinesia is the main cause, rather than increased saliva production.[133] Management strategies for drooling include chewing gum or sucking on hard candy, glycopyrrolate, ipratropium spray, atropine eye drops (anticholinergics), or botulinum toxin A or B injections to the salivary glands (efficacious and clinically useful by MDS evidence-based medicine recommendations).[10] Dysphagia has a pooled prevalence of about 35% with subjective testing, but objective testing demonstrates higher frequencies such as 82%, with obvious aspiration risk.[134] Dysphagia is attributed to bradykinesia and rigidity, but peripheral mechanisms in motor and sensory pharyngeal nerves also contribute.[135]

Constipation occurs in about 40% to 50% of PD patients, with 20% to 77% having decreased bowel movement frequency.[136] Constipation may be related to enteric nervous system dysfunction, central nervous system disease, medications, dietary changes, or limited physical activity. In addition, constipation has been suggested as a premotor feature, preceding motor symptoms by as many as 20 years.[137] Treatment of constipation in PD is similar to that for non-PD populations: increased dietary fiber and fluid intake and use of stool softeners or osmotic laxatives (polyethylene glycol [macrogol], lactulose, sorbitol). Lubiprostone has shown efficacy, with nausea as a common side effect; pyridostigmine and nizatidine effectiveness has only been discussed in case reports, and probiotics and prebiotic fiber are clinically useful.[138,139] Bypassing the gastrointestinal tract may useful for improved delivery and efficacy of PD medications such as with liquid levodopa formulations or parenteral routes, transdermal approaches (rotigotine patch), functional neurosurgery, apomorphine subcutaneous infusion, or percutaneous endoscopic infusion with a jejunal tube.[140]

Sexual dysfunction may occur in about 82% of PD patients.[141,142] Erectile dysfunction and ejaculatory impairment occurs in 79% of PD patients, being more common in those with depression, older age, comorbid pain, and PIGD phenotype.[143] A prospective study concluded that sexual activity in PD patients was associated with better motor and nonmotor outcomes and quality of life in men, suggesting that sexual health should be addressed.[144] However, hypersexuality as an ICD may occur in the context of dopamine agonist use; research suggests that PD patients with hypersexuality have reduced delay discounting of erotic rewards and abnormal reinforcing effects of levodopa when patients are confronted with erotic stimuli.[145,146] Sildenafil can be used for erectile dysfunction, although it may produce OH.[16] Sex therapy may help evaluate and treat the multiple factors underlying sexual dysfunction in PD patients and partners.[147]

VISUAL SYSTEM DISTURBANCES

Sensory system disturbances are often unrecognized and untreated, although 40% to 90% of PD patients will manifest some sensory symptoms during their disease.[148,149] Olfactory disturbances (hyposmia, anosmia), pain, and visual dysfunction are the most prominent sensory symptoms. Visual system changes in PD spans the retina tocortical brain regions. Deficits in visual acuity, color vision, eye movements, and complex visual tasks (judging distances or shape of objects) can affect motor function and increase susceptibility for hallucinations.[150] PD patients often complain of visual disturbances such as blurred vision when color stimuli are used (especially dark green, light blue, and dark red).[151] Convergence, binocular depth perception, and stereopsis are impaired in PD patients. Disturbances in visual acuity and color perception may reflect neurodegenerative changes in thalamus, posterior parietal lobe, and other visual pathways.[152] Reduced blink rates produce the classic "staring appearance" (hypomimia) in PD and can lead to dry eyes and reduced vision. Early parasympathetic dysfunction in PD is revealed by longer light reflex latencies and constriction times, with reduced contraction amplitude.[113] PD patients can present with disturbances of visuospatial orientation, facial recognition, and perception (eg, illusions, hallucinations), attributed to neurodegeneration within higher-order visuocognitive networks.[153] Management of visual issues in PD requires interdisciplinary work with eye-care practitioners to resolve specific visual deficits, use glasses or prisms, or other modalities.[9,151,154] Artificial tears can be used for dry eyes, and blepharospasm can be treated with botulinum toxin injections. Physical and occupational therapists can apply strategies to improve gaze control, visuospatial coordination, awareness, balance, and everyday function. Medications used in PD can have potential visual system side effects worth noting: anticholinergics (mydriasis, photophobia, dry eyes, decreased accommodation, anisocoria, blurred vision, anterior angle closure), dopamine agonists and other dopaminergic medications (hallucinations), and amantadine (mydriasis, blurred vision, hallucinations).[155]

MUSCULOSKELETAL AND SKIN DISTURBANCES

Musculoskeletal problems are more common in PD patients (45%–66.3%) than in the elderly population (4%–29%).[156,157] These problems are often undertreated and overlooked in PD patients in comparison with the general population.[158] Commonly involved body sites are the low back, knee, and shoulder. Previous pain occurs in 16.4% of patients at diagnosis, with 89% of this pain attributed to musculoskeletal problems. Shoulder problems associated with decreased arm swing and motion can be the presenting symptom of PD.[159] PD is associated with alterations in nociceptive processing at multiple levels, and one should recognize that some form of pain can occur in more than 80% of PD patients.[160,161] Osteoporosis is frequent in PD patients and complicates falls and fractures, which may lead to secondary motor and nonmotor complications.[162]

Dermatologic problems, such as seborrheic dermatitis and hyperhidrosis, also may accompany PD. Shiny and greasy skin can be identified as a premotor feature, and the lack of vasostability is related to autonomic dysfunction in the skin.[163] Antifungal shampoos (ketoconazole) applied to scalp and eyebrows can be efficacious.[164] An association between melanoma and PD has been found in some studies, prompting surveillance for cutaneous and ocular melanoma in PD patients.[165] A systematic review reports that levodopa can give rise to cutaneous complications (eg, malignant melanoma, allergic reactions, alopecia, vitiligo, skin hyperpigmentation, Laugier-Hunziker syndrome, Henoch-Schönlein syndrome, pseudobullous morphea, and scleroderma-like illness), although further study is needed.[166] Other drug-related skin reactions in PD include livedo reticularis with amantadine; contact dermatitis with rotigotine patch, and erythema, nodule formation, necrosis, and ulceration with subcutaneous apomorphine.[167] Suspension of the offending drug is usually effective in reversing drug-related adverse reactions.

DISCLOSURE

J.G. Goldman: Grants/research: Michael J. Fox Foundation, Parkinson's Foundation; Consulting: Acadia, Sunovion, WorldwideMed; Honoraria: American Academy of Neurology, International Parkinson's Disease and Movement Disorders Society, Parkinson's Foundation. C.M. Guerra None.

REFERENCES

1. Poewe W, Seppi K, Tanner CM, et al. Parkinson disease. Nat Rev Dis Primers 2017;3:17013.
2. Postuma RB, Berg D, Stern M, et al. MDS clinical diagnostic criteria for Parkinson's disease. Mov Disord 2015;30(12):1591–601.
3. Goldman JG, Postuma R. Premotor and nonmotor features of Parkinson's disease. Curr Opin Neurol 2014;27(4):434–41.
4. Berg D, Adler CH, Bloem BR, et al. Movement disorder society criteria for clinically established early Parkinson's disease. Mov Disord 2018;33(10):1643–6.
5. Fereshtehnejad SM, Postuma RB. Subtypes of Parkinson's disease: what do they tell us about disease progression? Curr Neurol Neurosci Rep 2017;17(4):34.
6. Konno T, Al-Shaikh RH, Deutschlander AB, et al. Biomarkers of nonmotor symptoms in Parkinson's disease. Int Rev Neurobiol 2017;133:259–89.
7. Marras C, Chaudhuri KR. Nonmotor features of Parkinson's disease subtypes. Mov Disord 2016;31(8):1095–102.
8. Titova N, Schapira AHV, Chaudhuri KR, et al. Nonmotor symptoms in experimental models of Parkinson's disease. Int Rev Neurobiol 2017;133:63–89.
9. Radder DLM, de Vries NM, Riksen NP, et al. Multidisciplinary care for people with Parkinson's disease: the new kids on the block! Expert Rev Neurother 2019;19(2):145–57.
10. Seppi K, Ray Chaudhuri K, Coelho M, et al. Update on treatments for nonmotor symptoms of Parkinson's disease-an evidence-based medicine review. Mov Disord 2019;34(2):180–98.
11. Broen MP, Narayen NE, Kuijf ML, et al. Prevalence of anxiety in Parkinson's disease: a systematic review and meta-analysis. Mov Disord 2016;31(8):1125–33.
12. Goodarzi Z, Mrklas KJ, Roberts DJ, et al. Detecting depression in Parkinson disease: a systematic review and meta-analysis. Neurology 2016;87(4):426–37.
13. Global Parkinson's Disease Survey (GPDS) Steering Committee. Factors impacting on quality of life in Parkinson's disease: results from an international survey. Mov Disord 2002;17:60–7.
14. Dobkin RD, Interian A. Improved understanding, detection, and management of neuropsychiatric complications: essential components to the optimal treatment of Parkinson's disease. Int Psychogeriatr 2019;31(1):1–4.
15. Martinez-Martin P, Rodriguez-Blazquez C, Forjaz MJ, et al. Neuropsychiatric symptoms and caregiver's burden in Parkinson's disease. Parkinsonism Relat Disord 2015;21(6):629–34.
16. Schrag A, Taddei RN. Depression and anxiety in Parkinson's disease. Int Rev Neurobiol 2017;133:623–55.
17. Dan X, Wang C, Zhang J, et al. Association between common genetic risk variants and depression in Parkinson's disease: a dPD study in Chinese. Parkinsonism Relat Disord 2016;33:122–6.
18. Lim EW, Tan EK. Genes and nonmotor symptoms in Parkinson's disease. Int Rev Neurobiol 2017;133:111–27.
19. Chagas MHN, Tumas V, Pena-Pereira MA, et al. Neuroimaging of major depression in Parkinson's disease: cortical thickness, cortical and subcortical volume, and spectroscopy findings. J Psychiatr Res 2017;90:40–5.
20. Won JH, Kim M, Park BY, et al. Effectiveness of imaging genetics analysis to explain degree of depression in Parkinson's disease. PLoS One 2019;14(2):e0211699.

21. Kim A, Kim HJ, Shin CW, et al. Emergence of non-motor fluctuations with reference to motor fluctuations in Parkinson's disease. Parkinsonism Relat Disord 2018;54:79–83.

22. Brun L, Lefaucheur R, Fetter D, et al. Non-motor fluctuations in Parkinson's disease: prevalence, characteristics and management in a large cohort of parkinsonian outpatients. Clin Neurol Neurosurg 2014;127:93–6.

23. Burn DJ, Landau S, Hindle JV, et al. Parkinson's disease motor subtypes and mood. Mov Disord 2012;27(3):379–86.

24. Brown RG, Landau S, Hindle JV, et al. Depression and anxiety related subtypes in Parkinson's disease. J Neurol Neurosurg Psychiatry 2011;82(7):803–9.

25. Bomasang-Layno E, Fadlon I, Murray AN, et al. Antidepressive treatments for Parkinson's disease: a systematic review and meta-analysis. Parkinsonism Relat Disord 2015;21(8):833–42 [discussion: 833].

26. Zhuo C, Xue R, Luo L, et al. Efficacy of antidepressant medication for depression in Parkinson disease: a network meta-analysis. Medicine (Baltimore) 2017; 96(22):e6698.

27. Menza M, Dobkin RD, Marin H, et al. A controlled trial of antidepressants in patients with Parkinson disease and depression. Neurology 2009;72(10):886–92.

28. Barone P, Poewe W, Albrecht S, et al. Pramipexole for the treatment of depressive symptoms in patients with Parkinson's disease: a randomised, double-blind, placebo-controlled trial. Lancet Neurol 2010;9(6):573–80.

29. Chaudhuri K, Martinez-Martin P, Antonini A, et al. Rotigotine and specific non-motor symptoms of Parkinson's disease: post hoc analysis of RECOVER. Parkinsonism Relat Disord 2013;19(7):660–5.

30. Antosik-Wojcinska A, Swiecicki L, Dominiak M, et al. Impact of STN-DBS on mood, drive, anhedonia and risk of psychiatric side-effects in the population of PD patients. J Neurol Sci 2017;375:342–7.

31. Espay AJ, Foster ED, Coffey CS, et al. Lack of independent mood-enhancing effect for dopaminergic medications in early Parkinson's disease. J Neurol Sci 2019;402:81–5.

32. Ryan M, Eatmon CV, Slevin JT. Drug treatment strategies for depression in Parkinson disease. Expert Opin Pharmacother 2019;20(11):1351–63.

33. Prediger RD, Matheus FC, Schwarzbold ML, et al. Anxiety in Parkinson's disease: a critical review of experimental and clinical studies. Neuropharmacology 2012;62(1):115–24.

34. Taylor J, Anderson WS, Brandt J, et al. Neuropsychiatric complications of Parkinson disease treatments: importance of multidisciplinary care. Am J Geriatr Psychiatry 2016;24(12):1171–80.

35. Berardelli I, Bloise MC, Bologna M, et al. Cognitive behavioral group therapy versus psychoeducational intervention in Parkinson's disease. Neuropsychiatr Dis Treat 2018;14:399–405.

36. Dobkin RD, Mann SL, Interian A, et al. Cognitive behavioral therapy improves diverse profiles of depressive symptoms in Parkinson's disease. Int J Geriatr Psychiatry 2019;34(5):722–9.

37. Dissanayaka NNW, Pye D, Mitchell LK, et al. Cognitive behavior therapy for anxiety in Parkinson's disease: outcomes for patients and caregivers. Clin Gerontol 2017;40(3):159–71.

38. Swalwell C, Pachana NA, Dissanayaka NN. Remote delivery of psychological interventions for Parkinson's disease. Int Psychogeriatr 2018;30(12):1783–95.

39. Wuthrich VM, Rapee RM. Telephone-delivered cognitive behavioural therapy for treating symptoms of anxiety and depression in Parkinson's disease: a pilot trial. Clin Gerontol 2019;42(4):444–53.

40. Nagy A, Schrag A. Neuropsychiatric aspects of Parkinson's disease. J Neural Transm (Vienna) 2019;126(7):889–96.

41. Marras C, Troster AI, Kulisevsky J, et al. The tools of the trade: a state of the art "how to assess cognition" in the patient with Parkinson's disease. Mov Disord 2014;29(5):584–96.

42. Weintraub D, Troster AI, Marras C, et al. Initial cognitive changes in Parkinson's disease. Mov Disord 2018;33(4):511–9.

43. Hanagasi HA, Tufekcioglu Z, Emre M. Dementia in Parkinson's disease. J Neurol Sci 2017;374:26–31.

44. Tramonti F, Bonfiglio L, Bongioanni P, et al. Caregiver burden and family functioning in different neurological diseases. Psychol Health Med 2019;24(1): 27–34.

45. Fengler S, Liepelt-Scarfone I, Brockmann K, et al. Cognitive changes in prodromal Parkinson's disease: a review. Mov Disord 2017;32(12):1655–66.

46. Williams-Gray CH, Mason SL, Evans JR, et al. The CamPaIGN study of Parkinson's disease: 10-year outlook in an incident population-based cohort. J Neurol Neurosurg Psychiatry 2013;84(11):1258–64.

47. Skorvanek M, Goldman JG, Jahanshahi M, et al. Global scales for cognitive screening in Parkinson's disease: critique and recommendations. Mov Disord 2018;33(2):208–18.

48. Aarsland D, Taylor JP, Weintraub D. Psychiatric issues in cognitive impairment. Mov Disord 2014;29(5):651–62.

49. Goldman JG, Holden SK, Litvan I, et al. Evolution of diagnostic criteria and assessments for Parkinson's disease mild cognitive impairment. Mov Disord 2018; 33(4):503–10.

50. Litvan I, Goldman JG, Troster AI, et al. Diagnostic criteria for mild cognitive impairment in Parkinson's disease: movement disorder society task force guidelines. Mov Disord 2012;27(3):349–56.

51. Martinez-Horta S, Kulisevsky J. Mild cognitive impairment in Parkinson's disease. J Neural Transm (Vienna) 2019;126(7):897–904.

52. Emre M, Aarsland D, Brown R, et al. Clinical diagnostic criteria for dementia associated with Parkinson's disease. Mov Disord 2007;22(12):1689–707 [quiz: 1837].

53. Anang JB, Gagnon JF, Bertrand JA, et al. Predictors of dementia in Parkinson disease: a prospective cohort study. Neurology 2014;83(14):1253–60.

54. Duncan GW, Firbank MJ, Yarnall AJ, et al. Gray and white matter imaging: a biomarker for cognitive impairment in early Parkinson's disease? Mov Disord 2016;31(1):103–10.

55. Seibert TM, Murphy EA, Kaestner EJ, et al. Interregional correlations in Parkinson disease and Parkinson-related dementia with resting functional MR imaging. Radiology 2012;263(1):226–34.

56. Fagan ES, Pihlstrom L. Genetic risk factors for cognitive decline in Parkinson's disease: a review of the literature. Eur J Neurol 2017;24(4). 561-e20.

57. Gratwicke J, Jahanshahi M, Foltynie T. Parkinson's disease dementia: a neural networks perspective. Brain 2015;138(Pt 6):1454–76.

58. David FJ, Robichaud JA, Leurgans SE, et al. Exercise improves cognition in Parkinson's disease: the PRET-PD randomized, clinical trial. Mov Disord 2015; 30(12):1657–63.

59. Hazamy AA, Altmann LJP, Stegemoller E, et al. Improved cognition while cycling in Parkinson's disease patients and healthy adults. Brain Cogn 2017;113:23–31.

60. Alvarado-Bolanos A, Cervantes-Arriaga A, Rodriguez-Violante M, et al. Impact of neuropsychiatric symptoms on the quality of life of subjects with Parkinson's disease. J Parkinsons Dis 2015;5(3):541–8.

61. Fenelon G, Soulas T, Zenasni F, et al. The changing face of Parkinson's disease-associated psychosis: a cross-sectional study based on the new NINDS-NIMH criteria. Mov Disord 2010;25(6):763–6.

62. Forsaa EB, Larsen JP, Wentzel-Larsen T, et al. A 12-year population-based study of psychosis in Parkinson disease. Arch Neurol 2010;67(8):996–1001.

63. Pagonabarraga J, Martinez-Horta S, Fernandez de Bobadilla R, et al. Minor hallucinations occur in drug-naive Parkinson's disease patients, even from the premotor phase. Mov Disord 2016;31(1):45–52.

64. Fernandez HH, Aarsland D, Fenelon G, et al. Scales to assess psychosis in Parkinson's disease: critique and recommendations. Mov Disord 2008;23(4): 484–500.

65. Voss T, Bahr D, Cummings J, et al. Performance of a shortened scale for assessment of positive symptoms for Parkinson's disease psychosis. Parkinsonism Relat Disord 2013;19(3):295–9.

66. Thomsen TR, Panisset M, Suchowersky O, et al. Impact of standard of care for psychosis in Parkinson disease. J Neurol Neurosurg Psychiatry 2008;79(12): 1413–5.

67. Pagonabarraga J, Kulisevsky J, Strafella AP, et al. Apathy in Parkinson's disease: clinical features, neural substrates, diagnosis, and treatment. Lancet Neurol 2015;14(5):518–31.

68. Reijnders JS, Scholtissen B, Weber WE, et al. Neuroanatomical correlates of apathy in Parkinson's disease: a magnetic resonance imaging study using voxel-based morphometry. Mov Disord 2010;25(14):2318–25.

69. Starkstein SE, Mayberg HS, Preziosi TJ, et al. Reliability, validity, and clinical correlates of apathy in Parkinson's disease. J Neuropsychiatry Clin Neurosci 1992; 4(2):134–9.

70. Weintraub D, Claassen DO. Impulse control and related disorders in Parkinson's disease. Int Rev Neurobiol 2017;133:679–717.

71. Weintraub D, Papay K, Siderowf A, et al. Screening for impulse control symptoms in patients with de novo Parkinson disease: a case-control study. Neurology 2013;80(2):176–80.

72. Biundo R, Weis L, Abbruzzese G, et al. Impulse control disorders in advanced Parkinson's disease with dyskinesia: the ALTHEA study. Mov Disord 2017; 32(11):1557–65.

73. Corvol JC, Artaud F, Cormier-Dequaire F, et al. Longitudinal analysis of impulse control disorders in Parkinson disease. Neurology 2018;91(3):e189–201.

74. Garcia-Ruiz PJ, Martinez Castrillo JC, Alonso-Canovas A, et al. Impulse control disorder in patients with Parkinson's disease under dopamine agonist therapy: a multicentre study. J Neurol Neurosurg Psychiatry 2014;85(8):840–4.

75. Voon V, Sohr M, Lang AE, et al. Impulse control disorders in Parkinson disease: a multicenter case–control study. Ann Neurol 2011;69(6):986–96.

76. Claassen DO, Stark AJ, Spears CA, et al. Mesocorticolimbic hemodynamic response in Parkinson's disease patients with compulsive behaviors. Mov Disord 2017;32(11):1574–83.

77. Mamikonyan E, Siderowf AD, Duda JE, et al. Long-term follow-up of impulse control disorders in Parkinson's disease. Mov Disord 2008;23(1):75–80.

78. Yu XX, Fernandez HH. Dopamine agonist withdrawal syndrome: a comprehensive review. J Neurol Sci 2017;374:53–5.

79. Kasemsuk C, Oyama G, Hattori N. Management of impulse control disorders with deep brain stimulation: a double-edged sword. J Neurol Sci 2017;374:63–8.

80. Videnovic A. Disturbances of sleep and alertness in Parkinson's disease. Curr Neurol Neurosci Rep 2018;18(6):29.

81. Suzuki K, Okuma Y, Uchiyama T, et al. Impact of sleep-related symptoms on clinical motor subtypes and disability in Parkinson's disease: a multicentre cross-sectional study. J Neurol Neurosurg Psychiatry 2017;88(11):953–9.

82. Porter B, Macfarlane R, Walker R. The frequency and nature of sleep disorders in a community-based population of patients with Parkinson's disease. Eur J Neurol 2008;15(1):50–4.

83. Schenck CH, Mahowald MW. REM sleep behavior disorder: clinical, developmental, and neuroscience perspectives 16 years after its formal identification in SLEEP. Sleep 2002;25(2):120–38.

84. Hogl B, Stefani A, Videnovic A. Idiopathic REM sleep behaviour disorder and neurodegeneration - an update. Nat Rev Neurol 2018;14(1):40–55.

85. Zhang J, Xu CY, Liu J. Meta-analysis on the prevalence of REM sleep behavior disorder symptoms in Parkinson's disease. BMC Neurol 2017;17(1):23.

86. Duarte Folle A, Paul KC, Bronstein JM, et al. Clinical progression in Parkinson's disease with features of REM sleep behavior disorder: a population-based longitudinal study. Parkinsonism Relat Disord 2019;62:105–11.

87. Boeve BF, Molano JR, Ferman TJ, et al. Validation of the Mayo Sleep Questionnaire to screen for REM sleep behavior disorder in a community-based sample. J Clin Sleep Med 2013;9(5):475–80.

88. Chahine LM, Daley J, Horn S, et al. Questionnaire-based diagnosis of REM sleep behavior disorder in Parkinson's disease. Mov Disord 2013;28(8):1146–9.

89. Stiasny-Kolster K, Mayer G, Schafer S, et al. The REM sleep behavior disorder screening questionnaire–a new diagnostic instrument. Mov Disord 2007;22(16): 2386–93.

90. Di Giacopo R, Fasano A, Quaranta D, et al. Rivastigmine as alternative treatment for refractory REM behavior disorder in Parkinson's disease. Mov Disord 2012; 27(4):559–61.

91. Sobreira-Neto MA, Pena-Pereira MA, Sobreira EST, et al. Chronic insomnia in patients with Parkinson disease: which associated factors are relevant? J Geriatr Psychiatry Neurol 2019;33(1):22–7.

92. Martinez-Martin P, Cubo-Delgado E, Aguilar-Barbera M, et al. A pilot study on a specific measure for sleep disorders in Parkinson's disease: SCOPA-sleep. Rev Neurol 2006;43(10):577–83 [in Spanish].

93. Trenkwalder C, Kohnen R, Hogl B, et al. Parkinson's disease sleep scale—validation of the revised version PDSS-2. Mov Disord 2011;26(4):644–52.

94. Humbert M, Findley J, Hernandez-Con M, et al. Cognitive behavioral therapy for insomnia in Parkinson's disease: a case series. NPJ Parkinsons Dis 2017;3:25.

95. Pierantozzi M, Placidi F, Liguori C, et al. Rotigotine may improve sleep architecture in Parkinson's disease: a double-blind, randomized, placebo-controlled polysomnographic study. Sleep Med 2016;21:140–4.

96. Yang H, Petrini M. Effect of cognitive behavior therapy on sleep disorder in Parkinson's disease in China: a pilot study. Nurs Health Sci 2012;14(4):458–63.

97. Mitterling T, Heidbreder A, Stefani A, et al. Natural course of restless legs syndrome/Willis-Ekbom disease: long-term observation of a large clinical cohort. Sleep Med 2015;16(10):1252–8.

98. Gonzalez-Latapi P, Malkani R. Update on restless legs syndrome: from mechanisms to treatment. Curr Neurol Neurosci Rep 2019;19(8):54.

99. Knie B, Mitra MT, Logishetty K, et al. Excessive daytime sleepiness in patients with Parkinson's disease. CNS Drugs 2011;25(3):203–12.

100. Tholfsen LK, Larsen JP, Schulz J, et al. Development of excessive daytime sleepiness in early Parkinson disease. Neurology 2015;85(2):162–8.

101. Abbott RD, Ross GW, White LR, et al. Excessive daytime sleepiness and subsequent development of Parkinson disease. Neurology 2005;65(9):1442–6.

102. Xiang YQ, Xu Q, Sun QY, et al. Clinical features and correlates of excessive daytime sleepiness in Parkinson's disease. Front Neurol 2019;10:121.

103. Bolitho SJ, Naismith SL, Salahuddin P, et al. Objective measurement of daytime napping, cognitive dysfunction and subjective sleepiness in Parkinson's disease. PLoS One 2013;8(11):e81233.

104. Videnovic A, Klerman EB, Wang W, et al. Timed light therapy for sleep and daytime sleepiness associated with Parkinson disease: a randomized clinical trial. JAMA Neurol 2017;74(4):411–8.

105. Postuma RB, Anang J, Pelletier A, et al. Caffeine as symptomatic treatment for Parkinson disease (Cafe-PD): a randomized trial. Neurology 2017;89(17):1795–803.

106. Breen DP, Vuono R, Nawarathna U, et al. Sleep and circadian rhythm regulation in early Parkinson disease. JAMA Neurol 2014;71(5):589–95.

107. van Wamelen DJ, Podlewska AM, Leta V, et al. Slave to the rhythm: seasonal differences in non-motor symptoms in Parkinson's disease. Parkinsonism Relat Disord 2019;63:73–6.

108. Mantovani S, Smith SS, Gordon R, et al. An overview of sleep and circadian dysfunction in Parkinson's disease. J Sleep Res 2018;27(3):e12673.

109. Baumann CR. Sleep-wake and circadian disturbances in Parkinson disease: a short clinical guide. J Neural Transm (Vienna) 2019;126(7):863–9.

110. Li S, Wang Y, Wang F, et al. A new perspective for Parkinson's disease: circadian rhythm. Neurosci Bull 2017;33(1):62–72.

111. De Pablo-Fernandez E, Tur C, Revesz T, et al. Association of autonomic dysfunction with disease progression and survival in Parkinson disease. JAMA Neurol 2017;74(8):970–6.

112. Nolano M, Provitera V, Manganelli F, et al. Loss of cutaneous large and small fibers in naive and l-dopa-treated PD patients. Neurology 2017;89(8):776–84.

113. Postuma RB, Gagnon JF, Pelletier A, et al. Prodromal autonomic symptoms and signs in Parkinson's disease and dementia with Lewy bodies. Mov Disord 2013;28(5):597–604.

114. Stankovic I, Petrovic I, Pekmezovic T, et al. Longitudinal assessment of autonomic dysfunction in early Parkinson's disease. Parkinsonism Relat Disord 2019;66:74–9.

115. Oh YS, Kim JS, Chung YA, et al. Orthostatic hypotension, non-dipping and striatal dopamine in Parkinson disease. Neurol Sci 2013;34(4):557–60.

116. Jost WH, Del Tredici K, Landvogt C, et al. Importance of ^{123}I-metaiodobenzylguanidine scintigraphy/single photon emission computed tomography for diagnosis and differential diagnostics of Parkinson syndromes. Neurodegener Dis 2010;7(5):341–7.

117. Strano S, Fanciulli A, Rizzo M, et al. Cardiovascular dysfunction in untreated Parkinson's disease: a multi-modality assessment. J Neurol Sci 2016;370:251–5.

118. Umehara T, Nakahara A, Matsuno H, et al. Predictors of postprandial hypotension in elderly patients with de novo Parkinson's disease. J Neural Transm (Vienna) 2016;123(11):1331–9.

119. Espay AJ, LeWitt PA, Hauser RA, et al. Neurogenic orthostatic hypotension and supine hypertension in Parkinson's disease and related synucleinopathies: prioritisation of treatment targets. Lancet Neurol 2016;15(9):954–66.

120. Gibbons CH, Schmidt P, Biaggioni I, et al. The recommendations of a consensus panel for the screening, diagnosis, and treatment of neurogenic orthostatic hypotension and associated supine hypertension. J Neurol 2017;264(8):1567–82.

121. Kaufmann H, Norcliffe-Kaufmann L, Hewitt LA, et al. Effects of the novel norepinephrine prodrug, droxidopa, on ambulatory blood pressure in patients with neurogenic orthostatic hypotension. J Am Soc Hypertens 2016;10(10):819–26.

122. Sharabi Y, Goldstein DS. Mechanisms of orthostatic hypotension and supine hypertension in Parkinson disease. J Neurol Sci 2011;310(1–2):123–8.

123. McDonald C, Winge K, Burn DJ. Lower urinary tract symptoms in Parkinson's disease: prevalence, aetiology and management. Parkinsonism Relat Disord 2017;35:8–16.

124. Zesiewicz TA, Evatt M, Vaughan CP, et al. Randomized, controlled pilot trial of solifenacin succinate for overactive bladder in Parkinson's disease. Parkinsonism Relat Disord 2015;21(5):514–20.

125. Giannantoni A, Conte A, Proietti S, et al. Botulinum toxin type A in patients with Parkinson's disease and refractory overactive bladder. J Urol 2011;186(3): 960–4.

126. Mock S, Osborn DJ, Brown ET, et al. The impact of pallidal and subthalamic deep brain stimulation on urologic function in Parkinson's disease. Neuromodulation 2016;19(7):717–23.

127. Sung HY, Park JW, Kim JS. The frequency and severity of gastrointestinal symptoms in patients with early Parkinson's disease. J Mov Disord 2014;7(1):7–12.

128. Braak H, de Vos RA, Bohl J, et al. Gastric alpha-synuclein immunoreactive inclusions in Meissner's and Auerbach's plexuses in cases staged for Parkinson's disease-related brain pathology. Neurosci Lett 2006;396(1):67–72.

129. Heintz-Buschart A, Pandey U, Wicke T, et al. The nasal and gut microbiome in Parkinson's disease and idiopathic rapid eye movement sleep behavior disorder. Mov Disord 2018;33(1):88–98.

130. Narozanska E, Bialecka M, Adamiak-Giera U, et al. Pharmacokinetics of levodopa in patients with Parkinson disease and motor fluctuations depending on the presence of *Helicobacter pylori* infection. Clin Neuropharmacol 2014; 37(4):96–9.

131. Fasano A, Visanji NP, Liu LW, et al. Gastrointestinal dysfunction in Parkinson's disease. Lancet Neurol 2015;14(6):625–39.

132. Sharma JC, Lewis A. Weight in Parkinson's disease: phenotypical significance. Int Rev Neurobiol 2017;134:891–919.

133. Karakoc M, Yon MI, Cakmakli GY, et al. Pathophysiology underlying drooling in Parkinson's disease: oropharyngeal bradykinesia. Neurol Sci 2016;37(12): 1987–91.

134. Kalf JG, de Swart BJ, Bloem BR, et al. Prevalence of oropharyngeal dysphagia in Parkinson's disease: a meta-analysis. Parkinsonism Relat Disord 2012;18(4): 311–5.

135. Suttrup I, Warnecke T. Dysphagia in Parkinson's disease. Dysphagia 2016; 31(1):24–32.

136. Knudsen K, Krogh K, Ostergaard K, et al. Constipation in Parkinson's disease: subjective symptoms, objective markers, and new perspectives. Mov Disord 2017;32(1):94–105.

137. Svensson E, Henderson VW, Borghammer P, et al. Constipation and risk of Parkinson's disease: a Danish population-based cohort study. Parkinsonism Relat Disord 2016;28:18–22.

138. Ondo WG, Kenney C, Sullivan K, et al. Placebo-controlled trial of lubiprostone for constipation associated with Parkinson disease. Neurology 2012;78(21): 1650–4.

139. Sakakibara R, Doi H, Sato M, et al. Nizatidine ameliorates slow transit constipation in Parkinson's disease. J Am Geriatr Soc 2015;63(2):399–401.

140. Ondo WG, Hunter C, Ferrara JM, et al. Apomorphine injections: predictors of initial common adverse events and long term tolerability. Parkinsonism Relat Disord 2012;18(5):619–22.

141. Hurt CS, Rixon L, Chaudhuri KR, et al. Barriers to reporting non-motor symptoms to health-care providers in people with Parkinson's. Parkinsonism Relat Disord 2019;64:220–5.

142. Ferrucci R, Panzeri M, Ronconi L, et al. Abnormal sexuality in Parkinson's disease: fact or fancy? J Neurol Sci 2016;369:5–10.

143. Deng X, Xiao B, Li HH, et al. Sexual dysfunction is associated with postural instability gait difficulty subtype of Parkinson's disease. J Neurol 2015; 262(11):2433–9.

144. Picillo M, Palladino R, Erro R, et al. The PRIAMO study: active sexual life is associated with better motor and non-motor outcomes in men with early Parkinson's disease. Eur J Neurol 2019;26(10):1327–33.

145. Bronner G, Aharon-Peretz J, Hassin-Baer S. Sexuality in patients with Parkinson's disease, Alzheimer's disease, and other dementias. Handb Clin Neurol 2015;130:297–323.

146. Girard R, Obeso I, Thobois S, et al. Wait and you shall see: sexual delay discounting in hypersexual Parkinson's disease. Brain 2019;142(1):146–62.

147. Bronner G, Korczyn AD. The role of sex therapy in the management of patients with Parkinson's disease. Mov Disord Clin Pract 2018;5(1):6–13.

148. Zhu M, Li M, Ye D, et al. Sensory symptoms in Parkinson's disease: clinical features, pathophysiology, and treatment. J Neurosci Res 2016;94(8):685–92.

149. Broen MP, Braaksma MM, Patijn J, et al. Prevalence of pain in Parkinson's disease: a systematic review using the modified QUADAS tool. Mov Disord 2012;27(4):480–4.

150. Weil RS, Schrag AE, Warren JD, et al. Visual dysfunction in Parkinson's disease. Brain 2016;139(11):2827–43.

151. Armstrong RA. Visual dysfunction in Parkinson's disease. Int Rev Neurobiol 2017;134:921–46.

152. Sun L, Zhang H, Gu Z, et al. Stereopsis impairment is associated with decreased color perception and worse motor performance in Parkinson's disease. Eur J Med Res 2014;19:29.

153. Jaywant A, Shiffrar M, Roy S, et al. Impaired perception of biological motion in Parkinson's disease. Neuropsychology 2016;30(6):720–30.

154. Radder DLM, Sturkenboom IH, van Nimwegen M, et al. Physical therapy and occupational therapy in Parkinson's disease. Int J Neurosci 2017;127(10): 930–43.

155. Armstrong RA. Visual signs and symptoms of Parkinson's disease. Clin Exp Optom 2008;91(2):129–38.

156. Fejer R, Ruhe A. What is the prevalence of musculoskeletal problems in the elderly population in developed countries? A systematic critical literature review. Chiropr Man Therap 2012;20(1):31.
157. Kim YE, Lee WW, Yun JY, et al. Musculoskeletal problems in Parkinson's disease: neglected issues. Parkinsonism Relat Disord 2013;19(7):666–9.
158. Kim YE, Kim HJ, Yun JY, et al. Musculoskeletal problems affect the quality of life of patients with Parkinson's disease. J Mov Disord 2018;11(3):133–8.
159. Ozturk EA, Kocer BG. Predictive risk factors for chronic low back pain in Parkinson's disease. Clin Neurol Neurosurg 2018;164:190–5.
160. Blanchet PJ, Brefel-Courbon C. Chronic pain and pain processing in Parkinson's disease. Prog Neuropsychopharmacol Biol Psychiatry 2018;87(Pt B):200–6.
161. Jost WH, Buhmann C. The challenge of pain in the pharmacological management of Parkinson's disease. Expert Opin Pharmacother 2019;20(15):1–8.
162. Metta V, Sanchez TC, Padmakumar C. Osteoporosis: a hidden nonmotor face of Parkinson's disease. Int Rev Neurobiol 2017;134:877–90.
163. Sariahmetoglu H, Soysal A, Sen A, et al. Forehead sympathetic skin responses in determining autonomic involvement in Parkinson's disease. Clin Neurophysiol 2014;125(12):2436–40.
164. Arsic Arsenijevic VS, Milobratovic D, Barac AM, et al. A laboratory-based study on patients with Parkinson's disease and seborrheic dermatitis: the presence and density of Malassezia yeasts, their different species and enzymes production. BMC Dermatol 2014;14:5.
165. Dalvin LA, Damento GM, Yawn BP, et al. Parkinson disease and melanoma: confirming and reexamining an association. Mayo Clin Proc 2017;92(7):1070–9.
166. Bougea A, Spantideas N, Katoulis A, et al. Levodopa-induced skin disorders in patients with Parkinson disease: a systematic literature review approach. Acta Neurol Belg 2019;119(3):325–36.
167. Skorvanek M, Bhatia KP. The skin and Parkinson's disease: review of clinical, diagnostic, and therapeutic issues. Mov Disord Clin Pract 2017;4(1):21–31.

Surgical Treatment of Parkinson Disease

Kyle T. Mitchell, MD[a],*, Jill L. Ostrem, MD[b]

KEYWORDS

- Parkinson disease • Functional neurosurgery • Stereotaxy • Deep brain stimulation
- Focused ultrasonography • Thalamotomy • Review

KEY POINTS

- Surgery improves quality of life and motor outcomes in Parkinson disease in carefully selected patients.
- Targeted brain lesions with Gamma Knife radiosurgery or focused ultrasonography can provide unilateral symptomatic relief in Parkinson disease without craniotomy, but long-term outcomes are less established.
- Deep brain stimulation is an effective but complex therapy that requires multidisciplinary management.
- Novel surgical methods, improved hardware, and advances in stimulation paradigms are transforming surgical treatment in Parkinson disease.

INTRODUCTION

Motor symptoms of Parkinson disease (PD) are typically managed with dopaminergic agents for several years after initial presentation. However, as the disease progresses, maximum medical management often proves inadequate because of development of medication-refractory symptoms, motor fluctuations, and/or medication-induced side effects that limit further efficacy. At this point, in carefully selected patients, surgical treatment with targeted lesions or deep brain stimulation (DBS) can improve quality of life and functional independence. This article discusses patient selection, surgical techniques, complications, and emerging therapies for the surgical treatment of PD.

INDICATIONS FOR SURGICAL TREATMENT OF PARKINSON DISEASE

When considering a surgical treatment of PD, having a high degree of diagnostic certainly is important. Given the lack of a confirmatory diagnostic biomarker, a clinical diagnosis of PD is made on pure clinical grounds. Atypical parkinsonian syndromes

---

[a] Duke University Movement Disorders Center, DUMC 3333, 932 Morreene Road, Durham, NC 27705, USA; [b] UCSF Movement Disorders and Neuromodulation Center, 1635 Divisadero Street Suite 520, Box 1838, San Francisco, CA 94115, USA
* Corresponding author.
E-mail address: kyle.mitchell@duke.edu

Neurol Clin 38 (2020) 293–307
https://doi.org/10.1016/j.ncl.2020.01.001
0733-8619/20/© 2020 Elsevier Inc. All rights reserved.
neurologic.theclinics.com

such as multiple system atrophy and progressive supranuclear palsy can mimic PD in their early stages in both symptoms and levodopa responsiveness. Outcomes of reported cases of DBS for atypical parkinsonism (whether intentional or caused by inaccurate diagnosis) have been poor, with transient improvement at best and rapid decline in most patients.[1] With rare exceptions, a 4-year disease duration is considered a minimum for surgical intervention to help ensure diagnostic accuracy.[2]

Once a PD diagnosis is confirmed by a movement disorders specialist, patients ideally meet several criteria to be considered surgical candidates. Both surgical lesions and DBS improve medication "on" time and reduce dyskinesia compared with optimized medical management.[3,4] As a result, moderate to advanced PD characterized by levodopa-responsive symptoms with motor fluctuations and/or dyskinesia is the primary indication for surgery. Per consensus opinion, clinicians may consider surgery for patients with motor fluctuations characterized by disabling "off" periods and functionally independent "on" periods.[5] Careful history taking, serial patient examinations in both on-medication and off-medication states, and self-reporting tools such as the Hauser diary all assist in defining relevant fluctuations.[6] Degree of levodopa responsiveness also guides patient selection. An improvement of at least 30% on the United Parkinson's Disease Rating Scale (UPDRS III) motor score or the updated version from the Movement Disorders Society (MDS-UPDRS III)[7] is a common minimum cutoff for surgery, because preoperative percentage improvement with levodopa is helpful in predicting surgical outcome.[8,9] In general, levodopa-nonresponsive symptoms are not expected to improve with surgery, with the exception of tremor.

There are several key exceptions to these criteria, particularly for patients in earlier stages of PD. Medication-limiting side effects such as excessive nausea, brittle dyskinesia, and dystonia prevent some patients from reaching the therapeutic dose needed for a robust motor improvement. If these patients have previously shown levodopa responsiveness at even low doses, surgery might still be considered. In addition, with the aim of preventing disability in high-functioning patients seeking to maintain employment or active lifestyles, DBS may be an option in earlier stages of PD even without significant disability. A large multicenter study showed improvement in quality of life compared with standard medical management in this subset of patients.[10] The goal of DBS in earlier stages of PD is extension of high-functioning status as opposed to more of a rescue therapy in later stages.

The most notable contraindication for surgery in PD is dementia. Some degree of cognitive impairment is nearly ubiquitous in PD, with measurable deficits in about one-third of newly diagnosed patients,[11] and 1 study showed a 6-fold risk of developing frank dementia at 4 years of follow-up compared with age-matched controls.[12] All potential surgical candidates should be evaluated with comprehensive preoperative neuropsychological testing to access risk, guide management, and counsel patients. Outcomes are generally poor in patients with dementia, and in some cases a worsening of cognition can occur in this more vulnerable population. Severe gait issues with prominent postural instability, common in later stages of PD, are also a relative contraindication to surgery. Patients with higher (worse) axial parkinsonism motor scores in the on-medication state show less improvement with DBS.[13] Any medical comorbidities that carry risk of hemorrhage, infection with delayed wound healing, or cardiovascular complications should also be carefully considered.

Further, clinicians must carefully assess patient expectations and priorities for surgery. One strategy is to ask the patients their top 3 reasons for DBS and then discuss whether or not each is a reasonable expected outcome for DBS. If an individual is most disabled by nonmotor complaints or symptoms that do not respond to levodopa, the surgery is less likely to improve quality of life regardless of motor benefit. Support at home and geographic access to specialists who can maintain and adjust the device over time are also important considerations. In our experience, a comprehensive risk/benefit analysis in a multidisciplinary team conference similar to surgical tumor boards helps consolidate information to make final decisions on surgical candidacy (**Fig. 1**).

TARGETED LESIONS FOR PARKINSON DISEASE

Surgical lesions with thermal pallidotomies and thalamotomies for complications of PD were first performed in the 1950s before medical management with levodopa became the standard of care. After a return in the 1990s,[14] lesioning procedures were put out of favor with the emergence of deep brain stimulation, and were limited to palliative use for patients who were deemed poor DBS candidates. Modern technology with use of direct image guidance and techniques that do not require craniotomy have led to a revival of surgical lesions as a treatment option for PD.

Gamma Knife radiosurgery has received mixed outcomes in recent years. This technique uses preoperative imaging of a skull-mounted frame for target localization followed by targeted radiation administration.[15] With a standardized radiosurgery dosing protocol to the ventral intermediate nucleus (VIM) thalamus, several groups have reported significant improvement in tremor with minimal side effects in PD.[15,16] However, results from Gamma Knife pallidotomy are overall poor, with no large studies and significant adverse events in several case series, which raises concern for overall underreporting of adverse events.[17,18] In general, Gamma Knife pallidotomy is not recommended, but thalamotomy can be considered for tremor in PD.[19]

MRI-guided focused ultrasonography (FUS) is a novel method that has shown promise for the treatment of movement disorders. Patients are placed in a stereotactic head frame with a mounted, MRI-compatible ultrasound transducer. After

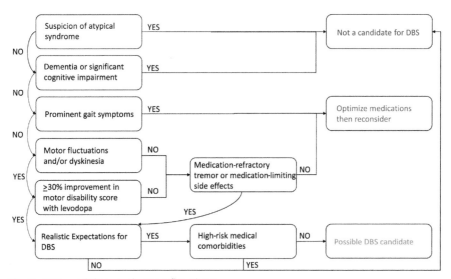

Fig. 1. DBS candidacy evaluation flowsheet.

direct targeting with MRI, ultrasonic energy is gradually increased to ablation temperatures at the target. The surgeon evaluates the lesion efficacy with patient-awake intraoperative clinical tremor assessments and assesses lesion size and location with MRI thermometry before higher-temperature permanent lesioning.[20] Results have been positive in essential tremor,[20] and exploratory studies in PD are ongoing. In small studies, unilateral FUS thalamotomy in tremor-dominant PD has proved safe and effective at tremor reduction[21] and improved quality of life with no observed detriment to mood or cognition.[22] Preliminary work on FUS pallidotomy for PD complicated by dyskinesia has revealed improved motor scores off medication and sustained reduction of dyskinesia at 1 year[23] (**Fig. 2**).

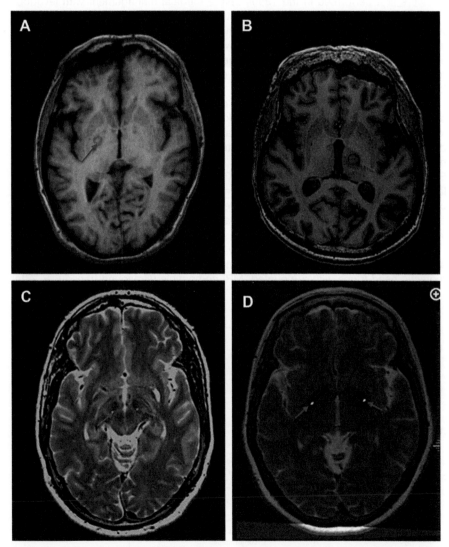

Fig. 2. Surgical brain targets. (*A*) MRI changes after successful pallidotomy (*red arrow*) (*B*) MRI changes after successful thalamotomy (*red arrow*) (*C*) DBS lead in bilateral subthalamic nucleus (*red arrows*) (*D*) DBS lead in bilateral globus pallidus pars interna (*red arrows*).

An obvious drawback to pallidotomy or thalamotomy regardless of method for PD is restriction to unilateral procedures caused by concern for significant and unpredictable side effects with bilateral lesioning. Inconsistency in lesion size and shape, particularly with Gamma Knife procedures,[15] also raises concerns about long-term efficacy and ability to mitigate complication risk. Although FUS is sometimes characterized as less invasive because of avoidance of craniotomy, a permanent subcortical lesion is created with reports of persistent gait or speech side effects in more than 10% of patients at 1 year.[20] Investigators have also noted waning benefit of FUS lesioning at 1 year, and DBS can be then considered as a rescue therapy in failed lesions.[20,24]

Surgical Lesion Key Points

- Thermal pallidotomy increases on time without dyskinesia.
- Gamma Knife and FUS lesions provide benefit without need for craniotomy.
- Gamma Knife pallidotomy has unpredictable outcomes and is not recommended.
- FUS thalamotomy improves tremor control but may have waning benefit over time.
- Lesioning procedures are best for unilateral or asymmetric symptoms in patients with poor access to care for maintenance of hardware or desire to avoid craniotomy or implanted devices.

DEEP BRAIN STIMULATION

DBS is the standard of care for appropriate candidates with PD. Large randomized controlled trials comparing DBS with medical management alone consistently show increased daily "on" time without dyskinesia, improved quality of life, and reduced motor disability scores with DBS.[3,10,25,26] After a thorough presurgical evaluation (outlined earlier) DBS care requires complex decision making by selecting the best surgical method, brain target, hardware, programming techniques, and complication management for a given patient. A multidisciplinary team is best equipped for successful long-term management.

Surgical Technique

Accurate surgical placement of stimulating electrodes, generally within 1 to 2 mm of an optimal target in the motor portion of subthalamic nucleus (STN) or globus pallidus pars interna (GPi), is crucial to the success of therapy. Several surgical techniques exist for DBS lead placement. In the microelectrode recording (MER)–guided, patient-awake method, the target is selected based on direct visualization with preoperative MRI. This targeted MRI then is fused with a computed tomography (CT) image of the patient with a calibrated frame or skull-mounted fiducials.[27] Operating suite software generates three-dimensional coordinates of the target in relation to these mounted fiducials. The surgeon then advances a microelectrode toward the intended target in submillimeter increments while recording specific physiologic neuronal markers to map out the targeted area and identify the ideal final lead location. Then, a permanent DBS stimulating electrode is placed along the trajectory and is tested for clinical benefit as well as side effect thresholds before being secured in the final position.[28]

Patient-awake, MER-guided lead placement is effective and was used in all of the pivotal DBS versus medical therapy trials; however, it is not appropriate for all patients. Some cannot tolerate awake surgery because of discomfort off dopaminergic medications or severe anxiety or claustrophobia. Direct image-guided surgery under general anesthesia offers an alternative. One approach involves using an interventional MRI (iMRI) localization method in which surgeons directly visualize lead placement to the intended target using serial real-time MRI scans in a diagnostic MRI suite (**Fig. 3**). Test stimulation is not performed, and the patient remains in the MRI gantry throughout the procedure.[29,30] This method has proved effective, with motor improvement similar to patient-awake surgery, requires fewer lead passes on average than MER-guided surgery, and is highly accurate, with a radial error of less than 1 mm in experienced centers.[31] Some groups have performed image-guided surgery in standard operating room suites with similar results by using intraoperative CT scans fused to preoperative MRI to indirectly confirm lead placement and guide adjustments.[32,33] Patient experience with DBS placement under general anesthesia has been positive, and many who elected iMRI-guided surgery report a nonspecific fear of being awake during neurosurgery as a deciding factor.[34]

Basal Ganglia Target Selection

The ideal DBS brain target (STN or GPi) selection in PD surgery is still debated (see **Fig. 2**). Some studies have shown greater improvement in secondary outcomes of off-medication motor disability[35,36] and bradykinesia[37] with STN stimulation compared with GPi, whereas many, including the aforementioned studies, showed no differences in overall motor outcomes between the targets.[38–40] Given a lack of robust evidence of significant motor differences between the targets, possible

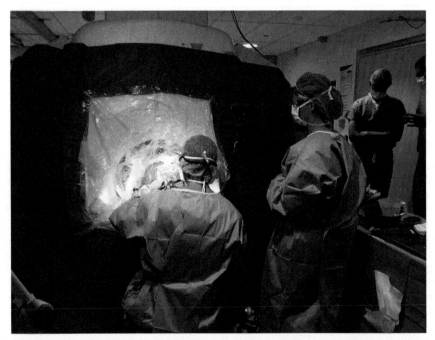

Fig. 3. Interventional MRI-guided DBS placement. The sterile surgical field is draped over the MRI bore. Real-time MRI is performed for direct visualization of lead placement in intended target. Corrections are made based on imaging by using trajectory adjustment dials that project out of the MRI bore. (*Courtesy of* Paul Larson, MD.)

cognitive and mood side effects are often considered. Greater decline in visuomotor processing speed,[38] verbal fluency,[40] and dementia rating scores[39] may occur after STN stimulation in contrast with GPi stimulation. Adverse mood effects of increased anger as well as stimulation-induced impulsivity have both been reported after STN DBS placement, although high-level evidence for direct mood comparison between the brain targets is lacking and dramatic examples are rare.[40,41] Nevertheless, consideration of preoperative mood and cognition as part of a thorough neuropsychiatric evaluation plays an important role in target selection.

STN DBS results in a greater reduction in dopaminergic medications compared with GPi DBS.[35,37,38] Patients receiving nonmotor mood benefits from medication may be better candidates for GPi stimulation. Those with dyskinesia caused by very-low-dose levodopa can be challenging to optimally program given the risk of STN DBS–induced dyskinesia and inability to further reduce medications. In contrast, the medication reduction offered by STN stimulation is preferred for patients with medication-limiting complications such as nausea, levodopa-induced dystonia, or drowsiness.[42] STN DBS also requires lower-energy stimulation for clinical effect on average, which likely prolongs implantable pulse generator (IPG) battery life[38] (**Table 1**).

In addition, the VIM thalamus is occasionally targeted for tremor-dominant PD, although benefit is limited to tremor alone, and degree of tremor control is not superior to the other targets.[43] In older, more cognitively borderline patients with mild overall parkinsonism but disabling tremor, unilateral VIM DBS can be considered because of possible lower risk of cognitive side effects[44] and hemorrhage and overall ease of surgery.[45]

Levodopa-refractory freezing of gait, a common disabling symptom in advanced PD, does not respond well to traditional targets and has prompted exploration of novel targets. Pedunculopontine nucleus DBS results have been mixed. A review of published case series revealed an overall modest improvement in freezing of gait but with variability in response with a significant portion of nonresponders and unclear impact on overall quality of life.[46] Dorsal cord stimulation is currently under investigation as a less invasive option for refractory gait symptoms in PD, with inconsistent benefit in small early studies.[47,48]

Table 1		
Target selection considerations in deep brain stimulation		
Target	**STN**	**GPi**
Features	• Requires antiparkinsonian medication reduction • Greater decline in some cognitive scales • Possible risk of greater stimulation-induced side effects (impulsivity, dyskinesia, dysarthria) • Greater motor benefit off medication • Average lower stimulation amplitudes	• Less antiparkinsonian medication reduction • Direct antidyskinesia effect • Simpler programming parameters
Pearls to help guide target determination	• Need for medication reduction to reduce side effects • Generally chosen for younger healthy patients with PD without cognitive or mood issues	• Antiparkinsonian medications providing significant nonmotor benefits • Less access to follow-up/greater ease of programming

Surgical Complications

It is important to understand common complications of DBS to guide informed consent and determine ways to mitigate risks in this elective neurosurgery. Cerebral hemorrhage, the most devastating complication, has an overall reported incidence between 0.5% and 3.3% per lead, with the highest estimate at 5% of all implanted patients.[45,49–51] However, permanent neurologic deficits from hemorrhage are less common, with incidence between 0.6% and 1.1% of patients.[45,51,52] Hypertension and advanced age are associated with a higher hemorrhage risk[51] and thalamic target with a lower risk.[45]

Infection of DBS hardware often requires at least partial device removal and loss of therapy during several weeks of antibiotic treatment. The largest studies show infection rates between 2.2% and 4.5% at the IPG site, cranial incisions, or extracranial wiring, with infections originating intracranially seldom reported.[53–55] Patients with thin skin and/or older devices are particularly predisposed to hardware erosion, resulting in system compromise caused by infection. IPG replacement because of expected battery depletion also carries a higher risk of infection than initial implantations[55,56] **(Fig. 4)**.

In addition, hardware failure, with short circuits between contacts or open circuits caused by disconnected contacts, occurs in about 5% of patients.[57,58] These complications are usually limited to 1 contact and can often be managed nonsurgically by programming adjacent unaffected contacts. Delayed lead migration out of the intended target caused by technical error, failure of lead anchoring, or patient manipulation (so-called twiddler's syndrome) requires surgical correction and occurred in more than 10% of patients in a large cohort.[59]

Programming Techniques/Hardware Choices

DBS programming is the determination of optimal settings for a given patient by adjusting stimulating contact configuration, amplitude, pulse width, and frequency. Using standard quadripolar DBS leads, clinicians typically perform initial programming

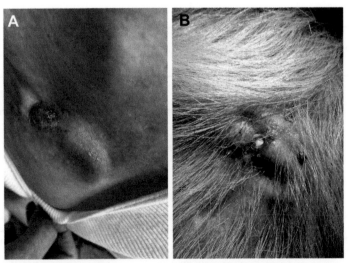

Fig. 4. DBS infections. (*A*) Induration and erythema at IPG site indicates hardware infection. (*B*) Chronic scalp erosion overlying DBS connector wire resulting in infection.

by assessing benefit for motor symptoms (ie, tremor, rigidity, bradykinesia) in the relative off-medication state and determining side effect thresholds for each contact. This monopolar review allows selection of the best contact and amplitude based on the therapeutic window. Fine tuning with bipolar stimulation, using multiple contacts, or adjustments of pulse width or frequency often follows in an attempt to optimize benefit while avoiding side effects caused by inadvertent stimulation of adjacent brain structures.

Novel DBS hardware for both lead configuration and IPG capabilities has vastly increased the number of possible stimulation parameters. New segmented 8-contact leads allow steering of stimulation toward a preferred direction in the motor portion of STN or GPi and away from side effect–inducing structures such as the internal capsule. Directional stimulation has shown promise in PD, allowing the expansion of the therapeutic window, and some clinicians prefer directional stimulation for chronic stimulation settings.[60–62] Additional device programming capabilities are being explored and include fractionation of current across multiple contacts using multiple-source current steering, lower pulse widths, and anodic stimulation.[63,64] Several of the newer-generation devices also offer rechargeable IPGs and MRI conditional compatibility. Given the multiple available DBS hardware options, clinician comfort with the programming platform and patient access to experienced technical support are also important considerations in device selection.[65]

The vast increase in permutations of DBS settings with newer devices creates a greater need for technology to assist programmers. Database-driven, probabilistic, image-guided programming software may ultimately assist in choosing the optimal stimulating contact.[66,67] Volume of tissue activation and tractography methods may guide novel programming algorithms, obviating a full monopolar review.[68] Local field

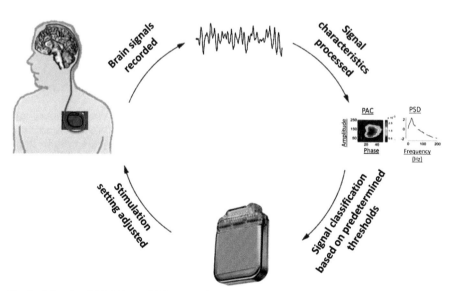

Fig. 5. Adaptive DBS. Using a bidirectional IPG, neural signals are recorded and processed. A programmed algorithm triggers stimulation changes as abnormal signals are encountered or predetermined signal thresholds are reached. Proposed signals for adaptive DBS include phase amplitude coupling (PAC) of neural oscillations and spontaneous neural activity plotted by power spectral density (PSD). (*Modified* with permission from Coralie DeHemptinne, PhD.)

potential recordings of pathologic basal ganglia oscillatory activity could also assist in contact selection and direction of stimulation.[69] In addition, development of automated programming based on objective, peripheral sensor–based measurement of symptoms to optimize DBS settings is also ongoing.[70,71]

Adaptive Deep Brain Stimulation

Traditional DBS delivers a continuous pattern of stimulation that requires manual adjustments to optimize therapy over time and does not adjust "on the fly" to varying needs for symptomatic relief, medication timing, sleep, or daily activities. Researchers are now designing adaptive stimulation paradigms to respond to neural and peripheral biomarkers providing targeted, individualized stimulation to treat specific symptoms. Cortical and subcortical local field potentials have revealed basal ganglia and motor cortex oscillatory activity that correlates with motor symptoms such as bradykinesia, rigidity, and treatment-induced dyskinesia.[72–75] Using a bidirectional device that records and stimulates simultaneously, programmed algorithms can switch on stimulation when needed and reduce stimulation when not based on crossing predefined thresholds of neural oscillatory activity.[76] Adaptive DBS has the potential to reduce side effects, prolong battery life, and perhaps provide greater efficacy than continuous stimulation[77,78] (**Fig. 5**).

SUMMARY

PD surgical approaches can provide symptomatic relief and improve quality of life in a carefully selected subset of patients. Surgical lesions and DBS therapy both increase motor "on" time when maximal medical management becomes insufficient. Novel surgical methods and stimulation techniques are transforming the field and advancing technology has the potential to improve future outcomes. Surgical decision making is complex, with determination of best surgical candidates, technique, complication management, hardware, and programming adjustments requiring a collaborative, multidisciplinary approach.

DISCLOSURE

K.T. Mitchell: Boston Scientific Corporation, 300 Boston Scientific Way, Marlborough, MA 01752. Type of support: consulting. Medtronic Corporation, 710 Medtronic Parkway, Minneapolis, MN 55432. Type of support: educational course grant. Rune Labs, Inc, 649 Irving St, San Francisco CA 94122. Type of support: consulting. J.L. Ostrem: Michael J. Fox Foundation, Grand Central Station, PO Box 4777, New York, NY 10163. Type of support: grant support. Boston Scientific Corporation, 300 Boston Scientific Way, Marlborough, MA 01752. Type of support: research support, training grant support. Medtronic Corporation, 710 Medtronic Parkway, Minneapolis, MN 55432. Type of support: training grant support/consulting. Cala Health, 875 Mahler Rd. # 145 Burlingame, CA 94010. Type of support: grant support for clinical trial. NIH-NINDS-RO1NS090913-01, PO Box 5801 Bethesda, MD 20824. Type of support: grant support. DOD Defense Advanced Research Projects Agency W911NF-14-2-00430, 675 N. Arlington Street, Arlington, VA 22203. Type of support: grant support. PCORI-FY16.782.002, 1828 L Street NW Suite 900, Washington DC 20036. Type of support: grant support. NIH-NINDS-UH3NS100544, PO Box 5801, Bethesda, MD 20824. Type of support: grant support. Biogen, 225 Binney Street, Cambridge, MA 02142. Type of support: grant support for clinical trial. Acadia Pharmaceuticals Inc, 3611 Valley Center Drive Suite 300, San Diego, CA 92130. Type of support: consulting.

REFERENCES

1. Shih LC, Tarsy D. Deep brain stimulation for the treatment of atypical parkinsonism. Mov Disord 2007;22(15):2149–55.
2. Hughes AJ, Daniel SE, Ben-Shlomo Y, et al. The accuracy of diagnosis of parkinsonian syndromes in a specialist movement disorder service. Brain 2002; 125(Pt 4):861–70.
3. Weaver FM, Follett K, Stern M, et al. Bilateral deep brain stimulation vs best medical therapy for patients with advanced Parkinson disease: a randomized controlled trial. JAMA 2009;301(1):63–73.
4. Vitek JL, Bakay RA, Freeman A, et al. Randomized trial of pallidotomy versus medical therapy for Parkinson's disease. Ann Neurol 2003;53(5):558–69.
5. Lang AE, Houeto JL, Krack P, et al. Deep brain stimulation: preoperative issues. Mov Disord 2006;21(Suppl 14):S171–96.
6. Hauser RA, Friedlander J, Zesiewicz TA, et al. A home diary to assess functional status in patients with Parkinson's disease with motor fluctuations and dyskinesia. Clin Neuropharmacol 2000;23(2):75–81.
7. Goetz CG, Tilley BC, Shaftman SR, et al. Movement Disorder Society-sponsored revision of the Unified Parkinson's Disease Rating Scale (MDS-UPDRS): scale presentation and clinimetric testing results. Mov Disord 2008;23(15):2129–70.
8. Kazumata K, Antonini A, Dhawan V, et al. Preoperative indicators of clinical outcome following stereotaxic pallidotomy. Neurology 1997;49(4):1083–90.
9. Charles PD, Van Blercom N, Krack P, et al. Predictors of effective bilateral subthalamic nucleus stimulation for PD. Neurology 2002;59(6):932–4.
10. Schuepbach WM, Rau J, Knudsen K, et al. Neurostimulation for Parkinson's disease with early motor complications. N Engl J Med 2013;368(7):610–22.
11. Kandiah N, Narasimhalu K, Lau PN, et al. Cognitive decline in early Parkinson's disease. Mov Disord 2009;24(4):605–8.
12. Aarsland D, Andersen K, Larsen JP, et al. Risk of dementia in Parkinson's disease: a community-based, prospective study. Neurology 2001;56(6):730–6.
13. Welter ML, Houeto JL, Tezenas du Montcel S, et al. Clinical predictive factors of subthalamic stimulation in Parkinson's disease. Brain 2002;125(Pt 3):575–83.
14. Laitinen LV, Bergenheim AT, Hariz MI. Leksell's posteroventral pallidotomy in the treatment of Parkinson's disease. J Neurosurg 1992;76(1):53–61.
15. Ohye C, Higuchi Y, Shibazaki T, et al. Gamma knife thalamotomy for Parkinson disease and essential tremor: a prospective multicenter study. Neurosurgery 2012;70(3):526–35 [discussion: 535–6].
16. Raju SS, Niranjan A, Monaco EA III, et al. Stereotactic radiosurgery for intractable tremor-dominant parkinson disease: a retrospective analysis. Stereotact Funct Neurosurg 2017;95(5):291–7.
17. Friedman JH, Epstein M, Sanes JN, et al. Gamma knife pallidotomy in advanced Parkinson's disease. Ann Neurol 1996;39(4):535–8.
18. Okun MS, Stover NP, Subramanian T, et al. Complications of gamma knife surgery for Parkinson disease. Arch Neurol 2001;58(12):1995–2002.
19. Martinez-Moreno NE, Sahgal A, De Salles A, et al. Stereotactic radiosurgery for tremor: systematic review. J Neurosurg 2018;1–12 [Epub ahead of print].
20. Elias WJ, Lipsman N, Ondo WG, et al. A randomized trial of focused ultrasound thalamotomy for essential tremor. N Engl J Med 2016;375(8):730–9.
21. Schlesinger I, Eran A, Sinai A, et al. MRI guided focused ultrasound thalamotomy for moderate-to-severe tremor in Parkinson's disease. Parkinsons Dis 2015;2015: 219149.

22. Sperling SA, Shah BB, Barrett MJ, et al. Focused ultrasound thalamotomy in Parkinson disease: nonmotor outcomes and quality of life. Neurology 2018;91(14): e1275–84.

23. Jung NY, Park CK, Kim M, et al. The efficacy and limits of magnetic resonance-guided focused ultrasound pallidotomy for Parkinson's disease: a Phase I clinical trial. J Neurosurg 2018;1–9 [Epub ahead of print].

24. Wang TR, Dallapiazza RF, Moosa S, et al. Thalamic deep brain stimulation salvages failed focused ultrasound thalamotomy for essential tremor: a case report. Stereotact Funct Neurosurg 2018;96(1):60–4.

25. Williams A, Gill S, Varma T, et al. Deep brain stimulation plus best medical therapy versus best medical therapy alone for advanced Parkinson's disease (PD SURG trial): a randomised, open-label trial. Lancet Neurol 2010;9(6):581–91.

26. Deuschl G, Schade-Brittinger C, Krack P, et al. A randomized trial of deep-brain stimulation for Parkinson's disease. N Engl J Med 2006;355(9):896–908.

27. Bot M, van den Munckhof P, Bakay R, et al. Analysis of stereotactic accuracy in patients undergoing deep brain stimulation using nexframe and the leksell frame. Stereotact Funct Neurosurg 2015;93(5):316–25.

28. Starr PA, Christine CW, Theodosopoulos PV, et al. Implantation of deep brain stimulators into the subthalamic nucleus: technical approach and magnetic resonance imaging-verified lead locations. J Neurosurg 2002;97(2):370–87.

29. Martin AJ, Larson PS, Ostrem JL, et al. Interventional magnetic resonance guidance of deep brain stimulator implantation for Parkinson disease. Top Magn Reson Imaging 2009;19(4):213–21.

30. Starr PA, Martin AJ, Ostrem JL, et al. Subthalamic nucleus deep brain stimulator placement using high-field interventional magnetic resonance imaging and a skull-mounted aiming device: technique and application accuracy. J Neurosurg 2010;112(3):479–90.

31. Ostrem JL, Ziman N, Galifianakis NB, et al. Clinical outcomes using ClearPoint interventional MRI for deep brain stimulation lead placement in Parkinson's disease. J Neurosurg 2016;124(4):908–16.

32. Brodsky MA, Anderson S, Murchison C, et al. Clinical outcomes of asleep vs awake deep brain stimulation for Parkinson disease. Neurology 2017;89(19): 1944–50.

33. Mirzadeh Z, Chapple K, Lambert M, et al. Parkinson's disease outcomes after intraoperative CT-guided "asleep" deep brain stimulation in the globus pallidus internus. J Neurosurg 2016;124(4):902–7.

34. LaHue SC, Ostrem JL, Galifianakis NB, et al. Parkinson's disease patient preference and experience with various methods of DBS lead placement. Parkinsonism Relat Disord 2017;41:25–30.

35. Odekerken VJ, van Laar T, Staal MJ, et al. Subthalamic nucleus versus globus pallidus bilateral deep brain stimulation for advanced Parkinson's disease (NSTAPS study): a randomised controlled trial. Lancet Neurol 2013;12(1):37–44.

36. Odekerken VJ, Boel JA, Schmand BA, et al. GPi vs STN deep brain stimulation for Parkinson disease: Three-year follow-up. Neurology 2016;86(8):755–61.

37. Anderson VC, Burchiel KJ, Hogarth P, et al. Pallidal vs subthalamic nucleus deep brain stimulation in Parkinson disease. Arch Neurol 2005;62(4):554–60.

38. Follett KA, Weaver FM, Stern M, et al. Pallidal versus subthalamic deep-brain stimulation for Parkinson's disease. N Engl J Med 2010;362(22):2077–91.

39. Weaver FM, Follett KA, Stern M, et al. Randomized trial of deep brain stimulation for Parkinson disease: thirty-six-month outcomes. Neurology 2012;79(1):55–65.

40. Okun MS, Fernandez HH, Wu SS, et al. Cognition and mood in Parkinson's disease in subthalamic nucleus versus globus pallidus interna deep brain stimulation: the COMPARE trial. Ann Neurol 2009;65(5):586–95.

41. Frank MJ, Samanta J, Moustafa AA, et al. Hold Your Horses: Impulsivity, Deep Brain Stimulation, and Medication in Parkinsonism. Science 2007;318(5854): 1309–12.

42. Ramirez-Zamora A, Ostrem JL. Globus pallidus interna or subthalamic nucleus deep brain stimulation for parkinson disease: a review. JAMA Neurol 2018; 75(3):367–72.

43. Parihar R, Alterman R, Papavassiliou E, et al. Comparison of VIM and STN DBS for Parkinsonian resting and postural/action tremor. Tremor Other Hyperkinet Mov (N Y) 2015;5:321.

44. Woods SP, Fields JA, Lyons KE, et al. Neuropsychological and quality of life changes following unilateral thalamic deep brain stimulation in Parkinson's disease: a one-year follow-up. Acta Neurochir (Wien) 2001;143(12):1273–7 [discussion: 1278].

45. Binder DK, Rau GM, Starr PA. Risk factors for hemorrhage during microelectrode-guided deep brain stimulator implantation for movement disorders. Neurosurgery 2005;56(4):722–32 [discussion: 722–32].

46. Thevathasan W, Debu B, Aziz T, et al. Pedunculopontine nucleus deep brain stimulation in Parkinson's disease: A clinical review. Mov Disord 2018;33(1):10–20.

47. Pinto de Souza C, Hamani C, Oliveira Souza C, et al. Spinal cord stimulation improves gait in patients with Parkinson's disease previously treated with deep brain stimulation. Mov Disord 2017;32(2):278–82.

48. Yadav AP, Nicolelis MAL. Electrical stimulation of the dorsal columns of the spinal cord for Parkinson's disease. Mov Disord 2017;32(6):820–32.

49. Xiaowu H, Xiufeng J, Xiaoping Z, et al. Risks of intracranial hemorrhage in patients with Parkinson's disease receiving deep brain stimulation and ablation. Parkinsonism Relat Disord 2010;16(2):96–100.

50. Ben-Haim S, Asaad WF, Gale JT, et al. Risk factors for hemorrhage during microelectrode-guided deep brain stimulation and the introduction of an improved microelectrode design. Neurosurgery 2009;64(4):754–62 [discussion: 762–3].

51. Zrinzo L, Foltynie T, Limousin P, et al. Reducing hemorrhagic complications in functional neurosurgery: a large case series and systematic literature review. J Neurosurg 2012;116(1):84–94.

52. Sansur CA, Frysinger RC, Pouratian N, et al. Incidence of symptomatic hemorrhage after stereotactic electrode placement. J Neurosurg 2007;107(5):998–1003.

53. Fenoy AJ, Simpson RK Jr. Management of device-related wound complications in deep brain stimulation surgery. J Neurosurg 2012;116(6):1324–32.

54. Sillay KA, Larson PS, Starr PA. Deep brain stimulator hardware-related infections: incidence and management in a large series. Neurosurgery 2008;62(2):360–6 [discussion: 366–7].

55. Fytagoridis A, Heard T, Samuelsson J, et al. Surgical replacement of implantable pulse generators in deep brain stimulation: adverse events and risk factors in a multicenter cohort. Stereotact Funct Neurosurg 2016;94(4):235–9.

56. Pepper J, Zrinzo L, Mirza B, et al. The risk of hardware infection in deep brain stimulation surgery is greater at impulse generator replacement than at the primary procedure. Stereotact Funct Neurosurg 2013;91(1):56–65.

57. Allert N, Jusciute E, Weirich O, et al. Long-term stability of short circuits in deep brain stimulation. Neuromodulation 2018;21(6):562–7.

58. Allert N, Jusciute E, Quindt R, et al. DBS electrodes with single disconnected contacts: long-term observation and implications for the management. Neuromodulation 2018;21(6):568–73.

59. Morishita T, Hilliard JD, Okun MS, et al. Postoperative lead migration in deep brain stimulation surgery: Incidence, risk factors, and clinical impact. PLoS One 2017;12(9):e0183711.

60. Steigerwald F, Muller L, Johannes S, et al. Directional deep brain stimulation of the subthalamic nucleus: A pilot study using a novel neurostimulation device. Mov Disord 2016;31(8):1240–3.

61. Dembek TA, Reker P, Visser-Vandewalle V, et al. Directional DBS increases side-effect thresholds-A prospective, double-blind trial. Mov Disord 2017;32(10): 1380–8.

62. Pollo C, Kaelin-Lang A, Oertel MF, et al. Directional deep brain stimulation: an intraoperative double-blind pilot study. Brain 2014;137(Pt 7):2015–26.

63. Timmermann L, Jain R, Chen L, et al. Multiple-source current steering in subthalamic nucleus deep brain stimulation for Parkinson's disease (the VANTAGE study): a non-randomised, prospective, multicentre, open-label study. Lancet Neurol 2015;14(7):693–701.

64. Kirsch AD, Hassin-Baer S, Matthies C, et al. Anodic versus cathodic neurostimulation of the subthalamic nucleus: a randomized-controlled study of acute clinical effects. Parkinsonism Relat Disord 2018;55:61–7.

65. Okun MS. Tips for choosing a deep brain stimulation device. JAMA Neurol 2019; 76(7):749–50.

66. D'Haese PF, Pallavaram S, Li R, et al. CranialVault and its CRAVE tools: a clinical computer assistance system for deep brain stimulation (DBS) therapy. Med Image Anal 2012;16(3):744–53.

67. Pallavaram S, Phibbs FT, Tolleson C, et al. Neurologist consistency in interpreting information provided by an interactive visualization software for deep brain stimulation postoperative programming assistance. Neuromodulation 2014;17(1): 11–5 [discussion: 15].

68. Anderson DN, Osting B, Vorwerk J, et al. Optimized programming algorithm for cylindrical and directional deep brain stimulation electrodes. J Neural Eng 2018;15(2):026005.

69. Telkes I, Viswanathan A, Jimenez-Shahed J, et al. Local field potentials of subthalamic nucleus contain electrophysiological footprints of motor subtypes of Parkinson's disease. Proc Natl Acad Sci U S A 2018;115(36):E8567–76.

70. Haddock A, Mitchell KT, Miller A, et al. Automated deep brain stimulation programming for tremor. IEEE Trans Neural Syst Rehabil Eng 2018;26(8):1618–25.

71. Heldman DA, Pulliam CL, Urrea Mendoza E, et al. Computer-guided deep brain stimulation programming for Parkinson's disease. Neuromodulation 2016;19(2): 127–32.

72. Kühn AA, Kupsch A, Schneider GH, et al. Reduction in subthalamic 8-35 Hz oscillatory activity correlates with clinical improvement in Parkinson's disease. Eur J Neurosci 2006;23(7):1956–60.

73. Kühn AA, Kempf F, Brücke C, et al. High-frequency stimulation of the subthalamic nucleus suppresses oscillatory beta activity in patients with Parkinson's disease in parallel with improvement in motor performance. J Neurosci 2008;28(24): 6165–73.

74. Swann NC, de Hemptinne C, Miocinovic S, et al. Gamma oscillations in the hyperkinetic state detected with chronic human brain recordings in Parkinson's disease. J Neurosci 2016;36(24):6445–58.

75. Eisinger RS, Cernera S, Gittis A, et al. A review of basal ganglia circuits and physiology: application to deep brain stimulation. Parkinsonism Relat Disord 2019;59:9–20.
76. Rouse AG, Stanslaski SR, Cong P, et al. A chronic generalized bi-directional brain-machine interface. J Neural Eng 2011;8(3):036018.
77. Little S, Pogosyan A, Neal S, et al. Adaptive deep brain stimulation in advanced Parkinson disease. Ann Neurol 2013;74(3):449–57.
78. Little S, Tripoliti E, Beudel M, et al. Adaptive deep brain stimulation for Parkinson's disease demonstrates reduced speech side effects compared to conventional stimulation in the acute setting. J Neurol Neurosurg Psychiatry 2016;87(12): 1388–9.

Current and Emerging Treatments of Essential Tremor

William George Ondo, MD

KEYWORDS

- Tremor • Essential tremor • Treatment • Botulinum toxin • Deep brain stimulation
- Thalamotomy

KEY POINTS

- Established treatments for tremor include the noncardiac selective beta-antagonists, primidone and topiramate.
- Deep brain stimulation of the ventral intermediate thalamus and stereotactic thalamotomy are robust established treatments for essential tremor; focused ultrasound thalamotomy is a newer technique that does not require physical penetration of the skull.
- Botulinum toxin injects, which weaken tremulous muscles, have been widely used for essential tremor, but injection techniques continue to be refined.
- Multiple investigational medications for essential tremor are being studied include the T-type calcium channel blockers and allosteric gamma-aminobutyric acid-A modulators.
- Several peripheral devices including alternating median radial nerve stimulation, a gyroscope glove, and counterweight devices continue to be refined.

INTRODUCTION

Essential tremor (ET), also known as benign ET, familial tremor, or senile tremor, is a common neurologic syndrome manifested by involuntary rhythmic oscillatory movement with volitional muscle action. Exact diagnostic criteria have varied modestly over time, and the clinical syndrome is likely pathophysiologically heterogeneous. The most recent tremor consensus tremor classification system emphasizes a 2-axis classification based on clinical characteristics (anatomy, frequency, quality, etc) and etiology (acquired, genetic, or idiopathic).[1] The condition is common, impacting up to 4% of all people, can occur at any age with bimodal peaks in the second and sixth decades, and gradually worsens over time.

The pathophysiology of ET is only partially illuminated. There is some understanding of culpable macrocircuitry, mostly based on functional PET/single photon emission computed tomography studies, functional MRI, tractography, transcranial stimulation,

Movement Disorders-Methodist Neurological Institute, Weill Cornel Medical School, 6560 Fannin Suite 1002, Houston, TX 77025, USA
E-mail address: wondo@houstonmethodist.org

Neurol Clin 38 (2020) 309–323
https://doi.org/10.1016/j.ncl.2020.01.002
0733-8619/20/© 2020 Elsevier Inc. All rights reserved.

neurologic.theclinics.com

and other electrophysiologic techniques.[2] However, there is very little understanding at the cellular level. The post mortem pathology of ET is inconsistent; variably being normal, demonstrating Lewy body pathology, cerebellar Purkinje cell degeneration,[3,4] and altered inferior olivary climbing fiber anatomy in the Purkinje cell layer.[5]

No currently available medication used for ET was specifically developed for this purpose. Recently, improved physiologic understanding, improved technology, and improved assessment techniques are facilitating rationally designed ET drug development and more sophisticated surgical and peripheral electromechanical treatments. This article reviews currently available and investigational pharmacologic (**Table 1**), device, and surgical treatments for ET.

Table 1
Pharmacologic treatments of ET

	Efficacy	Mechanism of Action	Daily Dose (mg) and Doses per Day	Common Side Effects
Ethanol	+++	GABAo	1 drink	Intoxication
Topiramate	+++	GABA0, CAI, Na, AMPA GABAs	50–400 2/d	Paresthesia, altered taste, weight loss, worse cognition
Primidone	+++	GABAo, Na	50–300 2–3/d	Sedation, dizzy, ataxia
Propranolol	+++	*Beta*	20–240 1–3/d	Fatigue, hypotension, bradycardia
Phenobarbital	++	GABAo, AMPA	30–180 1/d	Sedation, balance
Benzodiazepines	++	GABAo	Variable	Sedation, ataxia
Dihydropyridines Nicardipine nifedipine nimodipine	+	Ca^{2+}	Variable	Low BP, flushing
Gabapentin	+	Ca^{2+} $\alpha2\gamma$	300–3600 2–3/d	Sedation, dizziness, edema
Pregabalin	+	Ca^{2+} $\alpha2\gamma$	100–400 2–3/d	Sedation, dizziness, edema, weight gain
Zonisamide	+	Ca^{2+} LVA, Na	100–300 2/d	Malaise, weight loss
Levetiracetam	+	AMPA, GABAo, Na	500–3000 2/d	Agitation
Acetazolamide	+	CAI		Diuresis
CX-8998	++	Ca^{2+} T	Not available	Dizziness
PRAX-944	?	Ca^{2+} T	Not available	?
CAD-1883	?	PAM SK	Not available	?
Sage 324	?	GABAo	Not available	?

Abbreviations: AMPA, blocks glutamate release and/or inhibits AMPA (alpha-amino-3-hydroxy-5-methylisoxazole-4-propionic acid); Beta, blocks B1 and B2 adrenergic receptors; Ca^{2+} L, L-type (Ca_v1) antagonist; Ca^{2+} T, T type (Ca_v3) antagonist; Ca^{2+} $\alpha2\gamma$, inhibits the alpha-2 delta subunit of calcium channel blocker; Ca^{2+}, nonselective calcium channel inhibition, usually more affinity for Ca^{2+}.L; CAI, carbonic anhydrase inhibitor; GABAo, opens or potentiates GABA receptors; GABAr, inhibits GABA reuptake or metabolism; GABAs, increases GABA synthesis; NA, inhibits sodium channels; PAM SK, positive allosteric modulator of small conductance Ca^{2+} activated K^+ channels (SK channels).

ALCOHOLS

Ethanol is reported to decrease ET severity in approximately two-thirds of patients.[6] Improvement can be robust and rapid. Onset to tremor suppression typically takes 10 to 15 minutes and lasts 3 to 4 hours. A rebound tremor exacerbation is reported by many patients. Generally, the equivalent of a single drink is adequate in alcohol responders. Improvement is mostly derived from the central nervous system (CNS), based on weight loading studies and decreased cerebellar activity on PET after ingestion.[7] The exact cellular mechanism by which alcohol improves ET depression is unclear, but gamma-aminobutyric acid (GABA)ergic agonism and cellular decoupling are possible explanations, although ethanol's antitremor effect seems to be superior to those of other GABAergic medicines, including benzodiazepines.[8]

Octanol, an 8-carbon alcohol used as a food flavoring agent, is metabolized to octanoic acid, which is now thought to be its active metabolite. Several open-label and controlled studies have shown a short duration benefit (90–120 minutes) in tremor without problematic side effects[9–11] The medicine has minimal adverse effects and has a long established use at smaller doses in humans. Future development for tremor is unclear.

Sodium oxybate is a powerful sedating hypnotic used for catatonia. This agent is also reported to improve tremor, but is unlikely to have much clinical usefulness secondary to extreme sedation and abuse potential.[12]

BETA-ADRENERGIC ANTAGONISTS

Numerous trials have confirmed the efficacy of propranolol and other beta-blockers. The preponderance of evidences suggests that beta-blockers attenuate tremor predominately via a peripheral site, but drugs with good CNS penetration may be slightly superior. Beta-2 affinity (noncardiac selective) is required for maximal benefit. Agents with partial sympathomimetic properties such as pindolol and practolol do not improve tremor.

No agent to date is theoretically or empirically superior to propranolol (**Table 2**). Nadolol or satolol may offer equal efficacy with less CNS sedation. Nadolol, with a

Table 2
Beta-adrenergic antagonists

	Typical Dose Daily (mg)/ Frequency	Lipid Solubility	Sympathetic Activity	Beta-1 Activity	Beta-2 Activity	Tremor Efficacy
Propranolol	40–320/BID	+++	−	+	+	+++
Arotinolol	10–40/BID?	+	−	+	+	+++
Nadolol	80–240/qD	+++	−	+	+	+++
Sotolol	80–320/BID	+	−	+	+	+++
Timolol	10–20/BID	++	+/−	+	+	++
Metoprolol	100–200/BID	++	−	+	+/−	++
Atenolol	50–100/qD	+	−	+	+/−	+
Pindolol	10–30/BID	++	+	+	+	−

Comparative clinical trials: propranolol ≥ metoprolol (doses where metoprolol loses B1 selectivity), propranolol > atenolol, propranolol >> pindolol.
Abbreviations: BID, 2 times a day; qD, daily.

10- to 20-hour half-life, can also offer daily dosing. Most studies comparing propranolol to other beta-blockers have shown that subjects usually respond to both or neither study drug. Therefore, it is unlikely that patients will respond to another beta-blocker if propranolol is clearly ineffective.

Various trials and clinical consensus suggest that between 50% and 70% of patients with ET benefit from propranolol.[13] No clear clinical or physiologic factors consistently predict this response. Overall, propranolol decreases hand tremor amplitude by approximately 50% and also can improve head and voice tremor.[14] Tremor reduction occurs within 1 to 2 hours of ingestion making pro re nata dosing feasible. Efficacy seems to be dose dependent. Patients may prefer an extended release propranolol formulation over standard propranolol because of dosing convenience and mildly superior subjective efficacy.

Propranolol is generally well-tolerated, although adverse effects may continue to accrue over time. Patients most commonly complain of nonspecific weakness and fatigue. Other potential adverse reactions include weight gain, nausea, diarrhea, rash, impotence, depression and hypotension. Relative contraindications include insulin-dependent diabetes mellitus, reactive airway disease, heart block, and poorly controlled congestive heart failure. Moderate congestive heart failure may actually benefit from beta-adrenergic blockade; however, a cardiac consultation should be sought before the initiation of treatment in the setting of congestive heart failure.

PRIMIDONE AND OTHER BARBITURATES

Numerous open and controlled trials have consistently demonstrated that primidone improves subjective assessments, clinical assessments, and electrophysiologic measurements of tremor.[15] The overall efficacy of primidone seems to be comparable or slightly better than propranolol.[16] Head tremor probably improves less consistently.

In our experience, primidone tends to have a hit or miss effect. Clinical response to primidone does not seem to correlate with serum levels and further clinical improvement in doses of greater than 250 mg/d is unlikely.[16] A tremorlytic effect is observed within 1 hour of oral administration and peaks between 2 and 7 hours. Data concerning primidone's long-term efficacy is mixed, but over years, primidone gradually becomes less effective.

Primidone's actual mechanism of action is debated. Most assume a CNS effect, although there is little evidence supporting even this proposition. Recent theories have suggested an alteration of transmembrane calcium and sodium ion fluxes, similar to its proposed mode of action in epilepsy. Primidone, which is classified as a barbiturate, has relatively little effect on either GABA or glutamate receptors, although phenobarbital, a major metabolite of primidone increases the duration of GABA receptor opening, as opposed to increasing the frequency of openings, at distinct site on the GABA-A receptor. Phenobarbital itself has moderate tremorlytic properties, but less than primidone.[17] Primidone's initial half-life is 5 hours, but chronic administration increases this to about 10 hours.

Primidone can produce a variety of side effects when used in the ET population. Up to 50% of patients report acute side effects, usually with the first dose. Some of these adverse effects, predominately sedation, are dose related and can be lessened by initiating a low dose and titrating slowly. However, a subset of patients experience acute neurotoxic effects, resulting in dizziness, ataxia, and nausea. These symptoms can occur even at very low doses, but tend to resolve over time. We usually pretreat patients with 30 mg of phenobarbital for 3 consecutive nights before starting a dose of 25 mg of primidone at night.[18] This autoinduces the metabolism of primidone and improves the initial tolerability.

A novel extended release preparation of primidone is also being developed for ET (Osmotica), but no clinical data yet exist (personal communication, 2019). This system uses both immediate release and sustained release drug delivered through an osmotic pump system released through a semipermeable membrane.

TOPIRAMATE

Topiramate is a sulfamate substituted monosaccharide, with multiple mechanisms of actions. It inhibits voltage-gated sodium channels and thus suppresses action potentials associated with sustained repetitive cell firing, augments the inhibitory chloride ion influx mediated by GABA, increases endogenous GABA production, modestly inhibits carbonic anhydrase, and antagonizes the AMPA/kainate subtype of the glutamate receptor.

After initial reports of efficacy,[19] a large multicenter, 24-week, placebo-controlled, parallel trial confirmed the efficacy of topiramate in patients on either no other ET medication or 1 stable ET medication.[20] The 208-patient trial (still the largest ET trial) used a dose of 292 ± 129 mg/d (400 mg maximum). Observed tremor and functional scores improved on drug. Side effects were common, including confusion and word finding difficulties, altered taste, and paresthesia. More serious potential adverse events include kidney stones, reported in about 1% of chronic users, and ciliary edema, resulting in acute bilateral blurred vision. There are no comparative data, but efficacy of topiramate seems to be similar to that of primidone and beta-blockers. The worse side effect profile, especially in the elderly, tends to relegate it to a second line drug, but topiramate also treats epilepsy, headache, and obesity, so in certain patients it may be parsimonious. Extended release topiramate preparations exist but have not been formally tested in ET.

BENZODIAZEPINES

Benzodiazepines, especially clonazepam, are frequently used in the treatment of ET. These drugs potentiate GABA-A receptors, increasing inhibitory GABAergic effects, resulting in sedation, anxiolytic effects, and muscle relaxation. However, supporting clinical trial data for ET are minimal, with only alprazolam boasting a partially positive small controlled trial.[21] Given their familiarity and established, although not benign safety record, they will likely continue to be used. Clobazam is a novel long-acting 1, 5-benzodiazepine with somewhat unique GABA affinities and relatively little sedation that has not been assessed for ET.

ALPHA-2 DELTA CALCIUM CHANNEL ANTAGONISTS

Gabapentin is a structural analogue of GABA that antagonizes alpha-2-delta subunit of various calcium channels, resulting in reduced axonal release of glutamate and other neurotransmitters. The alpha-2-delta subunit is especially abundant in the spinal cord and thalamus. Several controlled clinical trials reported mixed results with gabapentin doses between 1200 and 3600 mg/d.[22–24] Anecdotally, results are modest but the drug is generally well-tolerated. An extended release preparation and a prodrug (gabapentin enacarbel) exist, but have not been tested in tremor. Pregabalin is another widely available alpha-2-delta antagonist used to treat pain. Small controlled trials have also reported mixed results for tremor.[25–27]

OTHER ANTIEPILEPTIC MEDICATIONS

Zonisamide improves the tremor of Parkinson's disease. Several open-label trials showed modest efficacy in ET, and one 4-week, 20 subject controlled parallel study of 200 mg/d zonisamide versus placebo showed improved accelerometry scores and numerically superior Fahn-Tolosa-Martin scale improvement (43% vs 16%,; $P = .16$).[28] Three patients discontinued the drug owing to somnolence. A recent meta-analysis concluded there were insufficient data to recommend zonisamide for tremor.[29]

Levetiracetam, which binds to the synaptic vesicle protein-2, has shown mixed results in small tremor trials. One 4-week, 10 subject open-label study that evaluated doses of up to 1500 mg 2 times a day reported modestly improved clinical ratings.[30] Another 24 patient, placebo-controlled, single dose study (1000 mg) demonstrated improved tremor, as measured by accelerometry and several functional tests 1 to 3 hours after the orally administered dose.[31] A planned 45 participant controlled trial was stopped after 15 participants when an interim analysis found no suggestion of benefit.[32] The drug is well-tolerated, but efficacy is modest at best. Brivaracetam, which has higher synaptic vesicle protein-2 affinity and is approved for seizure treatment, has not been formally evaluated for ET.

Glutamate is the most common excitatory neurotransmitter and has wide brain distribution. The main receptors for glutamate are kainate, N-methyl-D-aspartate, and alpha-aminon-3-hydroxy-5-methylisoxazole-4-proprionic acid (AMPA). Topiramate, levetiracetam and phenobarbital all modestly effect AMPA receptors. Perampanel, a relatively new antiepileptic drug, markedly and specifically inhibits AMPA receptors, but has not been tested in tremor.

CALCIUM CHANNEL BLOCKERS

Flunarizine, a piperazine derivative diphenylalkylamine slow channel calcium channel blocker, demonstrated clinical and electrophysiologic efficacy, at 10 mg/d, in one 15 subject placebo-controlled crossover trial,[33] but not in another trial for refractory patients.[34] Flunarizine commonly causes parkinsonism and so should be used with caution. Nicardipine demonstrated short-term accelerometry amplitude reduction over placebo but failed to sustain statistical improvement over a 1-month period.[35] A separate placebo-controlled trial comparing propranolol 160 mg/d with nicardipine 1 mg/kg/d reported that both medications were superior to placebo, but that propranolol tended to show greater efficacy than nicardipine on a clinical scale.[36] Nimodipine, another dihydropyridine-sensitive calcium channel blocker was superior to placebo at 30 mg 4 times a day in a small, controlled, crossover trial using accelerometry and subjective reporting.[37] Ethosuximide, a moderate affinity T-type calcium blocker, did not show benefit in a small trial.[38] Despite these data, available calcium blockers have not been widely used for tremor. Several novel T-type calcium blockers are currently under investigation (discussed elsewhere in this article).

MISCELLANEOUS ORAL MEDICATIONS

Other drugs reported to improve tremor include methazolamide, the antidepressant mirtazapine, low-dose theophylline (higher doses cause tremor), clozapine, clonidine, and trazadone.[13,39] Despite long-standing availability none of these agents have gained wide acceptance for ET.

INVESTIGATIONAL ORAL AGENTS

T-type calcium channel blocking medications are being investigated for ET. T-type (ie, low voltage, and Cav3) calcium channels are predominately neuronal and have minimal cardiovascular impact. They are especially abundant in the thalamus, cerebellum, and cortex; are thought to play a role in rhythmic neuronal firing; and can mitigate spontaneous action potentials in vitro by altering the resting membrane potential.[40]

CX-8998 (CAVION/Jazz) is a highly selective Cav3 antagonist with good CNS penetration and a 10- to 13-hour half-life, previously tested for schizophrenia. In preclinical trials, CX-8998 improved harmaline and GABA-A knockout tremor models.[41]

A 95-subject, phase II trial randomized CX-8998 (10 mg 2 times a day) 1:1 against placebo for 28 days (Late breaking MDS Abstract, 2018). Participants (18–75 years) could concurrently take 1 other stable ET drug, except primidone. Efficacy points included a videotaped centrally rated blinded TETRAS[42] performance scale, locally done TETRAS performance scale, subjective TETRAS activities of daily living scale, clinical global impressions, and accelerometry. Safety data in this study, and previous studies, were generally good; however, dropout secondary to adverse events was 17% in CX-8998 versus 6% in placebo in this trial. Dizziness most separated from placebo (42% vs 21%). The locally rated TETRAS performance ($P<.05$), TETRAS activities of daily living section ($P<.05$), and clinical global impressions ($P<.05$) favored the drug, whereas centrally rated TETRAS performance and accelerometry did not. The compound was recently purchased by Jazz Pharmaceuticals (Dublin, Ireland) and future studies are planned.

PRAX-944 (Praxis Precision Medicines, Cambridge, MA) is also a T-type calcium channel blocker that has been shown to interrupt burst and rhythmic firing in several animal models.[43] Preliminary human safety data are unremarkable. A phase II multicenter ET trial is ongoing in Australia. PRAX-944 is also being evaluated for epilepsy.

CAD-1883 (Cadent Therapeutics, Cambridge, MA) is a positive allosteric modulation of small conductance Ca^{2+} activated K^+ channels (SK channels) currently undergoing a phase II trial for ET. SK channels are activated by increasing intracellular Ca^{2+} concentrations and play a central role in neuronal repolarization after a spike and in the fast component of the after-hyperpolarization.[44,45] They seem to regulate somatic excitability and have been most studied in the context of synaptic plasticity.

ET may be caused by, or at least associated with, hypersynchronized firing of Purkinje cells in the cerebellar cortex.[46] Because SK channels mediate after-hyperpolarization and burst termination in cerebellar Purkinje cells, modulation of the SK channel could restore a normalized firing pattern and reduce tremor by desynchronizing Purkinje cell output.

The starting chemical points for CAD-1883 contained a 1,3-pyrimidyl chemical core similar to CyPPA, a modestly potent SK positive allosteric modulation.[45] From this, CAD-1883 was then engineered, and has increased SK positive allosteric modulation affinity, good oral bioavailability, brain penetration, metabolic stability, and limited off-target activity. The drug modulates cerebellar Purkinje cell firing in mouse brain slices and reduces forepaw and axial tremor in the harmaline-induced rat model of tremor (Kuo, personal communication, 2018) CAD-1883 also decreases measures of ataxic gait in a mouse model of hereditary ataxia, supporting the potential for the treatment of spinocerebellar ataxia and related diseases.

In phase I controlled trials with healthy volunteers, CAD-1883 was well-tolerated at doses of up to 1200 mg/d, demonstrated no food or sex effect, and achieved steady-state plasma concentrations several-fold higher than the level projected to be required for efficacy based on animal models. A large multicenter, placebo-controlled trial is currently evaluating the drug in ET.

Sage Therapeutics (Cambridge, MA) has developed a series of allosteric modulators of GABA-A receptors, several of which have been evaluated for ET. These drugs potentiate both synaptic and extrasynaptic receptors. Physiologically, this class reduces occipital beta activity, a possibly biomarker for tremor. Brexanolone (intravenous) and Sage 217 (oral) both moderately reduced accelerometry power in short open label trials (personal communication). Adverse events were mostly modest: dizziness, somnolence, and hypotension. However, future tremor studies are not planned for either drug. Sage 324, an oral allosteric modulator with a longer half-life is currently being investigated in a small multicenter ET trial, and a larger phase II trial is planned. This class is also in further development for status epilepticus and depressive disorders. Brexanolone was recently approved for post partum depression in the United States.

BOTULINUM TOXIN INJECTIONS

Botulinum toxin A and B (BoNT) successfully treat a variety of involuntary movements. The toxins cleave one of the SNARE proteins (SNAP-25 for type A, and synaptobrevin for type B) and thus inhibit acetylcholine release into the neuromuscular junction, resulting in diminished neurotransmitter release and motor weakness. The typical duration of effect is 3 to 4 months. Currently there are 4 widely available BoNT: 3 type A toxins (ona-, inco-, and abobotulinum toxin A), and 1 type B (rimabotulinum toxin B). The goal is to weaken the muscle generating tremor without inducing functional weakness.

Numerous open-label studies and a few controlled trials have reported benefits of BoNT for hand tremor associated with ET, but also for PD, dystonic tremor, and to a lesser extent cerebellar outflow tremor.[47] In ET, open-label studies that allow for flexible dosing demonstrate greater subjective benefits and improved quality-of-life scores. Treatment requires individualized muscle selection necessitating a good understanding of anatomy. The role of electromyographic and ultrasound guidance to improve injection accuracy is not clearly established, but may improve the efficacy to side effect ratio in some cases. Computerized kinematic tremor analysis guidance localization has also been advocated.[48] There are no prospective comparative trials evaluating either different injection techniques or different toxins in ET.

Head tremor in ET may respond particularly well to BoNT, although there are limited controlled data.[49] In general, posterior muscles such as the capitus splenius are most targeted. Vocal cord injections (thyroarytenoid, cricothyroid, or thyrohyoid muscles) can variably improve voice tremor to a similar degree overall as propranolol.[14] Vocal cord injections are done via electromyography or direct visualization and muscle selection, especially whether to inject a smaller dose bilaterally or larger dose unilaterally, is individualized.

In this author's experience, BoNT often effectively treats head tremor, jaw tremor, and hand tremor that oscillates mostly around the wrist. Larger amplitude proximal arm tremors and tremor oscillating around finger joints (metacarpophalangeal, and proximal and distal interphalangeal joints) are more difficult secondary to functional weakness side effects. Currently, the high cost of BoNT and lack of regulatory approval impedes more widespread use. A large multicenter, controlled trial of incobotulinum toxin A for ET is planned.

DEEP BRAIN STIMULATION AND THALAMOTOMY

When tremor amplitude becomes very large, pharmacologic agents are seldom adequate. This population, and those refractory to other agents, justify surgical intervention either with deep brain stimulation (DBS) into the ventral intermediate (VIM) thalamus or CNS lesioning. VIM DBS is a long-established treatment for ET and will not be reviewed in detail. DBS into the subthalamic nucleus and zona incerta are less established for ET. The exact mechanism of action is debated, but the high-frequency stimulation clinically mimics a lesion to the same area, rather than stimulating that area as the name suggests. Currently, 3 different systems are widely available (Medtronic [Dublin, Ireland], Abbvie/Abbott [North Chicago, IL], Boston Scientific [Marlborough, MA]). Lead configuration varies among the devices, with some allowing greater fidelity in field location, but no prospective clinical comparisons trials have been performed.

The efficacy of VIM DBS for ET is robust and often dramatic. Although formal prospective comparisons of DBS with best medical management have not been done, there is little doubt that DBS offers a greater treatment effect size, at least for severe tremor. Numerous series have reported marked contralateral tremor reduction in 68% to 100% of patients.[50] Head and voice tremor also improve, but this improvement may not be as robust. Although some reduction of effect has been seen over years, overall efficacy remains superior to baseline more than a decade later.[51] Thalamic stimulation has the advantage of being reversible and adjustable to the needs of the patient. This device also seems to be safer to use bilaterally, or in conjunction with a contralateral thalamotomy. Many people report transient paresthesias. Bilateral implantation commonly results in dysarthria, and subjective balance difficulties, which sometimes limit efficacy. Serious surgical complications are uncommon.

Stereotaxic radiofrequency thalamotomy is also a safe and effective treatment of ET, used for almost 70 years. One large prospective study comparing VIM DBS with thalamotomy found that they were equally effective, but that DBS had a better safety profile.[52] So, although stereotactic thalamotomy is faster, cheaper, and requires only minimal subsequent care, traditional radiofrequency thalamotomy has been little used over the past 2 decades.

Recently, 1 group reported a marked benefit of ET after unilateral laser thalamotomy.[53] Localization is MRI guided using the ClearPoint stereotactic system (ClearPoint Neuro, Inc, Irvine, CA). The procedure requires electrode penetration into the VIM thalamus, similar to traditional radiofrequency thalamotomy, but instead of electric generated thermal ablation, uses a laser, potentially resulting in more consistent and accurate localization. A 13-subject open-label trial for tremor (8 with ET) showed a mean 62% decrease in target limb tremor scores maintained at 3 to 17 months. The device is commercially available and used mostly in neuro-oncology.

Gamma knife thalamotomy uses extracranial cobalt radiation from a circular collimator to create a lesion, thus obviating the need for surgical craniotomy. It has been used in ET for many years and some open-label data report good long-term results,[54] although the only blinded trial did not show benefit.[55] The functional lesion can take months to develop and targeting cannot be refined, so fidelity is not consistent, sometimes resulting in permanent neurologic deficits.

A potentially more accurate and localizing linear accelerator radiosurgery technique is called virtual cone, which uses a multi-leaf collimator.[56] The VIM is targeted with 130 Gy delivered through a high-definition multileaf collimator. The radiation is delivered in 20 half-arches with the goal of creating a 4-mm sphere. A single case presented in abstract had "complete" relief of unilateral tremor.

Recently, focused ultrasound (FUS) lesioning has been developed to create highly targeted brain lesioning. The device (Exablate, InSightec, Haifa, Israel) uses up to 1080 transcranial, synchronized ultrasound waves that coalesce to create a targeted thermal lesion (**Fig. 1**). The procedure is done in an MRI scanner and lesion location can be adjusted in almost real time by slightly heating the area, then identifying it on a specially sequenced MRI. The lesion can then be adjusted in any dimension before increasing power enough to raise temperature to 55°C for approximately 40 seconds, making a permanent lesion. The partial warming often also decreases tremor, thus

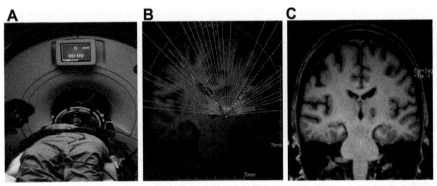

Fig. 1. (*A*) Exablate device with procedure done in MRI. (*B*) Computer-simulated targeting into the VIM nucleus. (*C*) Postprocedure lesion.

adding a physiologic assessment similar to DBS intraoperative stimulation, before permanent lesioning. Target fidelity based on postoperative MRI is excellent, usually within 1 mm of the planned target.

A large, sham-controlled, well-blinded clinical trial demonstrated marked tremor reduction in the targeted arm.[57] Adverse events were modest, usually transient sensory disturbance with rare cases of dysarthria. Potential loss of effect over time has been a concern, but a recent 4-year open-label report showed continued benefit.[58] Repeat procedures are also possible.[59] No prospective FUS versus DBS trial exists, but retrospective data and published study comparisons show equal efficacy and an overall equal adverse event burden.[60] FUS seems to be cost effective, especially compared with DBS, and the device is currently approved by US regulatory agencies for ET.[61] Bilateral FUS VIM lesioning trials are ongoing, but this procedure is not yet recommended. The same device is also used for lesions in the globus pallidus internus (GPI) and subthalamic nucleus for dystonia and Parkinson's disease.

Although incisionless, FUS creates a permanent lesion so is not noninvasive. It requires patients to completely shave their head and, importantly, about 8% of the population is not eligible secondary to skull thickness and lack of skull windows, which in eligible patients might also mitigate efficacy.[62] Potential high initial costs to purchase the device, and relatively modest reimbursement, compared with DBS, have limited its use.

NOVEL PERIPHERAL ELECTRIC AND MECHANICAL HAND TREMOR TREATMENTS

Peripheral nerve stimulation can create field potentials in the brain and has been used for many years to treat pain. Alternating peripheral nerve stimulation is thought to impact CNS neural circuits involved in ET.[63] The Cala ONE is a small wrist-worn device that delivers current alternating over the medial and radial nerve at a frequency synced to the patient's tremor. The device voltage is titrated up as tolerated and typically worn for 40 min/d.

A short, 77-subject, single treatment, sham-controlled trial showed improved TETRAS and simulated activities of daily living scores, but not improved spiral ratings, immediately after stimulation in the target limb.[64] A large, 3-month open-label study also showed improved examination and activities of daily living scales (personal communication). About 20% of subjects had some irritation at the electrode site, the only common AE. The Cala ONE device is available in 2020.

Low-frequency transcranial magnetic stimulation to the cerebellum[65,66] and supplementary motor area[67] have shown modest or no benefit in short term trials. The treatments consist of daily sessions of 1 Hz stimulation for weeks. Adverse events seem to be negligible.

Simple limb weighting may dampen tremor, but generally does not improve function secondary to loss of coordination and dexterity. Accelerometer engineered eating utensils, which shift the utensil tip opposite to the immediate hand tremor vector to lessen the total displacement of the tip, have been developed and are generally preferred to simple weighted devices.[68] Several of these devices are currently marketed.

Spring operated counterbalance dampening devices (5 micron) are being tested in humans with mixed results (personal communication). Currently, the size of these devices when strapped to the wrist makes use awkward. They also need to be mechanically matched to individual tremor frequencies.

A gyroscope glove which dampens movement in all directions is being developed for hand tremor (Gyrogear) but published data are lacking (personal communication).

Specific devices to physically dampen tremor while writing have also been developed but are not available commercially.

SUMMARY

Current ET treatments include oral medications, botulinum injects, CNS surgical interventions, and peripheral devices. Based on systematic review of 64 studies of treatment for ET, the MDS Task Force on Tremor and the MDS Evidence Based Medicine Committee concluded that propranolol, primidone, and topiramate were clinically useful; alprazolam and botulinum toxin type A were classified as possibly useful; and unilateral ventralis intermedius thalamic DBS, radiofrequency thalamotomy, and MRI-guided FUS thalamotomy were considered possibly useful.[69] Although these are effective in many cases, additional treatment options are clearly needed. For the first time, a number of pharmacologic, and electrical and mechanical devices are being developed specifically for ET.

DISCLOSURE

President of Tremor Research Group, which has consulted with CAVION, Cadent, Sage, and Merz. Dr W. G. Ondo has received Consultant fees: Amneal, ACADIA, Jazz, Sunovion, CADENT, InSightec Speaking fees: TEVA, USWorldMeds, Acorda, Neurocrine, ACADIA, Kyowa, ADAMAS Grant support: Biogen, Amneal, Sun, Revance, Lundbeck, Sonovion, Dystonia Coalition, RLS Foundation.

REFERENCES

1. Bhatia KP, Bain P, Bajaj N, et al. Consensus Statement on the classification of tremors. From the task force on tremor of the International Parkinson and Movement Disorder Society. Mov Disord 2018;33(1):75–87.

2. Buijink AW, van der Stouwe AM, Broersma M, et al. Motor network disruption in essential tremor: a functional and effective connectivity study. Brain 2015; 138(Pt 10):2934–47.

3. Erickson-Davis CR, Faust PL, Vonsattel JP, et al. "Hairy baskets" associated with degenerative Purkinje cell changes in essential tremor. J Neuropathol Exp Neurol 2010;69(3):262–71.

4. Rajput AH, Adler CH, Shill HA, et al. Essential tremor is not a neurodegenerative disease. Neurodegener Dis Manag 2012;2(3):259–68.

5. Louis RJ, Lin CY, Faust PL, et al. Climbing fiber synaptic changes correlate with clinical features in essential tremor. Neurology 2015;84(22):2284–6.

6. Koller WC, Biary N. Effect of alcohol on tremors: comparison with propranolol. Neurology 1984;34(2):221–2.

7. Boecker H, Wills AJ, Ceballos-Baumann A, et al. The effect of ethanol on alcohol-responsive essential tremor: a positron emission tomography study. Ann Neurol 1996;39(5):650–8.

8. Zeuner KE, Molloy FM, Shoge RO, et al. Effect of ethanol on the central oscillator in essential tremor. Mov Disord 2003;18(11):1280–5.

9. Bushara KO, Goldstein SR, Grimes GJ Jr, et al. Pilot trial of 1-octanol in essential tremor. Neurology 2004;62(1):122–4.

10. Voller B, Lines E, McCrossin G, et al. Dose-escalation study of octanoic acid in patients with essential tremor. J Clin Invest 2016;126(4):1451–7.

11. Shill HA, Bushara KO, Mari Z, et al. Open-label dose-escalation study of oral 1-octanol in patients with essential tremor. Neurology 2004;62(12):2320–2.

12. Frucht SJ, Bordelon Y, Houghton WH, et al. A pilot tolerability and efficacy trial of sodium oxybate in ethanol-responsive movement disorders. Mov Disord 2005; 20(10):1330–7.

13. Ondo WG. Essential tremor: treatment options. Curr Treat Options Neurol 2006; 8(3):256–67.

14. Justicz N, Hapner ER, Josephs JS, et al. Comparative effectiveness of propranolol and botulinum for the treatment of essential voice tremor. Laryngoscope 2016;126(1):113–7.

15. Zesiewicz TA, Elble RJ, Louis ED, et al. Evidence-based guideline update: treatment of essential tremor: report of the Quality Standards subcommittee of the American Academy of Neurology. Neurology 2011;77(19):1752–5.

16. Koller WC, Vetere-Overfield B. Acute and chronic effects of propranolol and primidone in essential tremor. Neurology 1989;39(12):1587–8.

17. Sasso E, Perucca E, Calzetti S. Double-blind comparison of primidone and phenobarbital in essential tremor. Neurology 1988;38(5):808–10.

18. Kanner AM, Parra J, Frey M. The "forgotten" cross-tolerance between phenobarbital and primidone: it can prevent acute primidone-related toxicity. Epilepsia 2000;41(10):1310–4.

19. Connor GS. A double-blind placebo-controlled trial of topiramate treatment for essential tremor. Neurology 2002;59(1):132–4.

20. Ondo WG, Jankovic J, Connor GS, et al. Topiramate in essential tremor: a double-blind, placebo-controlled trial. Neurology 2006;66(5):672–7.

21. Gunal DI, Afsar N, Bekiroglu N, et al. New alternative agents in essential tremor therapy: double-blind placebo-controlled study of alprazolam and acetazolamide. Neurol Sci 2000;21(5):315–7.

22. Ondo W, Hunter C, Vuong KD, et al. Gabapentin for essential tremor: a multiple-dose, double-blind, placebo-controlled trial. Mov Disord 2000;15(4):678–82.

23. Gironell A, Kulisevsky J, Barbanoj M, et al. A randomized placebo-controlled comparative trial of gabapentin and propranolol in essential tremor. Arch Neurol 1999;56(4):475–80.

24. Pahwa R, Lyons K, Hubble JP, et al. Double-blind controlled trial of gabapentin in essential tremor. Mov Disord 1998;13(3):465–7.

25. Zesiewicz TA, Sullivan KL, Hinson V, et al. Multisite, double-blind, randomized, controlled study of pregabalin for essential tremor. Mov Disord 2013;28(2): 249–50.

26. Ferrara JM, Kenney C, Davidson AL, et al. Efficacy and tolerability of pregabalin in essential tremor: a randomized, double-blind, placebo-controlled, crossover trial. J Neurol Sci 2009;285(1–2):195–7.

27. Zesiewicz TA, Ward CL, Hauser RA, et al. A pilot, double-blind, placebo-controlled trial of pregabalin (Lyrica) in the treatment of essential tremor. Mov Disord 2007;22(11):1660–3.

28. Zesiewicz TA, Ward CL, Hauser RA, et al. A double-blind placebo-controlled trial of zonisamide (zonegran) in the treatment of essential tremor. Mov Disord 2007; 22(2):279–82.

29. Bruno E, Nicoletti A, Filippini G, et al. Zonisamide for essential tremor. Cochrane Database Syst Rev 2017;(8):CD009684.

30. Ondo WG, Jimenez JE, Vuong KD, et al. An open-label pilot study of levetiracetam for essential tremor. Clin Neuropharmacol 2004;27(6):274–7.

31. Bushara KO, Malik T, Exconde RE. The effect of levetiracetam on essential tremor. Neurology 2005;64(6):1078–80.

32. Elble RJ, Lyons KE, Pahwa R. Levetiracetam is not effective for essential tremor. Clin Neuropharmacol 2007;30(6):350–6.

33. Biary N, al Deeb SM, Langenberg P. The effect of flunarizine on essential tremor. Neurology 1991;41(2 (Pt 1)):311–2.

34. Curran T, Lang AE. Flunarizine in essential tremor. Clin Neuropharmacol 1993; 16(5):460–3.

35. Garcia Ruiz PJ, Garcia de Yebenes Prous J, Jimenez Jimenez J. Effect of nicardipine on essential tremor: brief report. Clin Neuropharmacol 1993;16(5): 456–9.

36. Mitsuda M, Nomoto M, Iwata S. Effects of beta-blockers and nicardipine on oxotremorine-induced tremor in common marmosets. Jpn J Pharmacol 1999; 81(2):244–6.

37. Biary N, Bahou Y, Sofi MA, et al. The effect of nimodipine on essential tremor. Neurology 1995;45(8):1523–5.

38. Gironell A, Marin-Lahoz J. Ethosuximide for essential tremor: an open-label trial. Tremor Other Hyperkinet Mov (N Y) 2016;6:378.

39. Sadeghi R, Ondo WG. Pharmacological management of essential tremor. Drugs 2010;70(17):2215–28.

40. Dreyfus FM, Tscherter A, Errington AC, et al. Selective T-type calcium channel block in thalamic neurons reveals channel redundancy and physiological impact of I(T)window. J Neurosci 2010;30(1):99–109.

41. Handforth A, Homanics GE, Covey DF, et al. T-type calcium channel antagonists suppress tremor in two mouse models of essential tremor. Neuropharmacology 2010;59(6):380–7.

42. Elble R, Comella C, Fahn S, et al. Reliability of a new scale for essential tremor. Mov Disord 2012;27(12):1567–9.

43. Cain SM, Tyson JR, Jones KL, et al. Thalamocortical neurons display suppressed burst-firing due to an enhanced Ih current in a genetic model of absence epilepsy. Pflugers Arch 2015;467(6):1367–82.

44. Adelman JP, Maylie J, Sah P. Small-conductance Ca2+-activated K+ channels: form and function. Annu Rev Physiol 2012;74:245–69.

45. Brown BM, Shim H, Christophersen P, et al. Pharmacology of small- and intermediate-conductance calcium-activated potassium channels. Annu Rev Pharmacol Toxicol 2020;60:219–40 [Epub ahead of print].

46. Lin CY, Louis ED, Faust PL, et al. Abnormal climbing fibre-Purkinje cell synaptic connections in the essential tremor cerebellum. Brain 2014;137(Pt 12):3149–59.

47. Mittal SO, Lenka A, Jankovic J. Botulinum toxin for the treatment of tremor. Parkinsonism Relat Disord 2019;63:31–41.

48. Samotus O, Lee J, Jog M. Personalized bilateral upper limb essential tremor therapy with botulinum toxin using kinematics. Toxins (Basel) 2019;11(2) [pii:E125].

49. Pahwa R, Busenbark K, Swanson-Hyland EF, et al. Botulinum toxin treatment of essential head tremor. Neurology 1995;45(4):822–4.

50. Flora ED, Perera CL, Cameron AL, et al. Deep brain stimulation for essential tremor: a systematic review. Mov Disord 2010;25(11):1550–9.

51. Paschen S, Forstenpointner J, Becktepe J, et al. Long-term efficacy of deep brain stimulation for essential tremor: an observer-blinded study. Neurology 2019; 92(12):e1378–86.

52. Schuurman PR, Bosch DA, Bossuyt PM, et al. A comparison of continuous thalamic stimulation and thalamotomy for suppression of severe tremor [see comments]. N Engl J Med 2000;342(7):461–8.

53. Harris M, Steele J, Williams R, et al. MRI-guided laser interstitial thermal thalamotomy for medically intractable tremor disorders. Mov Disord 2019;34(1):124–9.

54. Young RF, Li F, Vermeulen S, et al. Gamma Knife thalamotomy for treatment of essential tremor: long-term results. J Neurosurg 2010;112(6):1311–7.

55. Lim SY, Hodaie M, Fallis M, et al. Gamma knife thalamotomy for disabling tremor: a blinded evaluation. Arch Neurol 2010;67(5):584–8.

56. Popple RA, Wu X, Brezovich IA, et al. The virtual cone: a novel technique to generate spherical dose distributions using a multileaf collimator and standardized control-point sequence for small target radiation surgery. Adv Radiat Oncol 2018;3(3):421–30.

57. Elias WJ, Lipsman N, Ondo WG, et al. A randomized trial of focused ultrasound thalamotomy for essential tremor. N Engl J Med 2016;375(8):730–9.

58. Park YS, Jung NY, Na YC, et al. Four-year follow-up results of magnetic resonance-guided focused ultrasound thalamotomy for essential tremor. Mov Disord 2019;34(5):727–34.

59. Weidman EK, Kaplitt MG, Strybing K, et al. Repeat magnetic resonance imaging-guided focused ultrasound thalamotomy for recurrent essential tremor: case report and review of MRI findings. J Neurosurg 2019;1–8. https://doi.org/10.3171/2019.4. JNS 182694.

60. Harary M, Segar DJ, Hayes MT, et al. Unilateral thalamic deep brain stimulation versus focused ultrasound thalamotomy for essential tremor. World Neurosurg 2019;126:e144–52.

61. Li C, Gajic-Veljanoski O, Schaink AK, et al. Cost-effectiveness of magnetic resonance-guided focused ultrasound for essential tremor. Mov Disord 2019; 34(5):735–43.

62. D'Souza M, Chen KS, Rosenberg J, et al. Impact of skull density ratio on efficacy and safety of magnetic resonance-guided focused ultrasound treatment of essential tremor. J Neurosurg 2019;1–6. https://doi.org/10.3171/2019.2. JNS 183517.

63. Brittain JS, Cagnan H, Mehta AR, et al. Distinguishing the central drive to tremor in Parkinson's disease and essential tremor. J Neurosci 2015;35(2):795–806.

64. Pahwa R, Dhall R, Ostrem J, et al. An acute randomized controlled trial of noninvasive peripheral nerve stimulation in essential tremor. Neuromodulation 2019; 22(5):537–45.
65. Shin HW, Hallett M, Sohn YH. Cerebellar repetitive transcranial magnetic stimulation for patients with essential tremor. Parkinsonism Relat Disord 2019;64: 304–7.
66. Gironell A, Kulisevsky J, Lorenzo J, et al. Transcranial magnetic stimulation of the cerebellum in essential tremor: a controlled study. Arch Neurol 2002; 59(3):413–7.
67. Badran BW, Glusman CE, Austelle CW, et al. A double-blind, sham-controlled pilot trial of Pre-Supplementary Motor Area (Pre-SMA) 1 Hz rTMS to treat essential tremor. Brain Stimul 2016;9(6):945–7.
68. Sabari J, Stefanov DG, Chan J, et al. Adapted feeding utensils for people with parkinson's-related or essential tremor. Am J Occup Ther 2019;73(2). 7302205120p7302205121-7302205120p7302205129.
69. Ferreira JJ, Mestre TA, Lyons KE, et al. MDS evidence-based review of treatments for essential tremor. Mov Disord 2019;34(7):950–8.

Medical and Surgical Treatments for Dystonia

H.A. Jinnah, MD, PhD[a,b],*

KEYWORDS

- Botulinum toxin • Deep brain stimulation • Therapy • Torticollis • Blepharospasm
- Meige syndrome • Oromandibular dystonia

KEY POINTS

- The dystonias are defined by excessive muscle contractions leading to involuntary postures and/or repetitive abnormal movements.
- The clinical manifestations of the dystonias vary and are grouped according to 4 clinical characteristics, including age at onset, body region affected, changes over time, and whether or not there are relevant accompanying neurologic or medical features.
- The etiologies for the dystonias vary. Most adult-onset cases are idiopathic, whereas most childhood-onset cases have a discoverable cause. There are many known causes, both inherited and acquired.
- Treatments are tailored to the clinical manifestations and the etiology, if known. They include oral medications, botulinum toxin injections, and surgical procedures.

OVERVIEW

The dystonias are defined by excessive muscular contraction producing involuntary abnormal movements.[1] The clinical appearance of abnormal movements in the dystonias varies widely.[2] Many movements tend to be slow and twisting, often with sustained abnormal postures. Sometimes dystonic movements are quick or tremor-like. Whether slow or fast, dystonic movements are not random. They tend to recur in the same pattern. They also tend to be worsened by voluntary effort.

The dystonias may arise at any age, from infancy to late adulthood. They may affect muscles in almost any region of the body. Most dystonias are chronic. Some are static, some are progressive, and some have characteristic fluctuations over time. In some cases, dystonia is the only problem. For others, dystonia is one part of a more complex syndrome. Because of the remarkable variability in the clinical expression of dystonia, it is helpful to have a strategy for lumping and splitting them into related groups.

[a] Department of Neurology, Emory University School of Medicine, Suite 6305 Woodruff Memorial Building, Atlanta, GA 30322, USA; [b] Department of Human Genetics, Emory University School of Medicine, Suite 6305 Woodruff Memorial Building, Atlanta, GA 30322, USA
* 6305 Woodruff Memorial Building, Atlanta, GA 30322.
E-mail address: hjinnah@emory.edu

Neurol Clin 38 (2020) 325–348
https://doi.org/10.1016/j.ncl.2020.01.003
0733-8619/20/© 2020 Elsevier Inc. All rights reserved.

Currently, the clinical features important for the classification of dystonia include age at onset, body region affected, variation over time, and whether or not dystonia is combined with other relevant features (**Fig. 1**).[1,3]

Etiologies for dystonia are also quite varied.[4] Most are idiopathic, and a cause cannot be found, even after extensive diagnostic evaluation. Although a cause can only be found in the minority of cases, there are many potential causes, both acquired and inherited. Acquired causes of dystonia include medications or toxins, structural defects such as vascular events or space-occupying lesions, and infectious or other inflammatory processes. There also are many inherited causes for the dystonias. There are only a few genes associated with isolated dystonia, but there are more than 100 genes associated with combined dystonias.[5] Because there are so many etiologies for dystonia and most of them are quite rare, obtaining a definitive etiologic

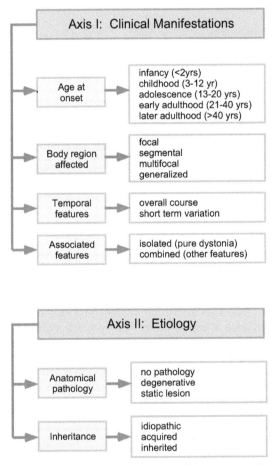

Fig. 1. Classification of the dystonias. The many types of dystonia are classified according to 2 axes. The first axis relates to clinical features. The main factors important for clinical classification include age at onset, body distribution, temporal features, and whether or not dystonia is combined with other neurologic or medical problems. The main factors important for etiologic classification include whether the disorder is associated with relevant brain pathology, and whether the disorder is acquired or inherited. However, a large proportion of cases remain idiopathic.

diagnosis can be challenging. However, an etiologic diagnosis is important because some of them have very specific treatments.

This article focuses on treatments for dystonia, both medical and surgical. Treatments are available for all types of dystonia. Most patients can benefit from symptomatic therapies, which include oral medications, local injections of botulinum toxin (BoNT), and surgical interventions. For some patients, there are specific treatments that target underlying disease mechanisms.

PATIENT EVALUATION
History and Examination

A thorough clinical evaluation is important for guiding therapeutic strategies. The basic overall strategy is described here. A more detailed approach is available in prior reviews.[4,6] The clinical evaluation begins with a careful history and examination, focusing on the 4 clinical features used to classify the dystonias into specific subgroups (**Fig. 2**). The age when dystonia first began provides a guide for potential etiologies. Those that begin in adults are more often idiopathic, whereas those that begin in children often have an identifiable cause.

The evolution of symptoms over time provides a further guide for potential etiologies. The adult-onset focal dystonias tend to evolve over a period of a few weeks

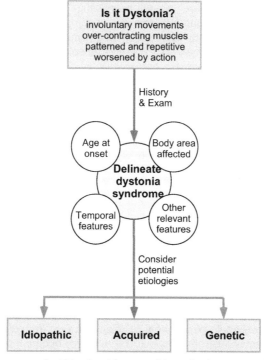

Fig. 2. Diagnostic approach. This algorithm provides a basic strategy for the diagnostic approach to most patients with dystonia. The initial step is to determine whether the disorder being considered is a type of dystonia, or something that may mimic dystonia. The next step is to use the history and examination to delineate the dystonia syndrome, using the main clinical features used for classification. The third step is to consider potential etiologies.

to a few years, and subsequent evolution is slower or hard to detect.[7–13] More rapid evolution over hours or days can point to a functional (psychogenic) cause, a drug effect such as a neuroleptic, a vascular or immunologic event, or an inherited disorder such as the syndrome of rapid-onset dystonia-parkinsonism syndrome. Diurnal fluctuations are characteristic of dopa-responsive dystonia, whereas sudden attacks are more characteristic of the paroxysmal dyskinesias.

The history and examination should also address if dystonia is the only problem, or if there are other relevant problems that are part of a recognizable syndrome.[4] The term *isolated dystonia* (previously called *primary dystonia*) refers to a disorder where dystonia is the only problem.[1,3] Because tremor occurs in approximately one-half of all patients with dystonia, it is allowed in the current definition of isolated tremor. The term *combined dystonia* is used when dystonia is one part of a more complex syndrome that includes other relevant neurologic or medical problems. For example, dystonia combined with myoclonus can point to one group of etiologies, whereas dystonia combined with liver disease might point to a different group of etiologies.[4]

Finally, the body region affected is important to define because it provides an important guide to the therapeutic approach. For example, BoNT often is the treatment of first choice for focal dystonias, and oral medications or surgery are more often used for generalized dystonias.

Laboratory Investigations

For most adult-onset dystonias, laboratory investigations depend on body area affected, temporal features, and any relevant accompanying problems. For most adult-onset focal or segmental dystonias, diagnostic testing is often unfruitful. Electromyography (EMG) often shows excessive muscle activity, but it is not usually conducted because the findings are not specific to dystonia. Brain imaging is not required, although laryngoscopy is useful to rule out structural defects of the vocal cords in the laryngeal dystonias.[14] Brain imaging can be useful to exclude a structural process for hemidystonia and generalized dystonia. Brain imaging can also be helpful for in adult-onset patients when there are additional neurologic features or unusually rapid progression. Genetic testing is not required in idiopathic adult-onset cases, but should be considered if there are other affected family members or the dystonia is part of a syndrome that points to a specific inherited disorder.

For most early-onset dystonias (children and young adults), laboratory testing is almost always conducted, because there is a greater likelihood of finding a cause. Brain imaging is valuable, because it can point to specific structural defects, or specific gray or white matter diseases. The accompanying clinical features and temporal evolution may point to specific syndromes, which can be evaluated by specific tests of blood, urine, or cerebrospinal fluid. Genetic testing should be considered when the clinical evaluation points to a specific syndrome that is inherited or when there are multiple affected family members. When there is a clear correlation between the clinical syndrome and a specific genetic disorder, it is reasonable to conduct focused genetic tests. If the clinical syndrome can be explained by multiple different genes, a dystonia gene panel or clinical exome is more efficient. Serial genetic testing of individual genes should be avoided, because the cost of 2 to 3 individual genes is often more expensive than a panel that includes nearly 100 genes. It is important to know that commercially available clinical gene panels vary dramatically. Some include all genes known to cause any type of dystonia (~100 genes), whereas others are selective for only the most common ones (10–12 genes). Recent studies have shown that the larger panels can achieve a molecular diagnosis for 10% to 30% of patients with dystonia, especially in early-onset cases.[15]

If a definitive diagnosis is not obtained after appropriate testing, it is useful to remember the test of time. Patients should be reevaluated in follow-up, and the diagnosis reconsidered if and when the initial clinical phenotype evolves.

NONPHARMACOLOGIC TREATMENT OPTIONS
Counseling

Counseling is important for 3 reasons. First, many patients with dystonia experience a diagnostic odyssey in which they have described their symptoms to multiple doctors over several years without getting a clear diagnosis.[16–19] They often try multiple treatments that produce little or no benefit. This process creates the impression that they have some mysterious and incurable disorder. Some counseling is helpful to address this incorrect impression. Patients may be directed to several online resources for more information (**Table 1**).

Table 1
Online resources for dystonia

Type of Dystonia	Source	Address
Blepharospasm and oromandibular syndrome	Benign Essential Blepharospasm Research Foundation	blepharospasm.org
All types of dystonia	Dystonia Coalition	rarediseasenetwork.org/cms/dystonia
All types of dystonia	Dystonia Medical Research Foundation	dystonia-foundation.org
All types dystonia	National Institute of Neurologic Disorders and Stroke	ninds.nih.gov/disorders/dystonias
Laryngeal dystonia	National Spasmodic Dysphonia Association	dysphonia.org
Cervical dystonia	National Spasmodic Torticollis Association	spasmodictorticollis.org

The second important reason for counseling is that there is a high risk of depression and anxiety in many types of dystonia.[20] There also is significant social withdrawal owing to embarrassment from overtly stigmatizing symptoms. These problems should be discussed openly and addressed with appropriate referrals if necessary.

The third reason that counseling is important is that finding the ideal treatment regimen often is a trial and error process. Oral medications have unpredictable efficacy and frequent side effects, sometimes requiring serial testing with multiple options, each requiring dose titration. The BoNTs require customization of the dose pattern over several treatment cycles, which can take several months. Deep brain stimulation (DBS) requires fine tuning of the stimulator settings, sometimes for 6 to 12 months. The trial and error approach and the time required to optimize therapies can be frustrating for patients. An open discussion regarding this process is important so that patients have realistic expectations and do not abandon treatment efforts too early.

Physical Therapy

Patients with dystonia often ask for physiotherapy. These procedures seem very intuitive in view of the spasms and pain that result from excessive involuntary muscle contractions. Options frequently requested include strengthening of nondystonic muscles, "retaining" exercises, and stretching of tight muscles. Many small open trials of various physiotherapy methods have reported positive results for different types of dystonia, but the most rigorous studies have failed to demonstrate any lasting benefits.[21,22] Despite the absence of evidence, it is reasonable to offer physiotherapy according to specific patient needs, especially those with severe generalized dystonias who may develop contractures.

Complementary and Alternative Medicine

Patients also frequently ask about related procedures such as chiropractic therapy, yoga, meditation, other relaxation or stress reduction programs, acupuncture, and dry needling, and others.[23] Here again, there is little evidence for long-term benefit, although some patients enjoy these options. Usually there is no harm in these procedures, apart from chiropractic methods, which occasionally can be overly aggressive or painful.

PHARMACOLOGIC TREATMENT OPTIONS
Symptom-Based Drugs

Patients with dystonia are offered a wide variety of medications.[24-29] Evidence-based reviews have been published,[30,31] but none of the available agents has been tested in rigorously controlled clinical trials. Their use is driven largely by anecdotal experience and expert opinion. The available therapeutic options fall into 2 broad categories. These include symptomatic drugs that are useful for many types of dystonia (**Table 2**), and drugs that are useful only in special circumstances (**Table 3**).

Table 2
Oral medications for symptomatic treatment of dystonia

Group	Examples	Notes
Benzodiazepines	Alprazolam, chlordiazepoxide, clonazepam, diazepam	Typical side effects include impaired concentration, sedation, fatigue, impaired coordination, withdrawal reactions
Muscle relaxants	Carisoprodol, chlorzoxazone, cyclobenzeprine, metaxolone, methocarbamol, orphenadrine	Typical side effects vary by class, but most centrally acting muscle relaxants can cause some degree of sedation and fatigue
Antispasticity agents	Baclofen, tizanidine	Typical side effects include impaired concentration, sedation, fatigue, impaired coordination, dizziness, weakness, withdrawal reactions
Anticholinergics	Benztropine, biperidin, ethopropazine, ophenadrine, procyclidine, trihexyphenidyl	Typical side effects include impaired concentration, memory loss, fatigue, dry mouth and eyes, constipation, urinary retention, blurry vision
Levodopa	Carbidopa/levodopa, benserazide/levodopa	Typical side effects include nausea and orthostatic hypotension
Others	Cannabidiol, cyproheptidine, deutetrabenazine, gabapentin, lithium, mexilitine, nabilone, riluzole, tetrabenazine, valbenazine, zolpidem	These drugs have been reported to be useful in anecdotal reports, so they are not widely used

A large international survey of medication use across the adult-onset dystonias revealed the benzodiazepines to be the most commonly prescribed, followed by muscle relaxants, antispasticity drugs, anticholinergics, and dopamine-related drugs.[25] Among children with dystonia, the most commonly used medications included baclofen and trihexyphenidyl, followed by levodopa and diazepam.[29] The benzodiazepines are used by 10% to 30% of all cases, depending on the type of dystonia.[25,29] They include alprazolam, chlordiazepoxide, clonazepam, and diazepam. They seem to provide at least partial benefits for many patients. Common side effects are sedation and impaired concentration. Other side effects include confusion, depression, and dizziness. The benzodiazepines are known to be habit forming, and sudden discontinuation can lead to withdrawal effects. As a result, their use must be monitored carefully.

Antispasticity agents include baclofen and tizanidine (in addition to the benzodiazepines noted elsewhere in this article). They are used by 5% to 10% of adult dystonia patients,[25] and 40% to 50% of children with dystonia.[29] Baclofen is the most common. It is particularly popular in childhood, when there is coexisting spasticity, such as in cerebral palsy.[32] For both adults and children, the most common side effects are sedation and impaired concentration. Baclofen can also cause confusion or dizziness. At high doses, sudden discontinuation can lead to serious withdrawal effects. Baclofen also can be administered intrathecally, via indwelling pumps.[33] This approach minimizes nonspecific side effects. However, the pumps must be refilled from time to time, and occasionally fail or become infected. Unrecognized pump failures, for example, caused by a blockage in the tubing, can lead to serious withdrawal reactions.

Drugs that block acetylcholine receptors (muscarinic subtype) are at least partly effective for many subtypes of dystonia.[28,29] They include benztropine, biperidin, ethopropazine, orphenadrine, procyclidine, and trihexyphenidyl. Trihexyphenidyl is the most commonly used, and high doses are typically required. Although the anticholinergics were among the first to be recognized as useful across many types of dystonia, they are used by only 2% to 5% of adults with dystonia,[25] and 30 to 40% of children with dystonia.[29] A major limitation is that high doses are often required, and side effects become limiting as the dose is titrated. The most concerning side effects in adults involve problems with cognition, such as impaired concentration, memory loss, confusion, and sedation. Other frequent side effects include dry mouth or dry eyes, urinary retention, constipation, depression, blurry vision, and worsening of narrow-angle glaucoma. There are now multiple studies linking long-term anticholinergic use with dementia, raising concern for chronic use in adults with dystonia.[34] It is often claimed that children tolerate high doses better than adults, although impaired performance in school can be difficult to identify in young children,[35,36] and the risk of late life dementia after chronic early exposure is unknown. In 1 study, more than 50% of children taking trihexyphenidyl experienced dose-limiting side effects.[29]

Muscle relaxant drugs also intuitively seem attractive, because dystonia involves excessive muscle contractions leading to soreness. They are often prescribed by primary care providers and they are used by 5% to 10% of adult patients, but rarely in children. The drugs included in this category include carisoprodol, chlorzoxazone, cyclobenzeprine, metaxalone, methocarbamol, and others.[37] Side effects vary among these options, but all are centrally acting. As a result, some degree of sedation or fatigue is common, except perhaps for metaxolone. Carisoprodol is a controlled substance (schedule IV) and therefore requires special attention. Many patients seem to benefit at least partially, especially when there is pain and soreness from muscle spasms. However, patients should be counseled that most muscle relaxants have been approved for only short-term use (2–3 weeks), and the potential long-term effects of chronic use are not well-known.

Drugs for Special Circumstances

This category includes drugs that target a mechanism known to cause a specific type of dystonia. The most well-known in this class is levodopa, which is highly effective for dopa-responsive dystonia.[38–40] Because of its remarkable efficacy, a levodopa trial is mandatory for all children and young adults with unexplained dystonia, including those with a diagnosis of cerebral palsy. Children may respond to doses as low as one-half of a 25/100 mg tablet of carbidopa/levodopa 2 times daily. Larger doses are sometimes required, so an adequate trial must titrate the dose to 20 mg/kg daily divided across 3 to 4 daily doses for at least a month. It is not uncommon for adult neurologists to assume the care of children with cerebral palsy when

Table 3
Inherited dystonias with specific treatments

Treatment Strategy	Disorders
Removal of a toxic substance	Cerebrotendinous xanthomatosis Manganese transporter deficiencies Niemann-Pick type C Wilson's disease
Vitamins and/or cofactors	Abetalipoproteinemia Ataxia with vitamin E deficiency Biotin-thiamin responsive basal ganglia disease Cerebral folate deficiency Cobalamin deficiency Coenzyme Q10 deficiency Homocystinuria Pyruvate dehydrogenase deficiency
Avoidance of triggers	Alternating hemiplegia of childhood Biotin-thiamin responsive basal ganglia disease GLUT1 deficiency Glutaric aciduria Methylmalonic aciduria Propionic acidemia Rapid-onset dystonia-parkinsonism
Specific medications	AADC deficiency Dopa-responsive dystonia Episodic ataxia type 2 GLUT1 deficiency MOCS1 deficiency Paroxysmal kinesigenic dyskinesia
Dietary restrictions	Abetalipoproteinemia GLUT1 deficiency homocystinuria Maple syrup urine disease Methylmalonic aciduria Propionic acidemia

Abbreviation: AADC, aromatic L-amino acid decarboxylase deficiency.
  Further details regarding these disorders and their specific treatments can be found in a prior comprehensive review.[50]

they reach adulthood, and a repeat trial of levodopa is often required because of inadequate documentation of a levodopa trial, or inadequate dose titration. In addition to dopa-responsive dystonia, levodopa can sometimes be helpful for dystonia in other disorders. They are used in for dystonia occuring in ataxia telangiectasia, spinocerebellar ataxia type 3, Parkinson's disease, and others.[41,42] Levodopa is not typically used for the more common adult-onset focal dystonias,[43] although occasional patients do respond.[44]

Another well-known treatment strategy involving drugs that target a specific mechanism involves copper-lowering agents for Wilson's disease, which results from an inherited defect in a copper transporter leading to toxic copper accumulation.[45] Penecillamine and tetrathiomolybdenate are copper chelators that leech copper from the body, and zinc is a naturally occurring heavy metal that decreases copper absorption from the gastrointestinal tract. Treatment strategies depend on both severity and features of disease, and there remains significant controversy regarding the optimal approach.[46] A series of related disorders recently have been described with toxic manganese accumulation owing to manganese transporter defects. These disorders have a presentation very similar to Wilson's disease, and they respond to manganese chelators.[47–49]

Although many reviews addressing special treatments for specific forms dystonia focus on dopa-responsive dystonia and Wilson's disease, the list of options is much longer. A recent review described more than 30 inherited disorders with disease-specific treatments, and more than one-half of them included dystonia, either in isolation or as part of a multisystem disorder.[50] Only a few examples are highlighted here, with a more complete list of the disorders and their treatment approach is provided in **Table 3**. For example, several disorders that usually present in early childhood dystonia as one part of a multisystem syndrome can be treated by supplementation with vitamins or essential cofactors. Examples include biotin-thiamine–responsive basal ganglia disease, biotinidase deficiency, and ataxia with vitamin E deficiency. Other disorders can be managed with dietary changes. Examples include GLUT1 deficiency syndromes, maple syrup urine disease, and abetalipoproteinemia. Dystonic spasms in paroxysmal kinesigenic dyskinesia respond extraordinarily well to very low doses of carbamazepine and related anticonvulsants. Although all of these disorders are quite rare, early diagnosis is critical because treatments can be life-altering. For many, late diagnosis can lead to irreversible neurologic defects.

Another category of treatable dystonias include autoimmune disorders, some of which have identifiable antibodies (**Table 4**).[51,52] One of the most well-known examples is Sydenham's chorea, where chorea usually predominates. However, many children with Sydenham's chorea also have dystonic posturing, and dystonia may be the dominant problem. Antibacterial therapy is important. For most of the other disorders, typically dystonia is part of a multisystem disorder, sometimes combined with encephalopathy. Once again, early diagnosis is valuable because many are associated with underlying malignancy. Treatment of the malignancy is essential and may sometimes be combined with immunomodulatory agents.

LOCAL TREATMENT OPTIONS
Overview of Botulinum Toxins

The most common forms of dystonia emerge in adults and affect a limited number of muscles. The treatment of choice for many of these focal dystonias is local injection of

Table 4
Dystonia associated with antibodies

Antibody	Typical Age at Onset	Clinical Features	Association with Malignancy
AQP4	Children or adults	Tonic spasms may resemble paroxysmal dystonia; often combined with optic neuritis and/or myelitis	Sometimes
CV2 or CRMP5	Children or adults	Dystonia may be combined with chorea, parkinsonism, optic neuritis, myelitis, and encephalopathy	Frequent
D2R	Children	Dystonia may be combined with chorea or parkinsonism, in setting of encephalopathy that includes prominent behavioral and sleep disturbances	Not usually
GAD or amphiphysin	Adults	Stiff person syndrome may present with a syndrome that is, easily mistaken for dystonia	Occasional
GABA$_A$R	children or adults	dystonia may be combined with chorea ataxia, sometimes opsoclonus-myoclonus in setting of broader encephalopathy	Frequent
LGI1	Adults	Faciobrachial dystonic seizures may resemble paroxysmal segmental dystonia, often with encephalopathy and sleep disorder	Occasional
Ma2	Children or adults	Dystonia may be combined with parkinsonism and sleep disorder in setting of broader encephalopathy	Frequent
NMDAR	Children or adults	Dystonia may paroxysmal or combined with chorea, ataxia, myoclonus, parkinsonism, oculogyric crises in setting of broader encephalopathy	Frequent
Ri or ANNA-2	Adults	Dystonia may be combined with ataxia, myoclonus, rigidity, opsoclonus and cranial nerve signs of brainstem encephalitis	Frequent

Further details regarding these antibodies and associated clinical syndromes can be found in prior reviews.[51,52]

BoNT. These treatments can also be applied to the most troublesome areas among patients with broader muscle involvement in generalized dystonias, such as the abnormal head/neck movements or tight leg muscles often seen dyskinetic cerebral palsy.

The BoNTs are synthetic derivatives of naturally occurring toxins made by the bacterium *Clostridium botulinum*, the cause of botulism. Seven serotypes are known, and 2 have been developed as therapeutics, serotypes A and B (**Table 5**). The most commonly available formulations of serotype A include abobotulinumtoxinA (Dysport), incobotulinumtoxinA (Xeomin), and onabotulinumtoxinA (Botox). Serotype B is available as rimabotulinumtoxinB (Myobloc). Several less widely available formulations are available in specific parts of the world. Although doses vary among the BoNT products, their overall effects are similar.

For many types of dystonia, the BoNTs reduce abnormal movements, pain and spasms, and disability. The doses and muscles injected must be customized for each patient. Benefits emerge within 1 week, and they last for approximately

Table 5
Most commonly used BoNT preparations

	Onabotulinum toxinA	Abobotulinum toxinA	Incobotulinum toxinA	Rimabotulinu toxinB
Trade name	Botox	Dysport	Xeomin	Myobloc
Vial supplied	Vacuum dried	Freeze dried	Powder	Liquid
Doses available (U)	100, 200	300, 500	50, 100	1000, 2500, 5000
Storage temperature	Refrigerate	Refrigerate	Room temperature	Refrigerate
Dose equivalents[a]	1	2.5–3.0	1	40

[a] As the first BoNT approved by the US Food and Drug Administration, onabotulinumtoxinA was defined as having a standard strength of 1 unit. The approximate dose-equivalents for the others are compared against this value.

12 weeks.[53] The usefulness of BoNT has been summarized in several systematic and evidence-based reviews.[54–57] There are also many practical guides describing muscle selection and dosing.[58,59] Only the most common applications are described elsewhere in this article.

Cervical Dystonia (Torticollis)

Numerous studies have demonstrated the long-term efficacy of BoNT for cervical dystonia.[55,56,60] The BoNTs attenuate abnormal head movements, they reduce neck pain, and they improve overall quality of life. Although good responses can be achieved in the vast majority of patients with cervical dystonia, there are a few subtypes of cervical dystonia where it can be very difficult to get satisfactory results, such as those with prominent anterocollis, tremor-dominant cervical dystonia, or longstanding abnormal postures.[61,62]

Side effects are usually minor and transient. Dysphagia can result when large doses applied to anterior neck muscles (sternocleidomastoids and scalenes) spread to nearby muscles of swallowing in the pharynx. Neck extensor weakness (head drop) can occur when large doses are applied to posterior neck muscles (semispinalis capitus, splenius cervicus) that hold up the head. A systemic flu-like syndrome may also occur in a minority of patients.[63]

Craniofacial Dystonia (Blepharospasm and Meige Syndrome)

Many studies also have demonstrated the long-term efficacy of BoNT for blepharospasm.[55,60] The BoNTs reduce spasms of eye closure and excessive blinking, and they improve overall quality of life. The vast majority of patients see good effects, with only minor or transient side effects. Ptosis or diplopia can occur from spread of high doses applied to the upper middle eye region, or from inadvertent injections that are too deep and fall behind the fascial plane that separates anterior eyelid muscles (orbicularis oculi) from posterior muscles (levator palpebra and muscles controlling eye movements).

Patients with blepharospasm sometimes develop apraxia of eyelid opening, a phenomenon that refers to inability to open the eyes without apparent spasm. Eyelid opening apraxia may also be the sole manifestation of blepharospasm. This phenomenon may be caused by spasms of the eyelid muscles, which are not overtly visible on examination. Good responses are more difficult to achieve in these patients, unless the eyelid muscles are treated too.[64–66]

Approximately one-half of patients with blepharospasm experience spread of muscle spasms to the lower face, jaw, and/or tongue.[9,12,13] The combination of dystonia in the upper face and oromandibular regions is sometimes called Meige syndrome. Occasionally, the oromandibular regions are affected in isolation.[67,68] Although many neurologists are reluctant to treat the lower face and jaw, good outcomes can be achieved with proper dosing and muscle patterns.[68–71]

Limb Dystonias (Writer's Cramp)

The most common limb dystonias in adults involve the hand and/or arm and present as task-specific disorders such as writer's cramp and musician's dystonias. In children, the lower limb is more often involved, and most often results from cerebral palsy or an inherited disorder. Achieving satisfactory results for limb dystonias is possible, but not as straightforward as treatment of the craniofacial dystonias.[72] In the limbs, special attention must be directed toward distinguishing dystonic muscles from compensatory ones. The most common side effects from treating limb dystonias is weakness, which results from doses that are too high or treatment of compensatory muscles.

Laryngeal Dystonias (Spasmodic Dysphonia)

BoNTs are widely used for the treatment of the laryngeal dystonias.[73–75] Reliably good responses can be expected for the adductor spasmodic dysphonia, with reduction in voice breaks, reduction in speaking effort, and increased quality of life. A very common side effect is a hoarse or weak voice after treatment. Dysphagia is less common, but can be severe. Satisfactory responses are more challenging to obtain for abductor spasmodic dysphonia, or when involvement spreads to the pharyngeal or respiratory muscles.

SURGICAL TREATMENT OPTIONS

Surgical interventions can be offered when satisfactory responses cannot be achieved with BoNT and/or oral medications. The surgical options are grouped here into 2 main categories, namely, DBS and ablative procedures. In both cases, access to a multidisciplinary team of experts is required for patient selection and management of potential complications.

Deep Brain Stimulation

A thorough presurgical evaluation is valuable, because the outcomes of DBS depend on careful patient selection.[76–78] Etiology plays an important role in predicting outcomes, which are reliably good for some causes and reliably poor for others. It is often claimed that isolated dystonias respond more reliably to DBS than dystonias combined with other neurologic features. This view is oversimplified. For example, good outcomes are can be reliably anticipated for isolated dystonia caused by defects in the *TOR1A* gene, but outcomes for isolated dystonia caused by defects in *THAP1* gene are less predictable.[79] Good outcomes also can be expected for some combined dystonia syndromes such as myoclonus-dystonia (*SCGE* gene) and X-linked dystonia-parkinsonism (*TAF1* gene), but not for rapid-onset dystonia-parkinsonism (*ATP1A3* gene).[80]

The etiology also influences outcomes of DBS in acquired forms of dystonia. For example, reliably good outcomes can be anticipated for tardive dystonia owing to neuroleptics. In contrast, outcomes for dystonic cerebral palsy are less reliable.[35] Knowing etiologies, both genetic and acquired, is therefore critical for proper counseling regarding potential risks and benefits. Patients who have etiologies for their dystonia that are known to be associated with unpredictable outcomes should be counseled so they can make a fully informed decision.

Even when etiology cannot be determined, certain clinical characteristics predict outcomes from DBS. In general, patients with mobile dystonia fare better than those with fixed postures associated with underlying contractures. Patients with short disease durations fare better than those with longstanding dystonia. Patients who are younger fare better than those who are older, although very young patients (<12 years old) experience higher rates of complications such as migration of leads or infections of the equipment. Other characteristics associated with poorer outcomes from DBS include significant medical comorbidities that increase risk for any surgery, significant psychiatric comorbidities that increase risk for suicide or noncompliance, advanced or progressive dementia, patients who live far from a DBS center and may have difficulty with frequent travel, and dystonia syndromes that are combined with significant spasticity or ataxia.

With proper patient selection, long-term outcomes for DBS are good, with benefits lasting for many years.[81–83] Long-term complications are not uncommon, so close monitoring by the DBS team is important. For example, 1 study of 47 cases with dystonia owing to defects in the *TOR1A* gene followed for more than 10 years reported an 8.5% incidence of delayed equipment infections requiring antibiotic treatment or reoperation, an 8.5% incidence of equipment failure requiring reoperation, and a 4.3% incidence of reoperations to reposition electrodes.[84]

Ablation Procedures

Currently, DBS is the most commonly used surgical method for all subtypes of dystonia, because it is reversible and tunable. However, before DBS, specific brain regions were commonly ablated. Ablative procedures are experiencing a renaissance, because of steady improvements in delineating the subtypes of dystonia and brain regions where reliably good outcomes can be expected.[77,78] In fact, ablative procedures may be preferable to DBS in some circumstances.

Small lesions of the thalamus seem to be safe and reliable for certain task-specific dystonias of the upper limb.[85,86] With a permanent result that has few apparent side effects, such lesions may be preferable over DBS. There is less risk of infection with ablation, both immediately and in the long term. Ablation also may be preferred by particularly small or young patients who do not want the hassle of permanent indwelling DBS hardware. Permanent ablation may also be a reasonable option for patients who cannot make frequent return visits for DBS management, patients who cannot afford DBS surgery, or as a palliative procedure for progressive neurodegenerative disorders with severe disability.

The most common method for surgical ablation involves making an electrolytic lesion through a temporarily placed electrode. Focused ultrasound has recently been shown to be effective as an ablative tool for tremor, and some have advocated using it for dystonia too.[87] However, experience with focused ultrasound for dystonia is still limited, and outcomes seem to vary. Although focused ultrasound is sometimes claimed to be superior to traditional surgical methods because it is noninvasive, it is important to emphasize that it still produces a brain lesion, along with the usual potentially permanent side effects.

Ablative surgical procedures targeting peripheral nerves or nerve roots were commonly used for dystonia in the past and are still sometimes offered in some situations. Selective peripheral denervation can be done for patients with cervical dystonia for medically resistant patients who do not want DBS. Success rates for selective peripheral denervation are similar to those for DBS.[88,89] Typical side effects include local scarring, local muscle atrophy and weakness, dysphagia, and dysesthesia or hypoesthesia relating to destruction of sensory nerves to the neck.

Several related surgical procedures may be offered to patients with blepharospasm. They include suspension of the frontalis, surgical shortening of the levator palpebrae, removal of excess eyelid skin, and stripping of orbicularis oculi muscles.[90–92] Only a minority of patients with blepharospasm have these procedures, because they are offered only by a few centers. However, it is good to know about them because patients may ask. In general, experience is limited, and there are no methodical studies that address their long-term safety and efficacy.

Several surgical procedures are sometimes offered to patients with laryngeal dystonia as well.[93,94] Most of these aim at reorganizing the nerves or muscles of the larynx. Once again, experience is limited, and there are no large-scale studies demonstrating the long-term efficacy and safety of these procedures.

EXPERIMENTAL THERAPEUTICS AND THE FUTURE OF TREATMENT
Unmet Needs

Oral agents currently available have limited efficacy for most dystonias, except for a few subtypes of dystonia where there are mechanism-specific drugs. BoNT can be very effective, but it is not suitable for all types of dystonia. In addition, there has been increasing awareness that approximately one-third of patients discontinue BoNT.[95] Similarly, some patients with dystonia are not suitable surgical candidates or they do not want to undergo surgery. Because of the increasing awareness of a significant unmet need, and special incentives from the US Food and Drug Administration for developing new treatments for rare disorders, there has been an increase in enthusiasm for developing new treatments for different types of dystonia.[96]

Clinicaltrials.gov listed 161 active or recently completed interventional trials for dystonia in October 2019 (clinicaltrials.gov). Included were trials of oral agents, trials of a novel BoNT and different ways of using existing BoNTs, trials involving DBS, and trials involving noninvasive brain stimulation. For example, there are several ongoing or recently completed trials including ampicillin for dystonia caused by the TOR1A gene, cannabis for pediatric dystonias, levetiracetam for cervical or oromandibular dystonia, perampanel for cervical dystonia, sodium oxybate for laryngeal dystonia, and zonegran for myoclonus-dystonia.

Oral Medications

The anticholinergics have broad efficacy across many types of dystonias, but their use is limited by nonspecific side effects. Most of these drugs nonselectively target all 4 major subclasses of muscarinic receptors, and have off-target effects too. These observations have stimulated interest in developing anticholingerics that may have fewer side effects, by more specifically targeting the muscarinic receptor subtypes most likely to be relevant to dystonia.[97] There also has been increasing interest in the relationship between dystonia and Parkinson disease. Some levodopa-induced dyskinesias have a dystonic quality, so drugs being developed to treat these dyskinesias may be repurposed for some types of dystonia.[98]

In addition to the development of potential new drugs with broad symptomatic effects, the remarkable advances in delineating genetic mechanisms for rare subtypes of dystonia has opened the door to new mechanism-specific interventions. For example, pantothenate kinase–associated neurodegeneration has been linked with defects in the synthesis of coenzyme A and toxic accumulation of brain iron.[99] In a recent large double-blind, placebo-controlled trial, the iron chelator deferiprone significantly decreased brain iron stores in patients with this disorder.[100] Clinical improvement in dystonia was not clinically significant, but the duration of the trial may have been insufficient to detect a disease-modifying effect. Another large randomized double-blinded, placebo-controlled clinical trial using a synthetic precursor of coenzyme A was recently completed (clinicaltrials.gov NCT03041116), and additional trials are anticipated. It therefore seems likely that new mechanism-specific therapeutics will be available for this devastating disorder. Similar advances are occurring in other disorders.

Botulinum Toxins

A new formulation of BoNT (daxibotulinumtoxinA) is being evaluated in clinical trials now (clinicaltrials.gov NCT03608397). In addition to this potential new BoNT, there have been advances in our understanding of the optimal strategies for application of existing BoNTs. For example, the increasing awareness that approximately one-third of patients discontinue BoNT[95] has stimulated interest in better understanding the reasons for discontinuation. One of the main reasons given by patients is apparently poor efficacy, which is sometimes attributed to BoNT resistance. Although measurable titers of antibodies to BoNT can be detected in many patients who are treated with BoNT,[101] true immunologically mediated resistance has become quite uncommon with current manufacturing processes.[102] Instead, several studies have indicated that the more common reason for poor responses is due to inadequate dosing or suboptimal muscle selection.[61,103,104] Increasing awareness of the reasons for apparently poor efficacy has pointed to the need for more rigorous training in the optimal use of the BoNTs.

Another reason for poor patient satisfaction can be related to the duration of benefit of BoNT. Because the average duration of benefit is approximately 12 weeks, most patients are traditionally scheduled for retreatment at fixed intervals of 12 weeks.[105] However, 12 weeks is an average, and the range varies from 8 to 16 weeks. Providing a fixed interval of 12 weeks for all patients leads some to experience significant fluctuations in symptom severity, a phenomenon that has been dubbed the yo-yo effect.[96] Thus, there has been increasing appreciation that the dosing interval needs to be customized, along with the dose and muscle pattern.[106]

The need for EMG guidance during BoNT procedures has been controversial for a long time. Some experts advocate EMG for nearly all procedures, whereas others advocate reliance on the clinical examination. Available studies comparing outcomes with and without EMG are inconclusive.[56] In our experience, EMG is almost never required for blepharospasm, because subcutaneous injections readily diffuse to the thin underlying muscles of the face. EMG often is required for dystonia involving the hand, because of the large number of small muscles that are grouped closely together in the hand and forearm. EMG is required only in a minority of cases of cervical dystonia, for example, those with particularly thick necks, deep muscle involvement, or very complex movement patterns. More recently, ultrasound guidance has been gaining in popularity, because muscles can be more precisely visualized.[107] The place of ultrasound guidance for the various types of dystonia is still being explored.

Deep Brain Stimulation

Significant advances in DBS therapy are anticipated in the next few years. For example, the most common target for dystonia has been the internal segment of the globus pallidus. However, other targets are being explored now, such as the subthalamic nucleus.[108] As our understanding of the neuroanatomic basis of dystonia has expanded, targets outside of the basal ganglia are being considered as well.[109,110] The exploration of other targets may provide new surgical options for subtypes of dystonia that do not respond reliably to current strategies.

There have also been technological advances, including the development of batteries that have a longer lifespans or are rechargeable, and smaller impulse generators suitable for small children or those who are particularly thin. These advances will minimize reoperations and surgical complications. There have also been advances in directional electrodes that can be aimed more precisely at their targets to limit side effects from nonspecific stimulation. Adaptive stimulation that responds to specific physiologic triggers may also provide greater efficacy and extend battery life by delivering stimulation only when it is needed.[77,78] All of these advances are likely to improve long-term surgical outcomes.

In addition to DBS, there has been increasing interest in noninvasive brain stimulation techniques, including transcranial magnetic stimulation and transcranial direct current stimulation.[111] Some positive results have been reported for small and unblinded trials, and larger trials are planned.

PUTTING IT ALL TOGETHER

Simple algorithms that describe a universal approach for addressing all dystonias are challenging to construct, because of the remarkable heterogeneity of the dystonias. However, a basic algorithmic approach with some general principles can be provided (**Fig. 3**), with the caveat that real-life management must be done on a case-by-case basis.

A thorough diagnostic evaluation is an important starting place, including attention to all 4 of the factors relevant for clinical classification. These factors include age at onset, body region affected, temporal features, and associated features. Age at onset plays an important starting role. For most adults, dystonia is idiopathic, so extensive diagnostic testing is often not conducted. Instead, the approach to treatment depends more on body distribution. For focal and segmental dystonias, the BoNTs are the treatment of first choice, sometimes with adjunctive oral agents, especially for the troughs in the cyclical responses to BoNT over time. When BoNT plus oral agents are insufficient, DBS should be considered. Generalized and hemidystonias are uncommon in adults, and some additional diagnostic testing with brain MRI may be required. BoNT is rarely adequate, so oral agents and DBS play a more important role.

For children, some diagnostic testing is valuable because the chances of finding an etiology are greater, and certain populations have specific treatments. Brain imaging is important to disclose particularly categories of disease, such as focal defects or gray or white matter diseases. Other diagnostic tests will depend on the nature of the dystonia syndrome. All children and young adults should be given a trial of levodopa to address dopa-responsive dystonia. If patients do not respond to levodopa, other oral agents and BoNT can be considered. DBS can be considered when more conservative measures fail.

LONG-TERM OUTCOMES

Long-term prognoses vary among the different subtypes of dystonia. The most common subtypes include the adult-onset focal dystonias. For these patients, progression is most obvious in the first 3 to 6 months, although continued

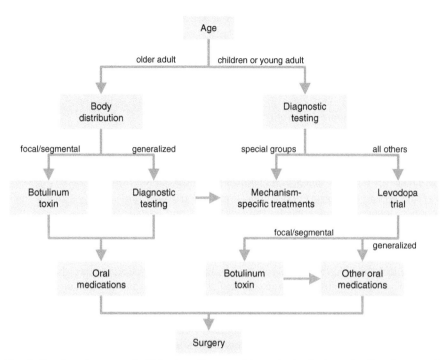

Fig. 3. Treatment approach. This algorithm provides a basic strategy for the therapeutic approach to most patients with dystonia. The clinical and etiologic evaluations are important, because They influence optimal treatments strategies. For children, diagnostic testing is essential because there is a greater likelihood of discovering a treatable cause. When a cause cannot be found, a trial of oral levodopa is conducted to rule out dopa-responsive dystonia. For adults, dystonia is more often idiopathic, so extensive workup is often not needed. Instead, the approach depends on body distribution. For the focal dystonias, BoNTs provide a useful starting point. Oral medications can be used, but often are not well-tolerated. Those who have unsatisfactory responses can be offered surgery. Generalized dystonias or dystonia combined with other neurologic problems in adults requires some additional diagnostic testing, to disclose a potentially treatable cause.

progression may occur for years.[7–13] The 5-year risk of spread from the originally affected area is 10% to 20% for cervical dystonia, limb dystonias, and laryngeal dystonias. The 5-year risk of spread for blepharospasm is approximately 50%. Complete remission occurs in 5% to 10% of the adult-onset focal dystonias, but remission usually is temporary.[112] Despite the chronic and sometimes progressive nature of the adult-onset focal dystonias, adequate symptom control is feasible in the majority with BoNT, oral medications, and rarely surgical intervention.

The childhood-onset dystonias are far less common. Progression to segmental and generalized dystonia is more frequent, and usually occurs over a period of several years. Further progression in adulthood is less common. For rare subtypes of the early-onset dystonias, there are specific mechanism-based oral medications that can have a dramatic effect, if started early.[50,51] When mechanism-specific treatments are not available, symptom-based oral medications and BoNT can be helpful, and surgical intervention is more frequently required.

SUMMARY

All dystonias are treatable. The majority benefit at least partly from symptom-based management, and several rare subtypes have specific treatments addressing the underlying disease mechanisms. For both adults and children, the list of treatment options is likely to grow in the near future, as ongoing research improves our ability to exploit existing therapies, and uncovers additional causes and biological mechanisms where new interventions can be designed.[96]

DISCLOSURE

H.A. Jinnah has active or recent grant support from the US government (National Institutes of Health), private philanthropic organizations (the Benign Essential Blepharospasm Research Foundation, Cure Dystonia Now) and industry (Cavion Therapeutics, Ipsen Pharmaceuticals, Retrophin Inc., and Revance). Dr H.A. Jinnah has also served on advisory boards or as a consultant for Allergan Inc., CoA Therapeutics, Medtronic Inc., and Retrophin Inc. He has received honoraria or stipends for lectures or administrative work from the American Academy of Neurology, the American Neurological Association, the Dystonia Medical Research Foundation, the International Neurotoxin Society, the International Parkinson's Disease and Movement Disorders Society, The Parkinson's Disease Foundation, and Tyler's Hope for a Cure. Dr H.A. Jinnah serves on the Scientific Advisory Boards for several private foundations including the Benign Essential Blepharospasm Research Foundation, Cure Dystonia Now, the Dystonia Medical Research Foundation, the Tourette Association of America, and Tyler's Hope for a Cure. He also is principal investigator for the Dystonia Coalition, which has received the majority of its support through NIH grants NS116025 and NS065701 from the National Institutes of Neurological Disorders and Stroke and previously grant TR 001456 from the Office of Rare Diseases Research at the National Center for Advancing Translational Sciences. The Dystonia Coalition has received additional material or administrative support from industry sponsors (Allergan Inc. and Merz Pharmaceuticals) as well as private foundations (The American Dystonia Society, Beat Dystonia, The Benign Essential Blepharospasm Foundation, Cure Dystonia Now, Dystonia Europe, Dystonia Inc., Dystonia Ireland, The Dystonia Medical Research Foundation, The Foundation for Dystonia Research, The National Spasmodic Dysphonia Association, and The National Spasmodic Torticollis Association).

REFERENCES

1. Albanese A, Bhatia K, Bressman SB, et al. Phenomenology and classification of dystonia: a consensus update. Mov Disord 2013;28:863–73.
2. Balint B, Mencacci NE, Valente EM, et al. Dystonia. Nat Rev Dis Primers 2018; 4:25.
3. Jinnah HA, Albanese A. The new classification for the dystonias: why was it needed and how was it accomplished? Mov Disord Clin Pract 2014;1:280–4.
4. Fung VS, Jinnah HA, Bhatia K, et al. Assessment of the patient with dystonia: an update on dystonia syndromes. Mov Disord 2013;28:889–98.
5. Jinnah HA, Sun YV. Dystonia genes and their biological pathways. Neurobiol Dis 2019;129:159–68.
6. Jinnah HA. The dystonias. Continuum (Minneap Minn) 2019;25(4):976–1000.
7. Esposito M, Fabbrini G, Ferrazzano G, et al. Spread of dystonia in patients with idiopathic adult-onset laryngeal dystonia. Eur J Neurol 2018;25:1341–4.

8. Norris SA, Jinnah HA, Espay AJ, et al. Clinical and demographic characteristics related to onset site and spread of cervical dystonia. Mov Disord 2016;31: 1874–82.
9. Svetel M, Pekmezovic T, Tomic A, et al. The spread of primary late-onset focal dystonia in a long-term follow up study. Clin Neurol Neurosurg 2015;132:41–3.
10. Martino D, Berardelli A, Abbruzzese G, et al. Age at onset and symptom spread in primary adult-onset blepharospasm and cervical dystonia. Mov Disord 2012; 27:1447–50.
11. Svetel M, Pekmezovic T, Jovic J, et al. Spread of primary dystonia in relation to initially affected region. J Neurol 2007;254:879–83.
12. Weiss EM, Hershey T, Karimi M, et al. Relative risk of spread of symptoms among the focal onset primary dystonias. Mov Disord 2006;21:1175–81.
13. Abbruzzese G, Berardelli A, Girlanda P, et al. Long-term assessment of the risk of spread in primary late-onset focal dystonia. J Neurol Neurosurg Psychiatry 2008;79:392–6.
14. Ludlow CL, Domangue R, Sharma D, et al. Consensus-based attributes for identifying patients with spasmodic dysphonia and other voice disorders. JAMA Otolaryngol Head Neck Surg 2018;144(8):657–65.
15. Powis Z, Towne MC, Hagman KDF, et al. Clinical diagnostic exome sequencing in dystonia: genetic testing challenges for complex conditions. Clin Genet 2019. https://doi.org/10.1111/cge.13657.
16. Macerollo A, Superbo M, Gigante AF, et al. Diagnostic delay in adult-onset dystonia: data from an Italian movement disorder center. J Clin Neurosci 2015;22: 608–10.
17. Creighton FXJ, Hapner ER, Klein AM, et al. Diagnostic delays in spasmodic dysphonia: a call for clinician education. J Voice 2015;29:592–4.
18. Bertram KL, Williams DR. Delays to the diagnosis of cervical dystonia. J Clin Neurosci 2015;25:62–4.
19. Tiderington E, Goodman EM, Rosen AR, et al. How long does it take to diagnose cervical dystonia? J Neurol Sci 2013;335:72–4.
20. Zurowski M, Marsh L, McDonald W. Psychiatric comorbidities in dystonia: emerging concepts. Mov Disord 2013;28:914–20.
21. De Pauw J, Van der Velden K, Meirte J, et al. The effectiveness of physiotherapy for cervical dystonia: a systematic literature review. J Neurol 2014;261(10): 1857–65.
22. Prudente CN, Zetterberg L, Bring A, et al. Systematic review of rehabilitation in focal dystonias: classification and recommendations. Mov Disord Clin Pract 2018;5:237–45.
23. Fleming BM, Schwab EL, Nouer SS, et al. Prevalence, predictors, and perceived effectiveness of complementary, alternative and integrative medicine in adult-onset primary dystonia. Parkinsonism Relat Disord 2012;18:936–40.
24. Jankovic J. Medical treatment of dystonia. Mov Disord 2013;28:1001–12.
25. Pirio Richardson S, Wegele AR, Skipper B, et al. Dystonia treatment: patterns of medication use in an international cohort. Neurology 2017;88:1–8.
26. Jinnah HA, Factor S. Diagnosis and treatment of dystonia. In: Jankovic J, editor. Neurologic clinics, vol. 33. Elsevier; 2015. p. 77–100.
27. Thenganatt MA, Jankovic J. Treatment of dystonia. Neurotherapeutics 2014;11: 139–52.
28. Greene P, Shale H, Fahn S. Experience with high dosages of anticholinergic and other drugs in the treatment of torsion dystonia. Adv Neurol 1988;50:547–56.

29. Lumsden DE, Kaminska M, Tomlin S, et al. Medication use in childhood dystonia. Eur J Paediatr Neurol 2016;20:625–9.
30. Albanese A, Barnes MP, Bhatia KP, et al. A systematic review on the diagnosis and treatment of primary (idiopathic) dystonia and dystonia plus syndromes: report of an EFNS/MDS-ES task force. Eur J Neurol 2006;13:433–44.
31. Balash Y, Giladi N. Efficacy of pharmacological treatment of dystonia: evidence-based review including meta-analysis of the effect of botulinum toxin and other cure options. Eur J Neurol 2004;11:361–70.
32. Greene P. Baclofen in the treatment of dystonia. Clin Neuropharmacol 1992;15:276–88.
33. Bonouvrie LA, Becher JG, Vles JSH, et al. The effect of intrathecal baclofen in dyskinetic cerebral palsy: the IDYS trial. Ann Neurol 2019;86(1):79–90.
34. Andre L, Gallini A, Montastruc F, et al. Association between anticholinergic (atropinic) drug exposure and cognitive function in longitudinal studies among individuals over 50 years old: a systematic review. Eur J Clin Pharmacol 2019;75(12):1631–44.
35. Fehlings D, Brown L, Harvey A, et al. Pharmacological and neurosurgical interventions for managing dystonia in cerebral palsy: a systematic review. Dev Med Child Neurol 2018;60:356–66.
36. Harvey AR, Baker LB, Reddihough DS, et al. Trihexyphenidyl for dystonia in cerebral palsy. Cochrane Database Syst Rev 2018;(5):CD012430.
37. See S, Ginzburg R. Choosing a skeletal muscle relaxant. Am Fam Physician 2008;78:365–70.
38. Wijemanne S, Jankovic J. Dopa-responsive dystonia–clinical and genetic heterogeneity. Nat Rev Neurol 2015;11:414–24.
39. Lee WW, Jeon BS. Clinical spectrum of dopa-responsive dystonia and related disorders. Curr Neurol Neurosci Rep 2014;14:461.
40. Kurian MA, Gissen P, Smith M, et al. The monoamine neurotransmitter disorders: an expanding range of neurological syndromes. Lancet Neurol 2011;10:721–33.
41. Charlesworth G, Mohire MD, Schneider SA, et al. Ataxia telangiectasia presenting as dopa-responsive cervical dystonia. Neurology 2013;81:1148–51.
42. Wilder-Smith E, Tan EK, Law HY, et al. Spinocerebellar ataxia type 3 presenting as an L-DOPA responsive dystonia phenotype in a Chinese family. J Neurol Sci 2003;213:25–8.
43. Lang AE. Dopamine agonists and antagonists in the treatment of idiopathic dystonia. Adv Neurol 1988;50:561–70.
44. Fan X, Donsante Y, Jinnah HA, et al. Dopamine receptor agonist treatment of idiopathic dystonia: a reappraisal in humans and mice. J Pharmacol Exp Ther 2018;365:20–6.
45. Bandmann O, Weiss KH, Kaler SG. Wilson's disease and other neurological copper disorders. Lancet Neurol 2015;14:103–13.
46. Sturm E, Piersma FE, Tanner MS, et al. Controversies and variation in diagnosing and treating children with Wilson disease: results of an international survey. J Pediatr Gastroenterol Nutr 2016;63:82–7.
47. Tuschl K, Meyer E, Valdivia LE, et al. Mutations in SLC39A14 disrupt manganese homeostasis and cause childhood-onset parkinsonism-dystonia. Nat Commun 2016;7:11601.
48. Tuschl K, Clayton PT, Gospe SM Jr, et al. Syndrome of hepatic cirrhosis, dystonia, polycythemia, and hypermanganesemia caused by mutations in SLC30A10, a manganese transporter in man. Am J Hum Genet 2012;90:457–66.

49. Quadri M, Federico A, Zhao T, et al. Mutations in SLC30A10 cause parkinsonism and dystonia with hypermanganesemia, polycythemia, and chronic liver disease. Am J Hum Genet 2012;90:467–77.
50. Jinnah HA, Albanese A, Bhatia KP, et al. Treatable inherited rare movement disorders. Mov Disord 2018;33:21–35.
51. Balint B, Vincent A, Meinck HM, et al. Movement disorders with neuronal antibodies: syndromic approach, genetic parallels and pathophysiology. Brain 2018;141:13–36.
52. Baizabal-Carvallo JF, Jankovic J. Movement disorders in autoimmune diseases. Mov Disord 2012;27:935–46.
53. Marsh WA, Monroe DM, Brin MF, et al. Systematic review and meta-analysis of the duration of clinical effect of onabotulinumtoxinA in cervical dystonia. BMC Neurol 2014;14:91.
54. Simpson DM, Blitzer A, Brashear A, et al. Assessment: botulinum neurotoxin for the treatment of movement disorders (an evidence-based review): report of the Therapeutics and Technology Assessment Subcommittee of the American Academy of Neurology. Neurology 2008;70:1699–706.
55. Simpson DM, Hallett M, Ashman EJ, et al. Practice guideline update summary: botulinum neurotoxin for the treatment of blepharospasm, cervical dystonia, adult spasticity, and headache: report of the guideline development Subcommittee of the American Academy of Neurology. Neurology 2016;86:1818–26.
56. Castelao M, Marques RE, Duarte GS, et al. Botulinum toxin type A therapy for cervical dystonia. Cochrane Database Syst Rev 2017;(12):CD003633.
57. Hallett M, Albanese A, Dressler D, et al. Evidence-based review and assessment of botulinum neurotoxin for the treatment of movement disorders. Toxicon 2013;67:94–114.
58. Truong D, Dressler D, Hallet M, et al. Manual of botulinum toxin. Cambridge (England): Cambridge University Press; 2009.
59. Jost W, Valerius KP. Pictoral atlas of botulinum toxin injection: dosage, localization, application. Berlin: Quintessence Publishing Company; 2008.
60. Jankovic J. Botulinum toxin: state of the art. Mov Disord 2017;32(8):1131–8.
61. Jinnah HA, Goodmann E, Rosen AR, et al. Botulinum toxin treatment failures in cervical dystonia: causes, management, and outcomes. J Neurol 2016;263:1188–94.
62. Ferreira JJ, Colosimo C, Bhidayasiri R, et al. Factors influencing secondary nonresponse to botulinum toxin type A injections in cervical dystonia. Parkinsonism Relat Disord 2015;21:111–5.
63. George EB, Cotton AC, Shneyder N, et al. A strategy for managing flu-like symptoms after botulinum toxin injections. J Neurol 2018;265:1932–3.
64. Esposito M, Fasano A, Crisci C, et al. The combined treatment with orbital and pretarsal botulinum toxin injections in the management of poorly responsive blepharospasm. Neurol Sci 2013;35:397–400.
65. Rana AQ, Shah R. Combination of blepharospasm and apraxia of eyelid opening: a condition resistant to treatment. Acta Neurol Belg 2012;112:95–6.
66. Aramideh M, Ongerboer de Visser BW, Brans JW, et al. Pretarsal application of botulinum toxin for treatment of blepharospasm. J Neurol Neurosurg Psychiatry 1995;59:309–11.
67. Termsarasab P, Tanenbaum DR, Frucht SJ. The phenomenology and natural history of idiopathic lower cranial dystonia. J Clin Mov Disord 2014;1:3.
68. Gonzalez-Alegre P, Schneider RL, Hoffman H. Clinical, etiological, and therapeutic features of jaw-opening and jaw-closing oromandibular dystonias: a

decade of experience at a single treatment center. Tremor Other Hyperkinet Mov (N Y) 2014;4:231.

69. Scorr LM, Silver MR, Hanfelt J, et al. Pilot single-blind trial of abobotulinumtoxinA in oromandibular dystonia. Neurotherapeutics 2018;15:452–8.

70. Nastasi L, Mostile G, Nicoletti A, et al. Effect of botulinum toxin treatment on quality of life in patients with isolated lingual dystonia and oromandibular dystonia affecting the tongue. J Neurol 2016;263:1702–8.

71. Moscovich M, Chen ZP, Rodriguez R. Successful treatment of open jaw and jaw deviation dystonia with botulinum toxin using a simple intraoral approach. J Clin Neurosci 2015;22:594–6.

72. Lungu C, Karp BI, Alter K, et al. Long-term follow-up of botulinum toxin therapy for focal hand dystonia: outcome at 10 years or more. Mov Disord 2011;26:750–3.

73. Watts CC, Whurr R, Nye C. Botulinum toxin injections for the treatment of spasmodic dysphonia. Cochrane Database Syst Rev 2004;(3):CD004327.

74. Patel AB, Bansberg SF, Adler CH, et al. The Mayo Clinic Arizona spasmodic dysphonia experience: a demographic analysis of 718 patients. Ann Otol Rhinol Laryngol 2015;124:859–63.

75. Blitzer A, Brin MF, Stewart CF. Botulinum toxin management of spasmodic dysphonia (laryngeal dystonia): a 12-year experience in more than 900 patients. Laryngoscope 2015;125:1751–7.

76. Hale AT, Monsour MA, Rolston JD, et al. Deep brain stimulation in pediatric dystonia: a systematic review. Neurosurg Rev 2018. https://doi.org/10.1007/s10143-018-1047-9.

77. Cury RG, Kalia SK, Shah BB, et al. Surgical treatment of dystonia. Expert Rev Neurother 2018;18:477–92.

78. Krack P, Martinez-Fernandez R, Del Alamo M, et al. Current applications and limitations of surgical treatments for movement disorders. Mov Disord 2017;32:36–52.

79. Bruggemann N, Kuhn A, Schneider SA, et al. Short- and long-term outcome of chronic pallidal neurostimulation in monogenic isolated dystonia. Neurology 2015;84:895–903.

80. Jinnah HA, Alterman R, Klein C, et al. Deep brain stimulation for dystonia: a novel perspective on the value of genetic testing. J Neural Transm (Vienna) 2017;124:417–30.

81. Tagliati M, Krack P, Volkmann J, et al. Long-term management of DBS in dystonia: response to stimulation, adverse events, battery changes, and special considerations. Mov Disord 2011;26(Suppl 1):S54–62.

82. Volkmann J, Wolters A, Kupsch A, et al. Pallidal deep brain stimulation in patients with primary generalised or segmental dystonia: 5-year follow-up of a randomised trial. Lancet Neurol 2012;11:1029–38.

83. Reese R, Gruber D, Schoenecker T, et al. Long-term clinical outcome in Meige syndrome treated with internal pallidum deep brain stimulation. Mov Disord 2011;26:691–8.

84. Panov F, Gologorsky Y, Connors G, et al. Deep brain stimulation in DYT1 dystonia: a 10-year experience. Neurosurgery 2013;73:86–93.

85. Horisawa S, Ochiai T, Goto S, et al. Safety and long-term efficacy of ventro-oral thalamotomy for focal hand dystonia: a retrospective study of 171 patients. Neurology 2019;92:e371–7.

86. Horisawa S, Taira T, Goto S, et al. Long-term improvement of musician's dystonia after stereotactic ventrooralthalamotomy. Ann Neurol 2013;74:648–54.

87. Krishna V, Sammartino F, Rezai A. A review of the current therapies, challenges, and future directions of transcranial focused ultrasound technology: advances in diagnosis and treatment. JAMA Neurol 2018;75:246–54.

88. Contarino MF, Van Den Munckhof P, Tijssen MA, et al. Selective peripheral denervation: comparison with pallidal stimulation and literature review. J Neurol 2014;261:300–8.

89. Ravindran K, Kumar N, Englot DJ, et al. Deep brain stimulation versus peripheral denervation for cervical dystonia: a systematic review and meta-analysis. World Neurosurg 2019;122:e940–6.

90. Georgescu D, Vagefi MR, McMullan TF, et al. Upper eyelid myectomy in blepharospasm with associated apraxia of lid opening. Am J Ophthalmol 2008;145: 541–7.

91. Grivet D, Robert PY, Thuret G, et al. Assessment of blepharospasm surgery using an improved disability scale: study of 138 patients. Ophthal Plast Reconstr Surg 2005;21:230–4.

92. Pariseau B, Worley MW, Anderson RL. Myectomy for blepharospasm 2013. Curr Opin Ophthalmol 2013;24:488–93.

93. Ludlow CL. Treatment for spasmodic dysphonia: limitations of current approaches. Curr Opin Otolaryngol Head Neck Surg 2009;17:160–5.

94. Ludlow CL, Adler CH, Berke GS, et al. Research priorities in spasmodic dysphonia. Otolaryngol Head Neck Surg 2008;139:495–505.

95. Jinnah HA, Comella CL, Perlmutter J, et al. Longitudinal studies of botulinum toxin in cervical dystonia: why do patients discontinue therapy? Toxicon 2018; 147:89–95.

96. Pirio Richardson S, Jinnah HA. New approaches to discovering drugs that treat dystonia. Expert Opin Drug Discov 2019;14(9):893–900.

97. Pisani A, Bernardi G, Ding J, et al. Re-emergence of striatal cholinergic interneurons in movement disorders. Trends Neurosci 2007;30:545–53.

98. Calabresi P, Standaert DG. Dystonia and levodopa-induced dyskinesias in Parkinson's disease: is there a connection? Neurobiol Dis 2019;132:104579.

99. Tello C, Darling A, Lupo V, et al. On the complexity of clinical and molecular bases of neurodegeneration with brain iron accumulation. Clin Genet 2018;93: 731–40.

100. Klopstock T, Tricta F, Neumayr L, et al. Safety and efficacy of deferiprone for pantothenate kinase-associated neurodegeneration: a randomised, double-blind, controlled trial and an open-label extension study. Lancet Neurol 2019; 18:631–42.

101. Albrecht P, Jansen A, Lee JI, et al. High prevalence of neutralizing antibodies after long-term botulinum neurotoxin therapy. Neurology 2019;92:e48–54.

102. Fabbri M, Leodori G, Fernandes RM, et al. Neutralizing antibody and Botulinum toxin therapy: a systematic review and meta-analysis. Neurotox Res 2015;25: 105–17.

103. Nijmeijer SW, Koelman JH, Standaar TS, et al. Cervical dystonia: improved treatment response to botulinum toxin after referral to a tertiary centre and the use of polymyography. Parkinsonism Relat Disord 2013;19:533–8.

104. Cordivari C, Misra VP, Vincent A, et al. Secondary nonresponsiveness to botulinum toxin A in cervical dystonia: the role of electromyogram-guided injections, botulinum toxin A antibody assay, and the extensor digitorum brevis test. Mov Disord 2006;21:1737–41.

105. Evidente VG, Pappert EJ. Botulinum toxin therapy for cervical dystonia: the science of dosing. Tremor Other Hyperkinet Mov (N Y) 2014;4:273.

106. Ojo OO, Fernandez HH. Is it time for flexibility in botulinum inter-injection intervals? Toxicon 2015;107:72–6.
107. Castagna A, Albanese A. Management of cervical dystonia with botulinum neurotoxins and EMG/ultrasound guidance. Neurol Clin Pract 2019;9:64–73.
108. Wagle Shukla A, Ostrem JL, Vaillancourt DE, et al. Physiological effects of subthalamic nucleus deep brain stimulation surgery in cervical dystonia. J Neurol Neurosurg Psychiatry 2018;89(12):1296–300.
109. Franca C, de Andrade DC, Teixeira MJ, et al. Effects of cerebellar neuromodulation in movement disorders: a systematic review. Brain Stimul 2018;11:249–60.
110. Horisawa S, Arai T, Suzuki N, et al. The striking effects of deep cerebellar stimulation on generalized fixed dystonia: case report. J Neurosurg 2019;1–5. https://doi.org/10.3171/2018.11.JNS182180.
111. Quartarone A, Rizzo V, Terranova C, et al. Therapeutic use of non-invasive brain stimulation in dystonia. Front Neurosci 2017;11:423.
112. Mainka T, Erro R, Rothwell J, et al. Remission in dystonia - Systematic review of the literature and meta-analysis. Parkinsonism Relat Disord 2019;66:9–15.

Medical and Surgical Treatments of Tourette Syndrome

Joohi Jimenez-Shahed, MD

KEYWORDS

- Tourette syndrome • Tics • Cognitive behavioral intervention for tics (CBIT)
- Alpha-2 agonists • Dopamine receptor blocking drugs
- Vesicular monoamine transporter type 2 inhibitors • Deep brain stimulation

KEY POINTS

- Tourette syndrome is a complex neuropsychiatric condition in which the main movement disorder is tics, although it is frequently accompanied by psychiatric comorbidities.
- Pharmacologic therapies can improve tic severity and frequency, but multiple treatment approaches may be required to sufficiently address tics and comorbidities, avoiding dose-limiting side effects.
- Nonpharmacologic therapies directed at tics can also be beneficial, but may offer lesser benefits when substantial comorbidities occur.
- Emerging pharmacologic approaches and surgical interventions, such as deep brain stimulation are being investigated to address issues of tolerability and refractory symptoms, respectively.

OVERVIEW: NATURE OF THE PROBLEM
Definition of Tics

Tics are involuntary or semi-voluntary, sudden, brief, intermittent, repetitive movements or muscle contractions (motor tics) or sounds (phonic tics) that can be classified as either simple or complex, and which occur on a background of normal activity or speech.[1,2] They often occur out of their normal context or in inappropriate situations, thereby calling attention to the affected person because of their exaggerated, forceful, and repetitive nature. They tend to follow a waxing and waning course,[2] in which old tics return or new tics develop without specific provocation or instigating factor. Other characteristic features of tics include:

- Association with a *premonitory sensation* (referred to as an "urge") before the motor or phonic tic occurs[3]

Movement Disorders Neuromodulation & Brain Circuit Therapeutics, Neurology, Icahn School of Medicine at Mount Sinai, Mount Sinai West, 1000 10th Avenue, Suite 10C, New York, NY 10019, USA
E-mail address: Joohi.Jimenez-Shahed@mountsinai.org

Neurol Clin 38 (2020) 349–366
https://doi.org/10.1016/j.ncl.2020.01.006
0733-8619/20/© 2020 Elsevier Inc. All rights reserved.

neurologic.theclinics.com

- o Examples: burning or itching of the eyes before an eye-blinking tic; throat "tick-ling" or discomfort before a throat-clearing tic; localized muscle tension before a shoulder-shrugging tic
- The sensation is temporarily *relieved* after performance of the movement or sound
  - o Patients may execute a tic or series of tics repeatedly until a "just right" feeling is achieved
- Tics (motor or phonic) can be transiently *suppressed*[4]
  - o Expression of tics can therefore vary in different environments (eg, school vs home)
  - o Prolonged suppression of tics may lead to an "inner tension" that results in a more dramatic burst of tics
- Tics are *suggestible*, meaning that mere discussion of tics and provoke their manifestation
- Tics may *improve* with intense concentration on a task or during distraction
- Tics may *worsen* with stress, fatigue, or excitement

Cause of Tics

Tourette syndrome (TS) is the most common cause of tics, but not all individuals with tics will meet diagnostic criteria (**Table 1**). In addition to these diagnostic classifications, secondary tics can occur as a component of other conditions (**Table 2**).

Recognizing Comorbidities in Tourette Syndrome

Although the diagnostic criteria for TS are based on the presence of tics, psychiatric and behavioral features are frequently present and are important to recognize (**Table 3**). Comorbidities, such as attention-deficit disorder or obsessive-compulsive

Table 1 Diagnostic categories for tics	
Tourette syndrome	• Two or more motor tics *and* at least 1 vocal tic, although they might not always happen at the same time. • Tics have been present for at least a year. The tics can occur many times a day (usually in bouts) nearly every day, or off and on. • Tics started before age 18 y. • Symptoms are not due to taking medicine or other drugs or due to having another medical condition that can cause tics.
Persistent (chronic) motor or vocal tic disorder	• One or more motor tics *or* vocal tics, but not both. • Tics occur many times a day nearly every day or on and off throughout a period of more than 1 y. • Tics started before age 18 y. • Symptoms are not due to taking medicine or other drugs, or due to having another medical condition that can cause tics.
Provisional tic disorder	• One or more motor tics *or* vocal tics. • Tics have been present for no longer than 12 mo in a row. • Tics started before age 18 y. • Symptoms are not due to taking medicine or other drugs, or due to having another medical condition that can cause tics.

Data from American Psychiatric Association., American Psychiatric Association. DSM-5 Task Force. *Diagnostic and statistical manual of mental disorders : DSM-5.* 5th ed. Washington, D.C.: American Psychiatric Association; 2013.

Table 2
Causes of secondary tics

Infections	Streptococcal encephalitis
Drugs	Prescription medications, eg, stimulants Recreational drugs, eg, cocaine
Brain trauma or injury	
Neurodegenerative disorders	Huntington disease Neuroacanthocytosis Neuronal degeneration with brain iron accumulation
Autism spectrum disorders	"Tourettism" that is separate from stereotypies or self-stimulatory behaviors
Chromosomal disorders	Down syndrome
Psychiatric disorders	Schizophrenia

Data from Mejia NI, Jankovic J. Secondary tics and tourettism. *Braz J Psychiatry.* 2005;27(1):11-17.

disorder (OCD) may influence tic severity when unaddressed or cause impairment or disability independently, such that identification and management of these features alongside tics are essential to the comprehensive approach to the patient with TS.[5]

Epidemiology and Natural History of Tourette Syndrome

Approximately 1% of children between the ages of 5 and 17 years has tics, whereas 1 out of every 160 children in that age range (0.6%) has TS.[6] TS does not appear to have any predilection for a particular race, ethnicity, or age group. Boys are approximately 3 to 4 times more likely than girls to display symptoms of TS.

   TS is typically considered a neurodevelopmental disorder that predominantly manifests in childhood and adolescence and tends to resolve or improve significantly by adulthood. Motor tics have a rostral to caudal manner of expression over time, with

Table 3
Prevalence of psychiatric and behavioral problems in Tourette syndrome

Obsessive-compulsive spectrum disorders	66.1% More common in girls
Attention-deficit/hyperactivity disorder	54.3% More common in boys
Mood disorders	29.8% More common in girls
Anxiety disorders (includes phobias, posttraumatic stress disorder)	29.7% More common in girls
Disruptive behavior disorders (eg, oppositional-defiant, conduct disorders)	29.7% More common in boys
Eating disorders (anorexia and bulimia)	2% More common in girls
Psychotic disorders	0.8%
Substance use disorders	6.2%
Night-time bedwetting and bowel movements	16.2%

Data from Hirschtritt ME, Lee PC, Pauls DL, et al. Lifetime prevalence, age of risk, and genetic relationships of comorbid psychiatric disorders in Tourette syndrome. *JAMA Psychiatry.* 2015;72(4):325-333.

a typical age at onset of 4 to 6 years.[7] Phonic tics may soon follow, first with simple vocalizations followed by complex words and/or phrases. It is worth noting that features of attention deficit may precede tic onset and OCD may be more likely to manifest after tics have become evident.[8]

Studies have demonstrated that the worst-ever time period for tics tends to be at 10 to 12 years.[9] Following this, approximately 50% of patients will experience resolution of tics by adulthood, 40% to 50% will have varying degrees of improvement, and about 5% to 10% of individuals will experience progressive worsening of tics past the teenage years.[10] During the period of tic expression, which spans important formative years, approximately one-fifth of individuals will suffer symptoms severe enough to compromise school functioning.[11] Once the period of severest tics has passed, comorbidities, such as OCD and attention-deficit/hyperactivity disorder (ADHD) may persist or worsen.[8]

PATIENT EVALUATION OVERVIEW

Correct identification of tic phenomenology using the characteristics described above is an important first step in the approach to TS. This should be followed by an assessment of tic severity, frequency, and impact on daily functions and activities. A basic tic inventory can be performed to understand the breadth and complexity of both motor and phonic tics. The Yale Global Tic Severity Score (YGTSS)[12,13] is the most widely used formal scale to assess tic severity and impairment (**Table 4**), but time constraints may limit its applicability in day-to-day patient management. In clinical trials, a reduction in the YGTSS Total Tic Score (TTS) of 35%, or 6 to 7 points, indicates a clinical treatment response.[14]

Along with these aspects, clinicians should include an assessment of treatment goals and preferences that may influence both treatment recommendations and adherence. When comorbidities are identified, a discussion with the patient and/or caregiver should be held to prioritize the most impairing features to tailor the treatment strategy to the individual patient's needs.[15]

The American Academy of Neurology has published the following level A and B recommendations with regards to the assessment of the patient with TS[16]:

Table 4
Components of the Yale Global Tic Severity Scale

	Components	Maximum Score
Total Tic Score (TTS)	Number	5 Vocal 5 Motor
	Frequency	5 Vocal 5 Motor
	Intensity	5 Vocal 5 Motor
	Complexity	5 Vocal 5 Motor
	Interference	5 Vocal 5 Motor
Tic Impairment Score (TIS)	n/a	50
Total YGTSS score	TTS + TIS	100

Data from Leckman JF, Riddle MA, Hardin MT, et al. The Yale Global Tic Severity Scale: initial testing of a clinician-rated scale of tic severity. *J Am Acad Child Adolesc Psychiatry.* 1989;28(4):566-573.

- Clinicians must evaluate functional impairment related to tics from the perspective of the patient and, if applicable, the caregiver.
- Clinicians should refer people with TS to resources for psychoeducation for teachers and peers, such as the Tourette Association of America.
- Clinicians should ensure an assessment for comorbid ADHD is performed in people with tics.
- Clinicians should evaluate the burden of ADHD symptoms in people with tics.
- Clinicians should ensure an assessment for comorbid OCD is performed in people with tics.
- Clinicians must ensure appropriate screening for anxiety, mood, and disruptive behavior disorders is performed in people with tics.
- Clinicians must inquire about suicidal thoughts and suicide attempts in people with TS and refer to appropriate resources if present.

MANAGEMENT GOALS

As with other disease states, the goal of therapy is to bring symptoms to the most manageable level and maximize tolerability and adherence to the recommended treatment regimen.[16] Treatment options and their potential risks and benefits should be reviewed. A clear explanation should be provided that, in most individuals, it will not be possible to achieve complete tic resolution, and that despite therapeutic intervention, tics can continue to wax and wane. The dynamic range of tic expression should be described and tips for alleviating environmental stressors and other potential triggers should be provided (**Box 1**). Parents and care providers should be taught to recognize both the presence of comorbidities and the interplay between them and tic severity. Psychoeducation about these and other issues plays a large role in the initial approach to patient management.

PHARMACOLOGIC TREATMENT OPTIONS
Dopamine Receptor Blocking Drugs

Dopamine receptor blocking drugs (DRBDs) remain the only treatments approved by the US Food and Drug Administration for the treatment of tics, including haloperidol, pimozide, and aripiprazole (**Table 5**). Although other DRBDs have been investigated, many have been shown to have efficacy similar to that of haloperidol.[17] However, this class of drugs can cause side effects, such as somnolence, weight gain, increased appetite, QT prolongation, and acute dystonic reactions.[18] Fluphenazine is a typical neuroleptic with probable anti-tic efficacy but with a more tolerable

---

Box 1
Strategies for managing environmental triggers of tic expression

If stress, anxiety, or boredom are associated with tic expression, then attempt to change the environment or activity

Maintain a regular sleep schedule

Learn to anticipate tic exacerbations

Try not to draw attention to tics, because negative reinforcement can worsen them

Reassure the child about tic expression

Educate and provide information to teachers, other school personnel or community members so they do not draw attention to tics

Table 5
Dopamine receptor blocking and depleting drugs in Tourette syndrome

Drug	Effective Dosing Range	Side Effects of Concern	Notable Benefits
Haloperidol	0.5–3 mg/d	Extrapyramidal symptoms, sedation, increased appetite	Up to 90% improvement in tics
Pimozide	1–6 mg/d	Similar to haloperidol, QT prolongation	
Aripirazole	2.5–20 mg/d	Weight gain, akathisia	May also help comorbid mood disorder in adults
Fluphenazine	0.25–3 mg/d (children) 2.5–10 mg/d (adults)	Little risk of weight gain	Better tolerated than haloperidol, little risk of weight gain
Risperidone	0.25–3 mg/d (children) 0.25–6 mg/d (adults)	Weight gain, hyperprolactinemia	May also help comorbid OCD and aggressive behavior
Olanzapine	2.5–20 mg/d	Weight gain	May also help comorbid aggression and OCD
Ziprasidone	5–10 mg/d (children)	Somnolence	
Tetrabenazine	50–150 mg/d	Somnolence, akathisia, depression	No risk of weight gain

Data from Refs.[15,17,19]

side effect profile, including little to no risk of weight gain. Atypical neuroleptics, such as risperidone and olanzapine may also help manage comorbid OCD and aggressive behaviors (see **Table 5**).

Novel drugs targeting the dopaminergic system, such as vesicular monoamine transporter type 2 inhibitors[20] and dopamine D1 antagonists[21,22] are under investigation for the management of tics in TS with the potential for a better tolerability profile than DRBDs. The use of novel VMAT2 inhibitors, such as deutetrabenazine (dTBZ) and valbenazine (VBZ) builds on the clinical experience using tetrabenazine for management of tics in TS.[23] Both of these drugs offer the potential advantages of reduced dosing frequency and the ability to maintain baseline DRBDs based on experience treating other hyperkinetic movement disorders, such as chorea associated with Huntington disease (dTBZ) and tardive dyskinesia (dTBZ + VBZ). In an open-label investigation of deutetrabenazine in 23 adolescent subjects with TS,[20] a mean dose of 32.1 mg reduced the TTS score by 37.6% from baseline. Randomized, double-blind, placebo-controlled trials are currently underway. Ecopipam, a D1 receptor antagonist, was studied in 40 child and adolescent subjects using a randomized, placebo-controlled crossover study design.[22] There was a greater relative tic reduction during active treatment compared with placebo at 30 days (−3.2 point reduction in the TTS). An open-label study in adults was also performed showing modest tic improvements (approximately 5-point reduction in the TTS).[21]

Alpha-2 Agonists

Alpha-2 agonists, such as clonidine and guanfacine are often recommended as first-line agents for tics, especially when mild (**Table 6**). Clonidine activates presynaptic

Table 6
Non-dopamine receptor blocking drug pharmacologic agents with evidence for tic improvement in Tourette syndrome

Drug Class	Drug Name	Dosing Range: Children	Dosing Range: Adults	Potential Side Effects
Alpha-2 agonists	Clonidine	0.025–0.3 mg/d	0.025–0.6 mg/d	Hypotension, bradycardia, sedation
	Guanfacine	0.5–3 mg daily	No specific recommendation	Hypotension, bradycardia, sedation, QTc prolongation
Antiepileptic drugs	Topiramate	1–9 mg/kg/d	50–200 mg/d	Paresthesias, cognitive slowing, kidney stones
GABA agonists	Clonazepam	No specific recommendation	Up to 6 mg/d	Somnolence, dependence
	Baclofen	10–40 mg/d		Somnolence

Data from Roessner V, Plessen KJ, Rothenberger A, et al. European clinical guidelines for Tourette syndrome and other tic disorders. Part II: pharmacological treatment. *Eur Child Adolesc Psychiatry.* 2011;20(4):173-196; and Pringsheim T, Doja A, Gorman D, et al. Canadian guidelines for the evidence-based treatment of tic disorders: pharmacotherapy. *Can J Psychiatry.* 2012;57(3):133-143.

autoreceptors in the locus coeruleus leading to reduced norepinephrine release and turnover, and guanfacine stimulates central alpha-2 adrenergic receptors leading to reduced sympathetic nerve impulses from the vasomotor center to the heart and blood vessels.[24] These drugs can be used to address ADHD in children, but clinical trials in TS have shown variable results in tic improvement. One well-designed randomized study of clonidine, methylphenidate, clonidine + methylphenidate, or placebo in patients with TS with comorbid ADHD showed that treatment regimens including clonidine improved both tics and hyperactive/impulsive aspects of ADHD to a statistically significant degree.[25] A meta-analysis of alpha-2 agonists in individuals with TS and ADHD[26] found a medium to large effect size on tics in patients with TS with comorbid ADHD but a small effect size when ADHD was absent. Therefore, it is recommended that use of alpha-2 agonists in patients with TS should be considered when comorbid ADHD is present, because both tics and hyperactivity/impulsivity can improve in these patients.

Antiepileptic Drugs

The 2 main antiepileptic drugs that have been investigated in TS included topiramate and levetiracetam. Topiramate enhances gamma-aminobutyric acid (GABA) type A receptor-mediated chloride flux thereby potentiating GABA-mediated inhibition, and levetiracetam enhances chloride ion influx at the GABA-A receptor by reducing the effect of zinc and beta carbolines. Of these 2 agents, topiramate has been demonstrated to reduce tics (see **Table 6**), but the clinical experience with levetiracetam has been less consistent.[15,19] At mean doses of 118 mg/d in a total of 29 subjects with TS, topiramate was shown in a double-blind placebo-controlled study[27] to reduce the TTS by 53.6% on average compared with 19.7% for placebo ($P = .0259$). Notably, side effects, such as somnolence/sedation and weight gain were absent. In a retrospective evaluation,[28] the mean stable dose of therapy in 41 subjects was 146.3 mg/d with 75% of individuals experiencing a moderate to marked degree of tic improvement on a global impression of response. Topiramate may therefore be an alternative to initiation of DRBDs for treatment of tics in individuals with TS.[15,19]

Gamma-Aminobutyric Acid Agonists

GABA agonists can induce widespread and nonspecific inhibition of synaptic transmission in the central nervous system. Clonazepam, which is a GABA-A agonist in the benzodiazepine class, carries risk of somnolence and dependence, and has not been well studied in clinical trials of TS or tic disorders.[15] Its benefit in TS may be indirect, for example, as an anxiolytic or soporific. Baclofen is a GABA-B agonist used for treatment of spasticity. Both a single open label and single small randomized trial have suggested tic improvement can be observed in children although more rigorous studies have not been performed.[15,19] Clonazepam and baclofen may be considered as adjunctive treatments for tics given the low level of evidence for their use.

Botulinum Toxin Injections

Botulinum toxin (BoNT) reduces muscle spasms and movements by blocking acetylcholine release at the neuromuscular junction, producing effects that can last approximately 12 weeks.[29] Evidence from 2 studies suggests efficacy for focal motor and phonic tics in patients with TS. In a randomized, double-blind controlled clinical trial of 18 subjects with simple motor tics,[30] facial, neck, or shoulder tics were treated and changes in tic frequency (tics/min) were measured using a video protocol. Dosing was according to investigator experience, using the same guidelines as management of dystonic movements in the same muscles. A 39% improvement in tics was seen with BoNT therapy compared with a 5.8% worsening with placebo. This study also investigated the premonitory urge and found relative reductions in this aspect of tics in patients under active treatment. Patients, however, did not report a change in symptoms.

In an open-label study of 30 patients with phonic tics,[31] 2.5 u of onabotulinumtoxin A was injected into each vocal cord, leading to a 93% improvement in vocalizations. Fifty percent of individuals were reported to be tic free and premonitory urges were also reduced. Side effects of BoNT therapy delivered in this manner can include transient weakness of injected muscles and hypophonia.

These data suggest that the frequency of problematic focal and/or simple tics, such as blepharospastic, cervical dystonic, or vocal tics and premonitory urges, can improve with BoNT injections. This treatment should be considered when problematic but amenable tics occur, or when insufficient benefit or dose-limiting side effects occur with pharmacologic therapies.[16,19]

NONPHARMACOLOGIC TREATMENT OPTIONS
Habit Reversal Training

Habit reversal training (HRT) in TS is comprised of 3 components: awareness training, competing response training, and relaxation therapy/anxiety management with social support and reward.[32] In awareness training, the patient is taught to detect their premonitory urges and the early movements that precede a tic. In competing response training, the patient identifies behaviors that are incompatible with expression of a particular tic, and is taught to implement them on early tic detection. Eight 1-hour sessions are standard. Good candidates are those who are cognitively mature enough to understand the therapy's goals, compliant with frequent clinic visits, and can practice the strategies at home. HRT has been shown to reduce tics by 18% to 37% in randomized controlled trials, including adults and children with TS.[33]

Cognitive Behavioral Intervention for Tics

Cognitive behavioral intervention for tics (CBIT) combines elements of HRT with psychoeducation and function-based behavioral interventions.[32] In CBIT, the third component of HRT (described above) is replaced with the teaching of functional interventions, such as making changes to day-to-day activities in ways that may help reduce tics. CBIT is also largely completed in 8 sessions.

A meta-analysis reviewing behavior therapies in TS found that HRT and CBIT can both help reduce tic severity with treatment effects that are similar to trials of pharmacologic agents, and are better than psychoeducation alone.[32] The odds ratio of a treatment response is 5.77 with a number needed to treat of 3. However, limitations exist: treatment effects may be lower with comorbid ADHD, and may be larger in older patients who can engage in a greater number of therapy hours. Furthermore, restricted access to such behavioral interventions may be due to the lack of proximity to qualified personnel. Recent evidence suggests that delivery of these interventions via telemedicine can be effective.[34,35] Long-term outcomes are not well studied.

Cannabis/Cannabinoids

For many years, small case series and anecdotal reports have suggested that cannabis-based products can alleviate tics in patients with TS, although it is as yet undetermined whether such effects are related to a direct anti-tic mechanism, improved anxiety or sleep, or an effect on comorbidities, such as ADHD and OCD.[36-38] Although often considered "natural," cannabis-based products are not without risk, and can cause dizziness, sleepiness, feeling "high," headache, red eyes, increased appetite, dry mouth, and decreased short-term memory and concentration.[37,39,40] More serious but less common effects can include psychosis, euphoria, and heightened anxiety.[41,42]

Limited clinical data exists about the use of delta-9-tetrahydrocannabinol (THC, the predominant psychoactive substance in marijuana) in patients with TS. A trial of 5 to 10 mg per day of THC in 12 adults with TS studied in a double-blind, placebo-controlled crossover design of a single dose demonstrated a significant reduction in self-reported measures of tic severity and global improvement with THC compared with placebo.[43] A 6-week, double-blind, placebo-controlled trial of 24 adults with TS also demonstrated a significant benefit of THC compared with placebo in some, but not all, of the outcomes assessed.[44] Seven subjects randomly assigned to THC who completed the study experienced significant reduction of their tic symptoms compared with placebo after the first 2 weeks of treatments that continued throughout the 6-week trial.

Despite these encouraging results, clinicians should be aware that cannabis-based compounds are regulated differently (or not at all) in each state, and the testing and verification of medical marijuana varies across states. Consistent or uniform dosing strategies are therefore not established. Safety of THC and related compounds in children and adolescents have not been ascertained, and concerns may exist.[45-47] Alternate strategies using THC and non-THC compounds that target the endocannabinoid system are currently being investigated in clinical trials for efficacy against tics in TS (www.clinicaltrials.gov: NCT03087201, NCT03247244, NCT03066193, NCT03058562). Until such a time that these treatments are available, clinicians should be aware of regional legislation governing access to and prescription of marijuana products as well as the potential risks and benefits, and counsel their adult patients with TS accordingly.

COMBINATION THERAPIES

The use of multiple treatment modalities and pharmacologic agents in the management of patients with TS is a well-accepted strategy, especially when managing comorbidities along with tics.[16,19] In some cases, the initial choice of pharmacologic agent can be chosen with an intent to address two TS-related features (eg, use of clonidine to simultaneously improve tics and ADHD), but at some point it may be required that additional agents for one or the other feature(s) are added. In addition, a combination of behavior therapy and pharmacologic agents may be necessary to effectively manage the full spectrum of tic expression in an individual patient, or even a combination of pharmacologic agents from different drug classes.[15] Of note, evidence-based guidelines for how to implement these combinations is lacking. However, a few general strategies should be considered:

- Avoid starting more than 1 agent at a time.
- Explore the full range of dosing for 1 agent (while assessing for side effects) before determining its effect and risks/benefits of ongoing therapy.
- Consider whether tic exacerbations are situational or environmental and can be addressed with psychoeducation before adding additional therapies.
- If the need for additional symptom control requires further pharmacologic adjustment or management, consider the need for continuation of the previous treatment before adding another one.

SURGICAL TREATMENT OPTIONS

A review of the literature regarding neurosurgical treatment of TS spanning 1960 to 2003[48] found reports of 65 cases of intractable TS treated with ablative surgical interventions but with little to no success and sometimes devastating complications. The first report of deep brain stimulation (DBS) for treatment of TS emerged in 1999 with a single case of a 42-year-old man treated with bilateral stimulation within the thalamic nuclei that attempted to replicate a previous lesioning approach described by Hassler and Dieckmann, that had met with relative success.[49] Since that initial report, the interest in using DBS to manage cases of refractory TS has grown, with multiple targets and stimulation approaches being investigated.[50] The 3 main targets that have emerged with the most supportive evidence of efficacy are the centromedian-parafascicular (CM-Pf) complex of the thalamus, the anteromedial globus pallidus interna (amGPi), and the posteroventral globus pallidus interna (pvGPi).

Despite encouraging results of marked tic improvement from numerous open-label reports, the randomized and blinded clinical trials of DBS in TS that have been reported to date have demonstrated less robust and differential effects in the blinded versus open-label phases of treatment (**Table 7**), highlighting the challenges in studying surgical treatments in this complex disorder and calling into question the best trial design to investigate efficacy.[51]

Although it is recognized that there are limited options for individuals with a poor response to traditional pharmacologic and behavioral therapies in TS (see section Treatment Resistance), the use of DBS remains investigational and should not be recommended without careful consideration of previous treatment trials and responses, severity and stability of comorbidities, risks/benefits of surgery, and the psychosocial and emotional well-being of the potential candidate. In an updated set of recommendations,[57] the Tourette Syndrome Association International Deep Brain Stimulation Database and Registry Study Group suggest the following inclusionary criteria for DBS candidacy in severe TS:

Table 7
Summary of randomized trials of deep brain stimulation in Tourette syndrome

Study	Target	Sample Size	Study Design	Open Label	Reduction in Total YGTSS (Blinded)	Reduction in Total YGTSS (Open Label)
Maciunas et al,[52] 2007	CM-Pf	5	Four 7-d randomized DBS conditions: right, left, bilat ON, bilat OFF	3 mo	6.45%	24.2%
Welter et al,[53] 2008	CM-Pf + GPi	3	Four 2-mo randomized conditions: bilat Gpi, bilat CM-Pf, Bilat CM-Pf + Gpi, sham (no) stim	Pt 1: 60 mo Pt 2: 33 mo Pt 3: 20 mo	Pt 1: 65% Pt 2: 96% Pt 3: 74% (all GPi stim only)	Pt 1: 82% (CM-Pf + GPi) Pt 2: not provided (GPi only) Pt 3: 74% (CM-Pf + GPi)
Ackermans et al,[54] 2011	CM Spv-Voi	6	Double-blind, randomized crossover trial (ON/OFF) × 3 mo in each condition	12 mo	37% (ON vs OFF)	49% (ON vs OFF)
Kefalopoulou et al,[55] 2015	Anteromedial GPi (N = 13) Posteroventral GPi (N = 2)	15	Double-blind, randomized crossover trial ON/OFF) × 3 mo in each condition	8–36 mo	15.3%	40.1%
Welter et al,[56] 2017	Anteromedial GPi	16	Double-blind, controlled, randomized to active vs sham DBS × 3 mo	6 mo	10.2%	39.9%

Abbreviations: bilat, bilateral; CM-Pf, centromedian-parafascicular complex; GPi, globus pallidus interna; Spv-Voi, substantia periventricularis-ventral oralis internus.

1. DSM-V diagnosis of TS by expert clinician
2. Age is not a strict criterion. Local ethics committee involvement for cases involving persons younger than 18 years, and for cases considered "urgent" (eg, impending paralysis from headsnapping tics)
3. Tic severity: YGTSS greater than 35/50
4. Tics are primary cause of disability
5. Tics are refractory to conservative therapy (failed trials of medications from 3 classes, CBIT offered)
6. Comorbid medical, neurologic, and psychiatric disorders are treated and stable 3 to 6 months
7. Psychosocial environment is stable
8. Demonstrated the ability to adhere to recommended treatments
9. Neuropsychological profile indicates candidate can tolerate demands of surgery, postoperative follow-up, and possibility of poor outcome

Because no comparative data exist, selection of the stimulation target will be left to the discretion of the DBS treatment team, and comprehensive assessment and documentation of symptoms both before and after stimulation are considered essential in this context. Further insight for treatment teams can be gained from the existing International Tourette Syndrome Deep Brain Stimulation Public Database and Registry,[58,59] in which improvements in tic scores were seen across targets (**Table 8**). Interestingly, the amGPi group (n = 18) demonstrated greater reduction in the YGTSS total score at 1 year compared with the thalamic group (n = 51) and pvGPi group (n = 17), although differences in patient selection, baseline patient characteristics, and treatment algorithms cannot be excluded. It should also be noted that the TTS of the YGTSS was not analyzed separately in this report. Adverse events in the entire cohort included stimulation-related adverse events (dysarthria in 6.3% and paresthesia in 8.2%), infections (2.5%), and intracerebral hemorrhage (1.3%). More long-term data to guide clinical care will become available as the registry continues.

TREATMENT RESISTANCE AND COMPLICATIONS
Treatment Resistance

Tics are often incompletely controlled with medications or nonpharmacologic approaches. Treatment goals should therefore be clearly discussed, including that there are no predictors of the magnitude of treatment response. However, although not formally defined, there are many possible reasons that a patient with TS may appear to be refractory to treatment,[60] including:

Table 8
Reduction in total Yale Global Tic Severity Score from baseline by target in the International Tourette Syndrome Deep Brain Stimulation Public Database and Registry

Target	6 mo (%)	12 mo (%)
All	40.1	45.1
CM-Pf	42.8	46.3
amGPi	44.9	50.5
pvGPi	19.8	27.7

Abbreviations: amGPi, anteromedial globus pallidus interna; CM-Pf, centromedian-parafascicular; pvGPi, posteroventral globus pallidus interna.

Data from Martinez-Ramirez D, Jimenez-Shahed J, Leckman JF, et al. Efficacy and Safety of Deep Brain Stimulation in Tourette Syndrome: The International Tourette Syndrome Deep Brain Stimulation Public Database and Registry. JAMA Neurol. 2018;75(3):353-359.

- Inadequate trial of appropriate pharmacologic agents (eg, dose too low or insufficiently titrated, duration of treatment too short, limited number of drug classes tried)
- Side effects and/or nonadherence to an appropriate pharmacologic agent
- Incorrect identification of movement phenomenology (eg, stereotypies or psychogenic movements mischaracterized as tics)
- Limited access to all available therapies (this may particularly true of behavioral therapies)
- Comorbid psychiatric condition(s) not addressed, but also contributing (or contributing more than tics) to disruptions in school/work, family, or social functioning.

Complications of Tourette Syndrome

There are no clear predictors of any single patient's clinical course and the individual phenotype may vary significantly among patients. Patients with TS, however, may request or require emergent evaluation for a variety of reasons, as follows:

Malignant Tourette syndrome

In a tertiary referral center, Cheung and colleagues[61] defined malignant TS as greater than 2 emergency room visits or greater than 1 hospitalization for TS symptoms or associated behavioral comorbidities. In a retrospective chart review, 5.1% of all patients with TS evaluated over a 3-year period met criteria. Hospital admissions or emergency room visits resulted from tic-related injuries, self-injurious behavior, uncontrollable violence and temper, and suicidal ideation/attempts. Individuals with malignant TS were significantly more likely to have a personal history of OCD or obsessive-compulsive behaviors (OCBs), suggesting that OCD/OCBs may play a central role in the development of "malignant" symptoms.

Coprolalia

Coprolalia is defined as vocal tics consisting of obscene words or phrases, and is more likely to occur with urges to have coprolalic behaviors, and in the presence of nonobscene socially inappropriate behaviors. The presence of more severe tics is the best predictor of coprolalia, and coprolalia correlates with significantly reduced quality of life.[62] When patients present urgently for management of this symptom feature, strategies for management include:

- Investigation into psychosocial factors that may have contributed to increasing/worsening symptoms
- Advancing drug therapy and/or behavior therapies
- Initiation of BoNT injections[31,63,64]

Tic "status"

Tic "status" is a term proposed by Kovacs and colleagues[65] to refer to an acute or subacute worsening in the hyperkinetic features of TS but with differing characteristics than the preexisting tics (eg, more severe, more complex, and longer-lasting). Other suggestive features may include:

- Severe systemic effects, such as cardiac/respiratory difficulties, autonomic dysregulation, or rhabdomyolysis
- Duration may be several minutes to several days (shortest reported duration was approximately 15 minutes)
- Cause may relate to withdrawal/cessation of anti-tic medications, comorbid infection, or severe psychological distress (eg, physical or emotional trauma)

- Notable exclusionary criteria include neuroleptic malignant syndrome, drug withdrawal-emergent movement disorders, and features suggestive of malignant TS
- Management strategies may include readministration of a previously discontinued drug, increasing doses of other baseline or alternate drugs, addition of benzodiazepines, such as clonazepam, or light/deep sedation

"Whiplash" tics

This complex tic refers to a repetitive and forceful, often dystonic, neck extension, flexion or rotation that has been described to produce cervical myelopathy, either by chronic repetitive trauma to the cervical cord, or due to acute disc herniation with cord compression.[66] A case of vertebral dissection has also been described. Rapid initiation of BoNT injections should be considered when whiplash tics are encountered to prevent neurologic sequelae.

EVALUATION OF OUTCOME, ADJUSTMENT OF TREATMENT, AND LONG-TERM RECOMMENDATIONS

Periodic evaluation with assessment of tic severity, frequency, and impairment is required to determine need for ongoing pharmacologic management, modifications to the treatment regimen, or introduction of new modalities. The presence and severity of comorbidities should be assessed at each visit. As children approach the worst-ever time period for tics, patients and families/caregivers should be counseled about this possibility, as well as the chance that symptoms will begin to improve afterward. During late adolescence, once tics have clearly begun to improve, it may be possible to begin weaning medications to determine whether they are still required. No particular guidelines exist, but to avoid the potential for significant symptom exacerbations, medications should be reduced gradually and one at a time. Even though tics may improve, adolescents and young adults may still continue to experience bothersome comorbidities, and these should continue to be assessed and managed as appropriate. Adults may experience recurrent tics after a period of latency, commonly in the context of stressors, such as substance use[67] or other life events.

SUMMARY

Effective management of tics in TS entails psychoeducation along with a discussion with patients, families, and/or caregivers about treatment goals and expectations. The presence and severity of psychiatric comorbidities should always be ascertained to determine if those symptoms require intervention. Careful selection of pharmacologic agents can possibly address more than 1 symptom concurrently. Nonpharmacologic treatments, such as behavior therapy should be considered and offered when appropriate. BoNT injections may be a useful adjunct in select cases to target particular tics. A thoughtful assessment of factors that may contribute to treatment refractoriness should be undertaken before considering surgical interventions for tic management, and patients/caregivers should be made aware that this procedure remains under investigation.

DISCLOSURE

Dr J. Jimenez-Shahed has received consulting fees from Medtronic, Boston Scientific, Abbott/St. Jude Medical, Teva, Nuvelution, and Bracket. She has received research funding from Medtronic, Abbott/St. Jude Medical, and Teva.

REFERENCES

1. Singer HS. Tics and Tourette syndrome. Continuum (Minneap Minn) 2019;25(4): 936–58.
2. Leckman JF, Bloch MH, Scahill L, et al. Tourette syndrome: the self under siege. J Child Neurol 2006;21(8):642–9.
3. Reese HE, Scahill L, Peterson AL, et al. The premonitory urge to tic: measurement, characteristics, and correlates in older adolescents and adults. Behav Ther 2014;45(2):177–86.
4. Verdellen CW, Hoogduin CA, Keijsers GP. Tic suppression in the treatment of Tourette's syndrome with exposure therapy: the rebound phenomenon reconsidered. Mov Disord 2007;22(11):1601–6.
5. Pringsheim T, Lang A, Kurlan R, et al. Understanding disability in Tourette syndrome. Dev Med Child Neurol 2009;51(6):468–72.
6. Scharf JM, Miller LL, Gauvin CA, et al. Population prevalence of Tourette syndrome: a systematic review and meta-analysis. Mov Disord 2015;30(2):221–8.
7. Jankovic J. Tourette's syndrome. N Engl J Med 2001;345(16):1184–92.
8. Bloch MH, Peterson BS, Scahill L, et al. Adulthood outcome of tic and obsessive-compulsive symptom severity in children with Tourette syndrome. Arch Pediatr Adolesc Med 2006;160(1):65–9.
9. Bloch MH, Leckman JF. Clinical course of Tourette syndrome. J Psychosom Res 2009;67(6):497–501.
10. Freeman RD, Tourette Syndrome International Database Consortium. Tic disorders and ADHD: answers from a world-wide clinical dataset on Tourette syndrome. Eur Child Adolesc Psychiatry 2007;16(Suppl 1):15–23.
11. Leckman JF, Zhang H, Vitale A, et al. Course of tic severity in Tourette syndrome: the first two decades. Pediatrics 1998;102(1 Pt 1):14–9.
12. Leckman JF, Riddle MA, Hardin MT, et al. The Yale Global Tic Severity Scale: initial testing of a clinician-rated scale of tic severity. J Am Acad Child Adolesc Psychiatry 1989;28(4):566–73.
13. Storch EA, Murphy TK, Geffken GR, et al. Reliability and validity of the Yale Global Tic Severity Scale. Psychol Assess 2005;17(4):486–91.
14. Storch EA, De Nadai AS, Lewin AB, et al. Defining treatment response in pediatric tic disorders: a signal detection analysis of the Yale Global Tic Severity Scale. J Child Adolesc Psychopharmacol 2011;21(6):621–7.
15. Roessner V, Plessen KJ, Rothenberger A, et al. European clinical guidelines for Tourette syndrome and other tic disorders. Part II: pharmacological treatment. Eur Child Adolesc Psychiatry 2011;20(4):173–96.
16. Pringsheim T, Okun MS, Muller-Vahl K, et al. Practice guideline recommendations summary: treatment of tics in people with Tourette syndrome and chronic tic disorders. Neurology 2019;92(19):896–906.
17. Huys D, Hardenacke K, Poppe P, et al. Update on the role of antipsychotics in the treatment of Tourette syndrome. Neuropsychiatr Dis Treat 2012;8:95–104.
18. Mogwitz S, Buse J, Ehrlich S, et al. Clinical pharmacology of dopamine-modulating agents in Tourette's syndrome. Int Rev Neurobiol 2013;112:281–349.
19. Pringsheim T, Doja A, Gorman D, et al. Canadian guidelines for the evidence-based treatment of tic disorders: pharmacotherapy. Can J Psychiatry 2012; 57(3):133–43.
20. Jankovic J, Jimenez-Shahed J, Budman C, et al. Deutetrabenazine in tics associated with Tourette syndrome. Tremor Other Hyperkinet Mov (N Y) 2016;6:422.

21. Gilbert DL, Budman CL, Singer HS, et al. A D1 receptor antagonist, ecopipam, for treatment of tics in Tourette syndrome. Clin Neuropharmacol 2014;37(1):26–30.

22. Gilbert DL, Murphy TK, Jankovic J, et al. Ecopipam, a D1 receptor antagonist, for treatment of tourette syndrome in children: a randomized, placebo-controlled crossover study. Mov Disord 2018;33(8):1272–80.

23. Tarakad A, Jimenez-Shahed J. VMAT2 inhibitors in neuropsychiatric disorders. CNS Drugs 2018;32(12):1131–44.

24. Rizzo R, Gulisano M, Cali PV, et al. Tourette syndrome and comorbid ADHD: current pharmacological treatment options. Eur J Paediatr Neurol 2013;17(5):421–8.

25. Tourette's Syndrome Study G. Treatment of ADHD in children with tics: a randomized controlled trial. Neurology 2002;58(4):527–36.

26. Weisman H, Qureshi IA, Leckman JF, et al. Systematic review: pharmacological treatment of tic disorders—efficacy of antipsychotic and alpha-2 adrenergic agonist agents. Neurosci Biobehav Rev 2013;37(6):1162–71.

27. Jankovic J, Jimenez-Shahed J, Brown LW. A randomised, double-blind, placebo-controlled study of topiramate in the treatment of Tourette syndrome. J Neurol Neurosurg Psychiatry 2010;81(1):70–3.

28. Kuo SH, Jimenez-Shahed J. Topiramate in treatment of Tourette syndrome. Clin Neuropharmacol 2010;33(1):32–4.

29. Pirazzini M, Rossetto O, Eleopra R, et al. Botulinum neurotoxins: biology, pharmacology, and toxicology. Pharmacol Rev 2017;69(2):200–35.

30. Marras C, Andrews D, Sime E, et al. Botulinum toxin for simple motor tics: a randomized, double-blind, controlled clinical trial. Neurology 2001;56(5):605–10.

31. Porta M, Maggioni G, Ottaviani F, et al. Treatment of phonic tics in patients with Tourette's syndrome using botulinum toxin type A. Neurol Sci 2004;24(6):420–3.

32. McGuire JF, Piacentini J, Brennan EA, et al. A meta-analysis of behavior therapy for Tourette syndrome. J Psychiatr Res 2014;50:106–12.

33. Dutta N, Cavanna AE. The effectiveness of habit reversal therapy in the treatment of Tourette syndrome and other chronic tic disorders: a systematic review. Funct Neurol 2013;28(1):7–12.

34. Conelea CA, Wellen BCM. Tic treatment goes tech: a review of TicHelper.com. Cogn Behav Pract 2017;24(3):374–81.

35. Jakubovski E, Reichert C, Karch A, et al. The ONLINE-TICS study protocol: a randomized observer-blind clinical trial to demonstrate the efficacy and safety of internet-delivered behavioral treatment for adults with chronic tic disorders. Front Psychiatry 2016;7:119.

36. Muller-Vahl KR, Kolbe H, Schneider U, et al. Cannabinoids: possible role in pathophysiology and therapy of Gilles de la Tourette syndrome. Acta Psychiatr Scand 1998;98(6):502–6.

37. Abi-Jaoude E, Chen L, Cheung P, et al. Preliminary evidence on cannabis effectiveness and tolerability for adults with Tourette syndrome. J Neuropsychiatry Clin Neurosci 2017;29(4):391–400.

38. Thaler A, Arad S, Schleider LB, et al. Single center experience with medical cannabis in Gilles de la Tourette syndrome. Parkinsonism Relat Disord 2019;61: 211–3.

39. Russo EB. Current therapeutic cannabis controversies and clinical trial design issues. Front Pharmacol 2016;7:309.

40. Muller-Vahl KR. Treatment of Tourette syndrome with cannabinoids. Behav Neurol 2013;27(1):119–24.

41. Drewe M, Drewe J, Riecher-Rossler A. Cannabis and risk of psychosis. Swiss Med Wkly 2004;134(45–46):659–63.

42. Grant CN, Belanger RE. Cannabis and Canada's children and youth. Paediatr Child Health 2017;22(2):98–102.
43. Muller-Vahl KR, Schneider U, Koblenz A, et al. Treatment of Tourette's syndrome with delta 9-tetrahydrocannabinol (THC): a randomized crossover trial. Pharmacopsychiatry 2002;35(2):57–61.
44. Muller-Vahl KR, Schneider U, Prevedel H, et al. Delta 9-tetrahydrocannabinol (THC) is effective in the treatment of tics in Tourette syndrome: a 6-week randomized trial. J Clin Psychiatry 2003;64(4):459–65.
45. Blest-Hopley G, Giampietro V, Bhattacharyya S. Residual effects of cannabis use in adolescent and adult brain—a meta-analysis of fMRI studies. Neurosci Biobehav Rev 2018;88:26–41.
46. Renard J, Rosen LG, Loureiro M, et al. Adolescent cannabinoid exposure induces a persistent sub-cortical hyper-dopaminergic state and associated molecular adaptations in the prefrontal cortex. Cereb Cortex 2017;27(2):1297–310.
47. Leishman E, Murphy M, Mackie K, et al. Delta(9)-Tetrahydrocannabinol changes the brain lipidome and transcriptome differentially in the adolescent and the adult. Biochim Biophys Acta Mol Cell Biol Lipids 2018;1863(5):479–92.
48. Temel Y, Visser-Vandewalle V. Surgery in Tourette syndrome. Mov Disord 2004; 19(1):3–14.
49. Vandewalle V, van der Linden C, Groenewegen HJ, et al. Stereotactic treatment of Gilles de la Tourette syndrome by high frequency stimulation of thalamus. Lancet 1999;353(9154):724.
50. Viswanathan A, Jimenez-Shahed J, Baizabal Carvallo JF, et al. Deep brain stimulation for Tourette syndrome: target selection. Stereotact Funct Neurosurg 2012; 90(4):213–24.
51. Jimenez-Shahed J. Design challenges for stimulation trials of Tourette's syndrome. Lancet Neurol 2015;14(6):563–5.
52. Maciunas RJ, Maddux BN, Riley DE, et al. Prospective randomized double-blind trial of bilateral thalamic deep brain stimulation in adults with Tourette syndrome. J Neurosurg 2007;107(5):1004–14.
53. Welter ML, Mallet L, Houeto JL, et al. Internal pallidal and thalamic stimulation in patients with Tourette syndrome. Arch Neurol 2008;65(7):952–7.
54. Ackermans L, Duits A, van der Linden C, et al. Double-blind clinical trial of thalamic stimulation in patients with Tourette syndrome. Brain 2011;134(Pt 3): 832–44.
55. Kefalopoulou Z, Zrinzo L, Jahanshahi M, et al. Bilateral globus pallidus stimulation for severe Tourette's syndrome: a double-blind, randomised crossover trial. Lancet Neurol 2015;14(6):595–605.
56. Welter ML, Houeto JL, Thobois S, et al. Anterior pallidal deep brain stimulation for Tourette's syndrome: a randomised, double-blind, controlled trial. Lancet Neurol 2017;16(8):610–9.
57. Schrock LE, Mink JW, Woods DW, et al. Tourette syndrome deep brain stimulation: a review and updated recommendations. Mov Disord 2015;30(4):448–71.
58. Martinez-Ramirez D, Jimenez-Shahed J, Leckman JF, et al. Efficacy and safety of deep brain stimulation in Tourette syndrome: the International Tourette Syndrome Deep Brain Stimulation Public Database and Registry. JAMA Neurol 2018;75(3): 353–9.
59. Deeb W, Rossi PJ, Porta M, et al. The International Deep Brain Stimulation Registry and Database for Gilles de la Tourette syndrome: how does it work? Front Neurosci 2016;10:170.

60. Kious BM, Jimenez-Shahed J, Shprecher DR. Treatment-refractory Tourette syndrome. Prog Neuropsychopharmacol Biol Psychiatry 2016;70:227–36.
61. Cheung MY, Shahed J, Jankovic J. Malignant Tourette syndrome. Mov Disord 2007;22(12):1743–50.
62. Eddy CM, Cavanna AE. 'It's a curse!': coprolalia in Tourette syndrome. Eur J Neurol 2013;20(11):1467–70.
63. Scott BL, Jankovic J, Donovan DT. Botulinum toxin injection into vocal cord in the treatment of malignant coprolalia associated with Tourette's syndrome. Mov Disord 1996;11(4):431–3.
64. Salloway S, Stewart CF, Israeli L, et al. Botulinum toxin for refractory vocal tics. Mov Disord 1996;11(6):746–8.
65. Kovacs N, Herold R, Janszky J, et al. Tics status: a movement disorder emergency: observations. J Neurol 2011;258(1):143–5.
66. Patterson AL, Choudhri AF, Igarashi M, et al. Severe neurological complications associated with Tourette syndrome. Pediatr Neurol 2016;61:99–106.
67. Schaefer SM, Chow CA, Louis ED, et al. Tic exacerbation in adults with tourette syndrome: a case series. Tremor Other Hyperkinet Mov (N Y) 2017;7:450.

Medical, Surgical, and Genetic Treatment of Huntington Disease

Christine M. Stahl, MD*, Andrew Feigin, MD

KEYWORDS

- Huntington disease • Vesicular monoamine transporter type 2 inhibitors
- Antipsychotic drugs • Deep brain stimulation • Antisense oligonucleotides

KEY POINTS

- Tetrabenazine and deutetrabenazine, vesicular monoamine transporter type 2 inhibitors, are the only Food and Drug Administration–approved drugs for Huntington disease (HD); both reduce chorea.
- Antipsychotic drugs, such as tiapride, olanzapine, and risperidone, are commonly used in the treatment of chorea and psychiatric symptoms of HD.
- Deep brain stimulation of the globus pallidus interna, but not the subthalamic nucleus, has been reported to be effective in treating medically refractory chorea in HD, although data are limited.
- RNA-based and DNA-based therapies targeting the production pathway of the neurotoxic mutant huntingtin protein are in development and may provide both symptomatic and disease-modifying treatment in HD.

INTRODUCTION

Huntington disease (HD) is a neurodegenerative disorder that is characterized by progressive motor dysfunction, behavioral changes, and cognitive decline. HD was first recognized as a clinical entity in 1872 by Dr George Huntington in his publication, "On Chorea," where he describes a "peculiar...hereditary chorea."[1] It was not until 1993, however, that the causative mutation was found following a decade of extensive investigation by a group of researchers. All HD patients have a CAG trinucleotide repeat expansion within the huntingtin gene on chromosome 4 that leads to the production of the mutant huntingtin protein (mHTT).[2] It is believed that the mHTT contributes to neuronal dysfunction and cell death, but the precise cellular and molecular mechanisms are not completely understood.[3]

NYU Langone Health, Marlene and Paolo Fresco Institute for Parkinson's and Movement Disorders, 222 East 41st Street, Floor 13, New York, NY 10017, USA
* Corresponding author.
E-mail address: christine.stahl@nyulangone.org

Neurol Clin 38 (2020) 367–378
https://doi.org/10.1016/j.ncl.2020.01.010
0733-8619/20/© 2020 Elsevier Inc. All rights reserved.

Clinical Features and Diagnosis

HD is inherited in an autosomal dominant pattern, but penetrance is variable and linked to the size of the CAG expansion. CAG repeat length between 10 and 26 is considered normal and over 40 is generally accepted because a repeat length always leading to the development of HD[4]; CAG repeats of 36 to 39 are associated with reduced penetrance. There is a growing body of evidence that individuals with CAG repeats in the intermediate range (27–35) may exhibit clinical, imaging, and pathologic manifestations of HD.[5] The average age of symptom onset is 40, though there is wide variability ranging from the first to the ninth decades of life.[6] Similar to HD penetrance, the age of symptom onset is related to the length of the CAG expansion, with longer repeat length associated with earlier age of onset.[7] Juvenile HD is defined as symptom onset at age less than 20, and in most cases CAG repeat lengths are over 55.[6] HD typically is diagnosed clinically with the presence of characteristic motor symptoms with or without psychiatric or cognitive manifestations, particularly if 1 of the parents was similarly affected. Now that the causative mutation is known, the suspected diagnosis can be confirmed by testing for the CAG repeat expansion.[6]

As discussed previously, HD is a disorder characterized by progressive motor dysfunction, behavioral changes, and cognitive impairment. This article briefly reviews the characteristic features of HD and then discusses the available treatment modalities.

Motor Symptoms

The phenomenology of motor dysfunction in HD is broad and can be subdivided into 2 categories: abnormal involuntary movements and impaired voluntary movements. The involuntary movements of HD are characterized primarily by chorea.[8] Chorea is most prominent in adult-onset HD and, in the early stages of the disease, typically is limited to the distal extremities and face. Over time, the chorea may spread more proximally.[6] The second category, impaired voluntary movements, includes bradykinesia, rigidity, dystonia, and incoordination. These symptoms predominate in earlier-onset HD, including juvenile HD, as well as in the later stages of adult-onset HD.[8] As the disease progresses, dysarthria and dysphagia become prominent and can lead to significant choking episodes. The most common cause of death in HD patients is pneumonia, usually related to aspiration.[9]

Although the abnormal movements of HD often are the first recognized symptom, the behavioral and cognitive symptoms of HD frequently are present well before the start of the motor manifestations.[6]

Behavioral and Psychiatric Symptoms

A variety of behavioral and psychiatric symptoms are seen in HD. The most common psychiatric condition is depression, which is present in approximately half of all HD patients. Anxiety, apathy, irritability, aggression, and psychosis also are seen in HD. Apathy, but not depression or anxiety, tends to linearly worsen with disease progression.[8] Suicide rates are elevated in HD and suicides occur most frequently in early symptomatic stages of HD, particularly when independence starts to decline.[6]

Cognitive Symptoms

Cognitive impairment in HD may begin prior to the motor symptoms; however, it is not always recognized at first, because symptoms may be mild. Cognitive deficits in HD may involve slowed processing speed as well as impaired attention, mental flexibility, planning, and visuospatial functions. Memory is less affected, and language is relatively preserved in HD, in contrast to Alzheimer disease. There often is an anosognosia of clinical deficits, involving unawareness of psychiatric and cognitive impairment as well as of involuntary movements or other movement disorders. This anosognosia can interfere with treatment because the patient does not see the need for such intervention. Over time, the cognitive decline progresses and dementia develops.[8]

TREATMENT

Currently, there are no disease-modifying treatments approved for HD. There are several pharmacologic and nonpharmacologic treatment modalities, however, that can improve the varied symptoms of HD as well as the quality of life of patients. Studies have demonstrated that the ideal care for HD patients is an interdisciplinary approach, including physical, occupational, and speech therapists, along with neurologists, psychiatrists, and psychologists.[10]

The following sections review the medical, surgical, and genetic treatments currently available.

Medical Treatment

Motor symptoms
Chorea Given the prominence of chorea in HD, much of the literature on the medical treatment of HD addresses reduction of chorea. It is hypothesized that chorea in HD is related to changes in the balance of glutamate and dopamine activity in basal ganglia circuitry.[11] Reducing dopamine neurotransmission has been observed to reduce chorea, and, as such, the primary drugs used for the chorea associated with HD are dopamine depleters and dopamine receptor blockers.[12]

The first step in treating chorea is to determine the appropriate time to start a medication. Because all available medications to date are symptomatic, these medications typically are not started until the chorea is bothersome to a patient or interfering with the patient's daily activities or safety.[13]

Tetrabenazine Tetrabenazine (TBZ), a dopamine depleter first designed in the 1950s to treat schizophrenia, was the first drug formally approved by the Food and Drug Administration (FDA) for treatment of HD chorea in 2008, following the results of the TETRA-HD study.[14,15] TBZ is a dopamine depleter that works via inhibition of the vesicular monoamine transporter type 2 (VMAT2) in the presynaptic terminals of dopaminergic neurons. VMAT2 facilitates transport of cytoplasmic dopamine into presynaptic vesicles. Therefore, inhibition of VMAT2 allows for increased degradation of dopamine by monoamine oxidases in the presynaptic terminal, leading to an overall depletion of dopamine.[15]

In the TETRA-HD study, which was a multicenter, double-blind, placebo-controlled trial in 84 HD patients randomized to TBZ or placebo for 12 weeks, there was a clear improvement of chorea in those on TBZ. The primary endpoint of the trial was a change from the baseline total chorea score of the Unified Huntington's Disease Rating Scale (UHDRS). The total chorea score assesses the severity of chorea present from 0 (absent) to 4 (marked/prolonged) in 7 body regions (face, Bucco-orolingual region, trunk, left and right upper extremities, and left and right lower extremities). The maximal score is 28.[16] In TETRA-HD, TBZ was titrated from 12.5 mg daily to the dose with greatest efficacy and tolerable side effects up to a maximal dose of 100 mg/d. TBZ has a half-life of 5 hours to 7 hours, because it is rapidly metabolized by the hepatic enzyme CYP2D6, so typically it is dosed 3 times daily.[17]

At 12 weeks, the TBZ group demonstrated a reduction of the total chorea score by 5.0 units, compared with a 1.5-unit decrease in the placebo group. Furthermore, there was a significant improvement in the TBZ group over placebo in the Clinical Global Impression

Scale - Global Improvement (CGI-I), with 69% of TBZ subjects reporting at least some improvement (CGI-I score ≤3) compared with only 24% of the placebo group.[14]

The main dose-limiting side effects reported were drowsiness, akathisia, parkinsonism, and depression. TBZ-related side effects typically are dose-related and improve with a reduced dose. In the TETRA-HD study, there was 1 suicide in the TBZ group, leading to the black box warning for TBZ, stating the drug is contraindicated in patients who are actively suicidal or with inadequately treated depression.[15] It is not clear, however, that depression underlies cases of TBZ-related suicide, and there is growing evidence it may be more correlated with impulsivity.[18]

Deutetrabenazine With the side-effect profile of TBZ and its required frequent dosing in mind, a novel VMAT2 inhibitor, deutetrabenazine, was designed. Deutetrabenazine replaces 6 hydrogen atoms in TBZ with 6 deuterium atoms, a heavier, nontoxic form of hydrogen. The deuterium-carbon bond is stronger than the normal hydrogen-carbon and thus is more slowly metabolized resulting in a longer half-life and less frequent and lower doses.

Deutetrabenazine's safety and efficacy in controlling chorea associated with HD was evaluated in the First-HD trial published in 2016. This study, which was a multicenter, double-blind, placebo-controlled trial, randomized 90 patients to deutetrabenazine or placebo. At 12 weeks, deutetrabenazine taken twice daily showed significant improvement of chorea, with a mean group decrease of total chorea score of 2.5 units compared with placebo. Furthermore, there was no significant difference between treatment groups with regard to adverse events, including sedation, depression, or suicidal ideation.[19] The results of the First-HD study lead to deutetrabenazine's FDA approval in 2017. Although there is no head-to-head study comparing TBZ and deutetrabenazine, a comparison of data from the TETRA-HD and First-HD studies showed deutetrabenazine was found to have an overall lower risk of moderate to severe adverse events, including agitation, akathisia, depression, drowsiness, and parkinsonism, compared with TBZ.[20]

Dopamine receptor blockers Dopamine receptor blockers, also referred to as antipsychotics or neuroleptics, are another class of medications frequently used to treat chorea in HD, particularly if there are comorbid psychiatric symptoms, including psychosis, depression, or aggressive behavior. According to an international survey of chorea treatment preferences among HD experts, a majority of clinicians from Europe preferred an antipsychotic as a first-line antichoreic drug, whereas there was an approximately equal divide between a preference for an antipsychotic versus TBZ in clinicians from North America and Australia.[21] Neuroleptics, however, especially typical antipsychotics (eg, haloperidol, pimozide, fluphenazine, and tiapride) may be associated with significant side effects, including weight gain, drowsiness, parkinsonism, and tardive dyskinesia, so their use requires close monitoring. Some atypical antipsychotics, which also block dopamine D2 receptors (eg, olanzapine, quetiapine, and risperidone), commonly are used to suppress chorea in HD, but these drugs have a similar side-effect profile to the typical antipsychotics.

Data on the efficacy of these drugs is mainly limited to case reports, small case series, or open-label studies, with few randomized controlled trials.[22,23] As such, the American Academy of Neurology (AAN) evidence-based guidelines for the treatment of chorea in HD published in 2011 did not find sufficient evidence to make recommendations regarding the use of dopamine blockers.[24] These guidelines, however, have been criticized by many HD experts for their focus on arbitrarily chosen criteria for chorea score improvement and adherence to data only from controlled clinical trials, resulting in recommendations that may not be representative of expert clinical experience.[25]

Atypical antipsychotics generally are preferred over typical antipsychotics due to the better side-effect profile. In a recent review of the literature in 2017, the investigators found that among HD experts tiapride (in Europe), olanzapine, and risperidone were the preferred first-line treatment of chorea, in addition to the VMAT-2 inhibitor TBZ.[22] The data on these 3 dopamine blockers, specifically, are reviewed.

Tiapride, a typical antipsychotic that is not available in the United States, is widely used in European countries. There were 2 randomized, placebo-controlled clinical trials from the 1980s evaluating the efficacy of tiapride in chorea reduction. The first, a randomized placebo-controlled, crossover study did not find a reduction of chorea in 22 HD patients given 300 mg/d for 2 weeks.[26] The second evaluated 29 HD patients receiving tiapride, 3 g/d over two 3-week periods, either preceded, interrupted, or followed by a 3-week placebo period. A reduction of chorea was reported; however, the study had some limitations, including a lack of a washout period, making the results difficult to interpret.[22,23,27] The not-yet published results of a recently completed single-center randomized controlled clinical trial in France comparing olanzapine and tiapride to TBZ (NEUROHD; NCT00632645).

Olanzapine, an atypical antipsychotic, was reported as the most commonly prescribed dopamine blocker for the motor and behavioral symptoms of HD in the United Kingdom, according to a 2008 survey.[28] A few small, open-label case series have demonstrated chorea reduction after treatment, although only 2 of the 3 reached statistical significance.[22]

Risperidone is an atypical antipsychotic but has a side-effect profile more similar to the typical antipsychotics with regard to developing drug-induced parkinsonism and tardive dyskinesia.[29] It also is used frequently in the treatment of chorea in HD, and, according to 1 survey of HD experts, is chosen as the first-choice antipsychotic drug by 43% of respondents.[21] Data on risperidone's efficacy are limited to case reports, case series, or retrospective studies, because there have been no clinical trials.[22]

Recently, Schultz and colleagues[30] have attempted to bridge the gap between expert opinion and evidenced-based medicine regarding the use of antipsychotics for chorea in HD. They retrospectively analyzed the Enroll-HD database and found that olanzapine and risperidone appeared to be at least comparable to TBZ in controlling chorea. There certainly is a need for larger-scale, randomized controlled investigations of antipsychotics for the treatment of chorea in HD.

Riluzole and amantadine As discussed previously, it has been suggested that an imbalance of dopamine and glutamate activity in the brain may underlie the development of chorea in HD, specifically that the overactivity of glutamate produces excitotoxicity-mediated changes in the striatum and cortex.[11] Several small studies have evaluated drugs that inhibit glutamate transmission, including riluzole and amantadine.

A multicenter, randomized, double-blind study of riluzole, a glutamate release inhibitor, demonstrated reduction of chorea in HD patients at 8 weeks with doses of 200 mg/d (but not 100 mg/d) compared with placebo. Riluzole, however, was not found to improve functional capacity and caused significant, although reversible, liver transaminase abnormalities.[31] More recently, in 2007, a larger randomized controlled trial of riluzole found no improvement of chorea over the 3-year study.[32]

Amantadine, a noncompetitive N-methyl-D-aspartic acid–type glutamate receptor antagonist, has been studied in a few small, randomized trials examining its effect on chorea reduction, with mixed results. In 1 study, an antichoreic effect was demonstrated with amantadine compared with placebo but often required doses as high as

400 mg/d.[33] In another randomized controlled study, however, amantadine failed to improve chorea scores, although most patients reported feeling subjectively better on amandatine.[34]

Both amantadine and riluzole have been recommended for the treatment of HD chorea (level B) in the 2011 AAN evidence-based guidelines; however, their use in HD according to expert opinion–based recommendations is controversial, as discussed previously.[25,35]

Other drugs investigated in Huntington disease Pridopidine, a dopamine stabilizer, has been studied extensively in HD, without meaningful clinical benefit.[36] The drug also has been found to have affinity to the sigma-1 receptor, located predominantly at the endoplasmic reticulum and mitochondrial and may activate neuroprotective pathways. Therefore, the drug may be studied in the future as a potential disease-modifying strategy.[37]

Other movement disorders Although chorea is the predominant movement disorder seen in HD, especially early in the disease course, dystonia, rigidity, and bradykinesia often emerge later as the disease progresses and these symptoms can have an impact on function and quality of life. Systemic medications, such as TBZ, baclofen, and benzodiazepines, are used to treat dystonia, and botulinum toxin injections may be useful for treating focal dystonia. For rigidity and bradykinesia, dopaminergic drugs, such as levodopa and dopamine agonists, can be effective.[10]

Additionally, fall prevention is critical in HD patients because falls are one of the strongest predictors of nursing home placement in HD.[38] There have been several small studies that report that physical therapy and exercise may improve gait and balance.[39,40]

Psychiatric and cognitive symptoms

Although the treatment of the motor features of HD often becomes a primary focus in the management of HD, the management of psychiatric and cognitive symptoms of HD is critical, because these symptoms can be more disabling to patients than the motor symptoms. As discussed previously, the anosognosia of clinical impairment that is often present in HD can interfere with implementing treatment.

Despite the importance of recognizing and treating psychiatric and cognitive symptoms, the data for HD-specific treatment are scarce, and there are few randomized clinical trials. For the psychiatric symptoms, however, including depression, anxiety, apathy, irritability/aggression, and psychosis, the results from case reports and case series support that standard treatment paradigms for these psychiatric symptoms appear to provide at least some benefit when applied to HD patients.[41,42] In 2018, Anderson and colleagues[43] published an expert-based consensus guideline on the clinical management of neuropsychiatric symptoms in HD, which can help bridge the gap, given the scarcity of available evidenced-based recommendations.

For mild depression without cognitive impairment, a trial of psychotherapy often is prescribed. If medication is required, however, given the overall tolerability of selective serotonin reuptake inhibitors (SSRIs) and serotonin-norepinephrine reuptake inhibitors (SNRIs), these drugs typically are considered first-line treatment choices. Addition of an antipsychotic may be necessary if psychotic symptoms are present with depression. Electroconvulsive therapy (ECT) has been used in some cases of treatment refractory severe depression. SSRIs and SNRIs also are first-line pharmacologic treatment of anxiety. Apathy remains a difficult symptom to treat in both HD and non-HD related cases, and currently there is no standard treatment of choice, although a trial of an antidepressant is reasonable, particularly when there is difficulty in separating depression from apathy. Irritability, aggression, and psychosis often require treatment with antipsychotics.[41–43]

Table 1 summarizes current symptomatic medications used in HD.

Surgical Treatment

Deep brain stimulation (DBS) poses particular challenges in HD, given the presence of both hyperkinetic and hypokinetic movements that predominate in different stages of the disease as well as the coexisting cognitive and neuropsychiatric manifestations of HD. Nonetheless, DBS has been explored in HD for the treatment of medically refractory chorea. The globus pallidus interna (GPi) is the most common target reported in the literature. Stimulation frequencies reported range from 40 Hz to 180 Hz, but 130 Hz is the most common.[44] The only randomized, double-blind controlled study of GPi stimulation in HD to date evaluated 4 subjects with adult-onset HD and 2 subjects with a juvenile variant. This study found no improvement in the juvenile patients but reported a 60% improvement in the chorea subscore on the UHDRS at 6 months postoperatively in the 4 adult-onset chorea predominant patients.[45] Similarly, several other small, prospective, open-label evaluations have found significant reduction of chorea with GPi stimulation.[46,47] Although chorea was reduced, however, in 6 advanced HD patients with GPi stimulation, Zittel and colleagues[47] found no improvement of other motor symptoms, such as bradykinesia, dystonia, or functional impairment. There currently is an ongoing European investigation of the efficacy of pallidal stimulation in overall motor function in HD in a multicenter, randomized, double-blind, parallel-group, sham-controlled trial (NCT02535884).

Despite promising results of improved chorea with GPi stimulation, the subthalamic nucleus (STN) has not been found to be an effective target for chorea in HD, although data are limited. In 1 case of DBS targeting both the bilateral GPi and STN, reduction of bradykinesia was observed; although pallidal stimulation suppressed chorea, there was no additional benefit to combined pallidal and STN stimulation.[48]

Genetic Treatment

To date, there are no disease-modifying treatments for HD. Preclinical studies in transgenic animal models of HD, however, have demonstrated that reducing the production

Table 1
Symptomatic medications for Huntington disease

Symptom	Medication	Evidence
Motor		
Chorea	Neuroleptic	Case series, expert opinion, small RCT[21,22,26]
	VMAT2 inhibitors	Large RCTs[14,19]
	Amantadine	RCT with conflicting outcomes[31,32]
	Riluzole	RCT with conflicting outcomes[34,36]
Parkinsonism	Dopaminergic medications	Case reports/series[57–59]
Psychiatric		
Depression	SSRI/SNRI, ECT	Expert opinion[42]
Anxiety	SSRI/SNRI, benzodiazepines	Expert opinion[43]
Agitation	SSRI/SNRI, benzodiazepines	Expert opinion[43]
Psychosis	Neuroleptic	Expert opinion[43]
Dementia	Acetylcholinesterase inhibitors	Small RCTs[60]

Abbreviation: RCT, randomized controlled trial.

of neurotoxic mHTT may reverse the neuropathology and motor/behavioral changes associated with the HD mutation.[49,50] These studies have led to several RNA-based and DNA-based strategies to knock down the production of mHTT in human HD, and these approaches have entered human clinical trials. Strategies that are now in human clinical trials include the use of antisense oligonucleotides (ASOs) and RNA interference (RNAi).

The huntingtin mRNA can be targeted by either ASOs or by RNAi, both of which lead to degradation of the mRNA and decreased levels of mHTT. ASOs are short sequences of single-stranded DNA designed to target and bind to specific mRNA sequences. The ASO-RNA hybrid is then degraded by normal cellular mechanisms. ASOs can be designed to be allele specific (ie, binding to only the mutant HD allele) or allele nonspecific (leading to the degradation of both mHTT mRNA and normal HTT mRNA). This in turn lowers the amount of HTT protein. ASOs, cannot cross the blood-brain barrier and must be delivered to the CSF, usually via lumbar puncture.[51] By contrast, RNAi utilizes double stranded RNA sequences that are complementary to HTT mRNA, and similar to ASOs bind mRNA leading to degradation and reduction in the target protein. Currently, RNAi therapies in development for HD are delivered via viral vector (current approaches are utilizing aden-associated virus (AAV)) to target regions in the brain (eg, striatum) through stereotactic neurosurgery.[52]

Several ASO therapies currently are in clinical trials for HD. A recently completed randomized, double-blind, multiple-ascending dose, phase I/II trial of an allele-nonspecific ASO demonstrated that this ASO, IONIS-HTTR$_X$, is safe and well tolerated when delivered intrathecally to early manifest HD patients. There was an observed dose-dependent reduction in mHTT up to approximately 40% in the cerebrospinal fluid at the conclusion of the 13-week treatment period.[53] An open-label extension has been offered to the study participants to continue to monitor safety and efficacy (NCT03342053). A large randomized, double-blind, placebo-controlled, phase III trial is now under way to investigate the efficacy of this therapy in adult patients with manifest HD (GENERATION-HD1; NCT03761849). In addition, 2 allele-specific ASOs (targeting only the mHTT) are being evaluated in 2 randomized, double-blind, placebo-controlled phase Ia/IIb trials in early manifest HD patients (PRECISION-HD1; NCT03225833 and PRECISION-HD2; NCT03225846). It remains unknown if the allele-nonspecific approach carries higher risk related to reduction of normal HTT.[54] Several RNAi approaches to HD also are entering human clinical trials.[55]

Other gene therapy approaches that hold promise for HD include zinc finger proteins that suppress DNA transcription and clustered, regularly interspaced, short palindromic repeats (CRISPR) with a CRISPR-associated system that can edit sequences of DNA.[52] These approaches remain in various stages of preclinical investigation and are beyond the scope of this review.

OTHER ONGOING DISEASE-MODIFYING CLINICAL TRIALS IN HUNTINGTON DISEASE

Increasing evidence suggests that neuroinflammatory responses may contribute to the progression of neurodegenerative disorders, including HD. Several therapies aimed at modulating the neuroinflammatory response are being evaluated in HD. In particular, semaphoring-4D (SEMA4D) is a transmembrane signaling protein that modulates a variety of processes central to neuroinflammation and neurodegeneration, and a monoclonal blocking antibody to SEMA4D has been shown to ameliorate neuropathologic changes and some cognitive signs in a transgenic mouse model of HD.[56] This has led to a large multicenter, randomized, double-blind, placebo-controlled trial of this monoclonal antibody (pepinemab) in HD

(SIGNAL; NCT02481674); this study has completed enrollment and results are expected at the end of 2020.

SUMMARY

HD is a neurodegenerative disorder characterized by progressive motor, behavioral, and cognitive decline caused by a CAG trinucleotide repeat expansion in the huntingtin gene on chromosome 4. Available medical and surgical treatments, including VMAT2 inhibitors, antipsychotics, and DBS, are limited to symptom management because there are no disease-modifying agents at this time. Emerging investigation of RNA-based and DNA-based therapies holds promise of providing both symptomatic relief and the first disease-modifying treatments for HD. Although these therapies are being sought, better symptomatic therapies are needed, especially to target the behavioral and cognitive manifestations of HD.

REFERENCES

1. Huntington G. On chorea. The medical surgical reporter: a weekly journal. The Medical Surgical Reporter 1872;26(15):317–21.
2. A novel gene containing a trinucleotide repeat that is expanded and unstable on Huntington's disease chromosomes. The Huntington's Disease Collaborative Research Group. Cell 1993;72:971–83.
3. Jimenez-Sanchez MLF, Underwood BR, Rubinsztein DC. Huntington's disease: mechanisms of pathogenesis and therapeutic strategies. Cold Spring Harb Perspect Med 2017;7 [pii:a024240].
4. ACMG/ASHG statement. Laboratory guidelines for Huntington disease genetic testing. The American College of Medical Genetics/American Society of Human Genetics Huntington Disease Genetic Testing Working Group. Am J Hum Genet 1998;62:1243–7.
5. Savitt D, Jankovic J. Clinical phenotype in carriers of intermediate alleles in the huntingtin gene. J Neurol Sci 2019;402:57–61.
6. Roos RA. Huntington's disease: a clinical review. Orphanet J Rare Dis 2010;5:40.
7. Andrew SE, Goldberg YP, Kremer B, et al. The relationship between trinucleotide (CAG) repeat length and clinical features of Huntington's disease. Nat Genet 1993;4:398–403.
8. Ross CA, Aylward EH, Wild EJ, et al. Huntington disease: natural history, biomarkers and prospects for therapeutics. Nat Rev Neurol 2014;10(4):204–16.
9. Heemskerk AW, Roos RA. Aspiration pneumonia and death in Huntington's disease. PLoS Curr 2012;4:RRN1293.
10. Testa CM, Jankovic J. Huntington disease: a quarter century of progress since the gene discovery. J Neurol Sci 2019;396:52–68.
11. Andre VM, Cepeda C, Levine MS. Dopamine and glutamate in Huntington's disease: a balancing act. CNS Neurosci Ther 2010;16(3):163–78.
12. Wyant KJ, Ridder AJ, Dayalu P. Huntington's disease-update on treatments. Curr Neurol Neurosci Rep 2017;17(4):33.
13. Jankovic J, Roos RA. Chorea associated with Huntington's disease: to treat or not to treat? Mov Disord 2014;29(11):1414–8.
14. Huntington Study Group. Tetrabenazine as antichorea therapy in Huntington disease: a randomized controlled trial. Neurology 2006;66(3):366–72.
15. Jankovic J, Clarence-Smith K. Tetrabenazine for the treatment of chorea and other hyperkinetic movement disorders. Expert Rev Neurother 2011;11(11):1509–23.

16. Unified Huntington's Disease Rating Scale: reliability and consistency. Huntington Study Group. Mov Disord 1996;11(2):136–42.
17. Mehanna R, Hunter C, Davidson A, et al. Analysis of CYP2D6 genotype and response to tetrabenazine. Mov Disord 2013;28(2):210–5.
18. Anderson KE, Gehl CR, Marder KS, et al. Comorbidities of obsessive and compulsive symptoms in Huntington's disease. J Nerv Ment Dis 2010;198(5):334–8.
19. Huntington Study Group, Frank S, Testa CM, et al. Effect of deutetrabenazine on chorea among patients with huntington disease: a randomized clinical trial. JAMA 2016;316(1):40–50.
20. Claassen DO, Carroll B, De Boer LM, et al. Indirect tolerability comparison of Deutetrabenazine and Tetrabenazine for Huntington disease. J Clin Mov Disord 2017;4:3.
21. Burgunder JM, Guttman M, Perlman S, et al. An international survey-based algorithm for the pharmacologic treatment of chorea in huntington's disease. PLoS Curr 2011;3:RRN1260.
22. Coppen EM, Roos RA. Current pharmacological approaches to reduce chorea in huntington's disease. Drugs 2017;77(1):29–46.
23. Bashir H, Jankovic J. Treatment options for chorea. Expert Rev Neurother 2018;18(1):51–63.
24. Armstrong MJ, Miyasaki JM, American Academy of N. Evidence-based guideline: pharmacologic treatment of chorea in Huntington disease: report of the guideline development subcommittee of the American Academy of Neurology. Neurology 2012;79(6):597–603.
25. Reilmann R. Pharmacological treatment of chores in Hungtington's disease - good clinical practice versus evidence-based guildline. Mov Disord 2013;28(8):1030–3.
26. Roos RA, Buruma OJ, Bruyn GW, et al. Tiapride in the treatment of Huntington's chorea. Acta Neurol Scand 1982;65(1):45–50.
27. Deroover J, Baro F, Bourguignon RP, et al. Tiapride versus placebo: a double-blind comparative study in the management of Huntington's chorea. Curr Med Res Opin 1984;9(5):329–38.
28. Priller J, Ecker D, Landwehrmeyer B, et al. A Europe-wide assessment of current medication choices in Huntington's disease. Mov Disord 2008;23(12):1788.
29. Komossa K, Rummel-Kluge C, Schwarz S, et al. Risperidone versus other atypical antipsychotics for schizophrenia. Cochrane Database Syst Rev 2011;(1):CD006626.
30. Schultz JL, Kamholz JA, Nopoulos PC, et al. Comparing risperidone and olanzapine to tetrabenazine for the management of chorea in huntington disease: an analysis from the enroll-HD database. Mov Disord Clin Pract 2019;6(2):132–8.
31. Huntington Study Group. Dosage effects of riluzole in Huntington's disease: a multicenter placebo-controlled study. Neurology 2003;61(11):1551–6.
32. Landwehrmeyer GB, Dubois B, de Yebenes JG, et al. Riluzole in Huntington's disease: a 3-year, randomized controlled study. Ann Neurol 2007;62(3):262–72.
33. Metman LV, Del Dotto P, LePoole K, et al. Amantadine for levodopa-induced dyskinesias: a 1-year follow-up study. Arch Neurol 1999;56(11):1383–6.
34. O'Suilleabhain P, Dewey RB Jr. A randomized trial of amantadine in Huntington disease. Arch Neurol 2003;60(7):996–8.
35. Mestre TA, Ferreira JJ. An evidence-based approach in the treatment of Huntington's disease. Parkinsonism Relat Disord 2012;18(4):316–20.

36. Reilmann R, McGarry A, Grachev ID, et al. Safety and efficacy of pridopidine in patients with Huntington's disease (PRIDE-HD): a phase 2, randomised, placebo-controlled, multicentre, dose-ranging study. Lancet Neurol 2019;18(2):165–76.

37. Bates GP, Dorsey R, Gusella JF, et al. Huntington disease. Nat Rev Dis Primers 2015;1:15005.

38. Wheelock VL, Tempkin T, Marder K, et al. Predictors of nursing home placement in Huntington disease. Neurology 2003;60(6):998–1001.

39. Vuong K, Canning CG, Menant JC, et al. Gait, balance, and falls in Huntington disease. Handb Clin Neurol 2018;159:251–60.

40. Bohlen S, Ekwall C, Hellstrom K, et al. Physical therapy in Huntington's disease–toward objective assessments? Eur J Neurol 2013;20(2):389–93.

41. Eddy CM, Parkinson EG, Rickards HE. Changes in mental state and behaviour in Huntington's disease. Lancet Psychiatry 2016;3(11):1079–86.

42. van Duijn E. Medical treatment of behavioral manifestations of Huntington disease. Handb Clin Neurol 2017;144:129–39.

43. Anderson KE, van Duijn E, Craufurd D, et al. Clinical management of neuropsychiatric symptoms of huntington disease: expert-based consensus guidelines on agitation, anxiety, apathy, psychosis and sleep disorders. J Huntingtons Dis 2018;7(3):355–66.

44. Hartmann CJ, Groiss SJ, Vesper J, et al. Brain stimulation in Huntington's disease. Neurodegener Dis Manag 2016;6(3):223–36.

45. Wojtecki L, Groiss SJ, Ferrea S, et al. A prospective pilot trial for pallidal deep brain stimulation in huntington's disease. Front Neurol 2015;6:177.

46. Gonzalez V, Cif L, Biolsi B, et al. Deep brain stimulation for Huntington's disease: long-term results of a prospective open-label study. J Neurosurg 2014;121(1): 114–22.

47. Zittel S, Tadic V, Moll CKE, et al. Prospective evaluation of Globus pallidus internus deep brain stimulation in Huntington's disease. Parkinsonism Relat Disord 2018;51:96–100.

48. Gruber D, Kuhn AA, Schoenecker T, et al. Quadruple deep brain stimulation in Huntington's disease, targeting pallidum and subthalamic nucleus: case report and review of the literature. J Neural Transm (Vienna) 2014;121(10):1303–12.

49. Yamamoto A, Lucas JJ, Hen R. Reversal of neuropathology and motor dysfunction in a conditional model of Huntington's disease. Cell 2000;101(1):57–66.

50. Lee CY, Cantle JP, Yang XW. Genetic manipulations of mutant huntingtin in mice: new insights into Huntington's disease pathogenesis. FEBS J 2013;280(18): 4382–94.

51. Rinaldi C, Wood MJA. Antisense oligonucleotides: the next frontier for treatment of neurological disorders. Nat Rev Neurol 2018;14(1):9–21.

52. Bashir H. Emerging therapies in Huntington's disease. Expert Rev Neurother 2019;1–13. https://doi.org/10.1080/14737175.2019.1631161.

53. Tabrizi SJ, Leavitt BR, Landwehrmeyer GB, et al. Targeting huntingtin expression in patients with huntington's disease. N Engl J Med 2019;380(24):2307–16.

54. Schulte J, Littleton JT. The biological function of the Huntingtin protein and its relevance to Huntington's disease pathology. Curr Trends Neurol 2011;5:65–78.

55. Miniarikova J, Evers MM, Konstantinova P. Translation of MicroRNA-based huntingtin-lowering therapies from preclinical studies to the clinic. Mol Ther 2018;26(4):947–62.

56. Southwell AL, Franciosi S, Villanueva EB, et al. Anti-semaphorin 4D immunotherapy ameliorates neuropathology and some cognitive impairment in the YAC128 mouse model of Huntington disease. Neurobiol Dis 2015;76:46–56.

57. Racette BA, Perlmutter JS. Levodopa responsive parkinsonism in an adult with Huntington's disease. J Neurol Neurosurg Psychiatry 1998;65(4):577–9.
58. Jongen PJ, Renier WO, Gabreels FJ. Seven cases of Huntington's disease in childhood and levodopa induced improvement in the hypokinetic–rigid form. Clin Neurol Neurosurg 1980;82(4):251–61.
59. Bonelli RM, Niederwieser G, Diez J, et al. Pramipexole ameliorates neurologic and psychiatric symptoms in a Westphal variant of Huntington's disease. Clin Neuropharmacol 2002;25(1):58–60.
60. Li Y, Hai S, Zhou Y, et al. Cholinesterase inhibitors for rarer dementias associated with neurological conditions. Cochrane Database Syst Rev 2015;(3):CD009444.

Treatment of Tardive Dyskinesia

Hassaan H. Bashir, MD, Joseph Jankovic, MD*

KEYWORDS

- Tardive dyskinesia • Tardive syndrome • VMAT2 inhibitors • Deutetrabenazine
- Valbenazine

KEY POINTS

- Tardive dyskinesia is a common movement disorder caused by treatment with antipsychotics ('neuroleptics') and other dopamine receptor blocking agents.
- The judicious use of dopamine receptor blocking agents is key to the prevention of tardive dyskinesia, reduction of disease burden, improvement in quality of life, and maintenance of remission.
- Deutetrabenazine and valbenazine are vesicular monoamine transporter 2 inhibitors approved by the FDA for the treatment of tardive dyskinesia, supported by high level evidence from pivotal clinical trials.
- Although evidence is limited, other treatment options can be considered in those who cannot tolerate or do not respond to vesicular monoamine transporter 2 inhibitors.
- Botulinum toxin or trihexyphenidyl can be considered for tardive dystonia and deep brain stimulation or electroconvulsive therapy can be considered for disabling symptoms refractory to other therapies.

INTRODUCTION AND OVERVIEW

The term, *tardive dyskinesia* (*TD*), originally was coined by Faurbye and colleagues[1] in their description of delayed-onset, persistent, rhythmic, stereotyped movements after exposure to dopamine receptor blocking agents (DRBAs). Initial studies focused on exposure to antipsychotics (or neuroleptics) but the DRBAs also include drugs used in the treatment of nausea (antiemetics), gastroparesis (promotility agents), and cough (antitussives). The original phenomenological descriptions focused on involuntary movements involving chiefly face, mouth, and tongue (orobuccolingual [OBL]), later classified as stereotypies; however, the phenomenology of TD gradually expanded to include other motor and nonmotor features.[2-4] This led to the concept of the tardive syndrome (TS), an umbrella term representing the full spectrum of hyperkinetic

Department of Neurology, Baylor College of Medicine, Parkinson's Disease Center and Movement Disorders Clinic, 7200 Cambridge, 9th Floor, Suite 9A, Houston, TX 77030-4202, USA
* Corresponding author.
E-mail address: josephj@bcm.edu

Neurol Clin 38 (2020) 379–396
https://doi.org/10.1016/j.ncl.2020.01.004
0733-8619/20/© 2020 Elsevier Inc. All rights reserved.
neurologic.theclinics.com

and hypokinetic movement disorders that include stereotypy, dystonia, akathisia, chorea, myoclonus, tics, tremor, parkinsonism, and gait disorders as well as ocular deviations, respiratory dyskinesia, and various sensory symptoms.[5,6] The use of the term, *extrapyramidal syndrome*, particularly popular among psychiatrists, is now strongly discouraged by experts for lack of clarity.[7]

The presentation of TS can vary from a mild, barely perceptible, orofacial movement or a feeling of irritation or a burning sensation in the mouth or genital area to a disabling and potentially even life-threatening condition that causes severe impairment in physical, mental, and social functioning.[8] Among the most serious forms of TS is status dystonicus as a complication of TD[9,10] and neuroleptic malignant syndrome.[11] TD has been associated with higher mortality among psychiatric patients.[12]

Epidemiologic studies have shown that TD is a common problem, associated with almost all DRBAs, except possibly clozapine.[13] Early studies of TD estimated prevalence rates among patients exposed to DRBAs ranging from 24% to 56% with an average closer to 20% to 30%.[14–16] In the era of typical (first-generation) antipsychotics, the risk of TD after exposure for 5 years was estimated to be 32%, 57% after 15 years and 68% after 25 years.[17] At first, the arrival of atypical (second-generation or third-generation) antipsychotics appeared to be associated with a lower risk of TD[18] (13.1% vs 32.4%); however, later studies did not confirm these findings.[19] The well-known Clinical Antipsychotic Trials of Intervention Effectiveness (CATIE) study, a large randomized clinical trial comparing effectiveness of typical and atypical antipsychotics in schizophrenia, failed to show decrease in TD with atypical antipsychotics.[20] A recent meta-analysis comparing typical and atypical antipsychotics across 41 studies between 2000 and 2015, estimated a mean prevalence of 25.3% for all treatment groups that was somewhat greater with typical antipsychotics (30%) versus atypical (20%) although the significance of this difference could not be determined because TD severity data were considered insufficient.[21] Unfortunately, prescribing rates for approved and off-label indications remain high and even may be increasing worldwide.[22] Antipsychotics are used frequently and inappropriately by physicians and allied professionals as an off-label treatment of depression, anxiety, insomnia, and other conditions.[23,24] This concerning trend highlights the importance of education about judicious use of antipsychotics.

Although the relationship of TD and antipsychotics is well established, drugs with the potential to cause TD also include antiemetics (metoclopramide, prochlorperazine, and promethazine), lithium, serotonin reuptake inhibitors (duloxetine and citalopram), tricyclic antidepressants (amoxapine and amitriptyline), and calcium channel blockers (cinnarizine and flunarizine).[3] Except for the antiemetics that act by blocking dopamine receptors, the other drugs appear to work through other mechanisms in causing TD. Compared with antipsychotics, however, the evidence for these drugs causing TD mostly are limited to case reports or case series.[25] A recent review of the literature found that rather than cause TD, both tricyclic antidepressants and selective serotonin reuptake inhibitors may unmask or exacerbate TD from prior or concurrent use of DRBAs, a possible priming effect.[26]

The exact cause of TD remains unknown although several theories have been proposed.[27] The mostly widely accepted theory is dopamine receptor supersensitivity, whereby chronic blockade of dopamine receptors leads to receptor up-regulation with subsequent postsynaptic supersensitivity. This theory is supported by the observation of reduction in TD when DRBA doses are increased and the exacerbation of TD with abrupt withdrawal of DRBAs (including a severe, potentially life-threatening variant known as withdrawal emergent dyskinesia).[28–32] This theory, however, does not explain the enduring symptoms of TD because the receptors would be expected to eventually down-regulate after DRBA discontinuation. It also does not explain the incidence of non-DRBAs causing TD. Alternatively, genetic factors, free radical damage, and aberrant, maladaptive synaptic plasticity also have been implicated in the pathophysiology of TD.[27]

Many risk factors have been identified for the development of TD.[33] Broadly, these are classified into modifiable and nonmodifiable factors. The modifiable include choice of DRBA, higher cumulative antipsychotic dose, prior acute dystonic reaction, diabetes, smoking, and alcohol/substance abuse, among others. The nonmodifiable include older age, female sex, white and African descent, intellectual disability, mood disorders, and genetic differences in antipsychotic metabolism.[27,33] An analysis of 189,415 patients treated with antipsychotics found the following predictors for the development of TD: age, diagnosis of schizophrenia, dosage of antipsychotic, and the presence of bipolar and related disorders.[34] Anticholinergics (eg, benztropine) frequently are coprescribed with antipsychotics by psychiatrists in an effort to reduce or prevent the onset of TD.[35] This practice is not supported, however, by evidence and even may precipitate or worsen TD.[36,37]

TD is an insidious, complex, and potentially devastating iatrogenic complication that has an impact on a substantial proportion of vulnerable patients; 2017 was a crucial year because it saw the approval of the first 2 medications to treat TD by the US Food and Drug Administration (FDA),[38] bringing renewed interest and much-needed investment in educating physicians, especially psychiatrists, in the diagnosis and treatment of TD. This article aims to provide the practicing neurologist with a succinct review of the treatment options for TD, with emphasis on recent developments.

MANAGEMENT GOALS

- Recognizing TD and effectively utilize rating scales, such as the Abnormal Involuntary Movement Scale (AIMS) to determine severity and monitor treatment response
- Initiating therapy with the highest level of evidence to reduce the signs and symptoms of TD
- Reducing deficits in physical, mental, and social functioning that are either a direct or indirect result of TD
- Minimize adverse effects (AEs) and the financial burden of treatment
- Emphasizing and promoting the judicious use of DRBAs
- Maintaining regular follow-up with frequent reassessments of the patient

GENERAL APPROACH

From the outset, the prevention of TD is of paramount importance. DRBAs should be avoided whenever possible by choosing alternative medication with lower or no risk of TD. If the use of a DRBA is necessary, then long-term treatment should be avoided whenever possible. Frequent reassessments must be utilized to determine if ongoing DRBA use is indicated and to remain vigilant for early symptoms and signs of TD. When TD is identified, DRBAs should be withdrawn slowly in patients who can tolerate it because abrupt withdrawal may worsen or precipitate TD (as well as the underlying psychiatric disorder when present).[29,39,40] Frequently, neurologists and psychiatrists must work together to provide multidisciplinary care to balance the risk of TD and management of underlying psychiatric illness. If patients require continued treatment, then every effort should be made to switch to medication with lower risk of TD. In the cases of antipsychotics, switching to clozapine or quetiapine may be considered because they have lower dopamine receptor affinity and relatively low risk of TD.[41,42] Pimavanserin, a nondopaminergic inverse serotonin agonist, is a novel antipsychotic approved for Parkinson disease psychosis[43] that also can be considered as an alternative, off-label treatment.[44] In cases of anti-emetics, those without dopamine receptor blocking activity should be considered first line (eg, ondansetron and trimethobenzamide). Even when the offending agent is withdrawn, remission rates may be as low as 13%.[45] This combination of increasing exposure rates and low remission rates highlights the need for effective treatment of TD. It also has led to the increased use of off-label treatments. Despite best efforts to minimize the risks of TD, a substantial proportion of patients will develop TD and require pharmacologic and/or surgical treatment. **Fig. 1** outlines a general approach to treatment of TD.

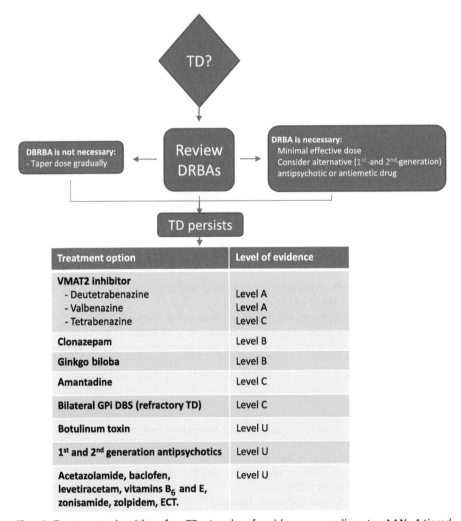

Fig. 1. Treatment algorithm for TD. Levels of evidence according to AAN 4-tiered scheme = level A (established as effective), level B (probably effective), level C (possibly effective), and level U (data inadequate)[55] (updated and modified).(*Adapted* from Bhidaya-siri R, Jitkritsadakul O, Friedman JH, Fahn S. Updating the recommendations for treatment of tardive syndromes: A systematic review of new evidence and practical treatment algo-rithm. J Neurol Sci. 2018;389:67-75; with permission.)

PHARMACOLOGIC TREATMENTS
Vesicular Monoamine Transporter Type 2 Inhibitors

Although the pathogenesis of TD is not fully understood, the finding that increased dopamine signaling plays an important role led to the pursuit of agents that could modulate signaling without directly blocking receptors. The vesicular monoamine transporters (VMATs) are transport proteins integrated into the synaptic vesicles of presynaptic neurons and exist as 2 isoforms, VMAT1 and VMAT2.[46] VMATs facilitate the transport of cytoplasmic monoamines (dopamine, histamine, norepinephrine, and serotonin) into presynaptic vesicles. In contrast to VMAT1, which is localized in both the central and peripheral nervous system, VMAT2 is found only in central presynaptic neurons.[46,47] Inhibition of VMATs thus reduces presynaptic storage and release of monoamines, particularly dopamine, which then are degraded by monoamine oxidase in the cytoplasm, resulting in presynaptic dopamine depletion.[13] Selective VMAT2 inhibition is preferred, because VMAT1 inhibitors, such as reserpine (a nonselective VMAT inhibitor used to treat hypertension and hyperkinetic movement disorders), are associated with multiple peripheral AEs such as bronchospasm, nausea, vomiting, hypotension, and nasal stuffiness.[47] Three selective VMAT2 inhibitors currently are available for the treatment of TD: tetrabenazine (TBZ), deutetrabenazine (DTBZ), and valbenazine (VBZ). **Table 1** provides a summarized comparison of these medications.

Tetrabenazine

TBZ originally was developed in the 1950s to treat psychosis and in 1971 it was introduced in the United Kingdom for the treatment of hyperkinetic movement disorders.[48] It was not until 2008 that it was approved in the United States for the treatment of Huntington chorea; however, it frequently is prescribed for off-label indications, including TD.[49]

Kazamatsuri and colleagues[50] reported the first clinical trial of TBZ in TD in 1972. This prospective, single-blind study of 24 chronic psychiatric patients with TD at

Table 1
Comparison of vesicular monoamine transporter type 2 inhibitors

Characteristic	Tetrabenazine (Xenazine)	Deutetrabenazine (Austedo)	Valbenazine (Ingrezza)
Mechanism of action	Reversible VMAT2 inhibitor	Reversible VMAT2 inhibitor	Reversible VMAT2 inhibitor
US FDA approval (y)	HD chorea (2008)	HD chorea (2017), TD (2017)	TD (2017)
Pivotal trials	TETRA-HD	First-HD, AIM-TD, ARM-TD	KINECT 2, KINECT 3
Active metabolites	Yes	Yes	Yes
Half-life	5–7 h	9–10 h	15–22 h
Dose range (recommended)	12.5–100 mg/d	6–48 mg/d	40–80 mg/d
Safety data	>40 y	>2 y	>2 y
AE profile	1. Sedation 2. Parkinsonism 3. Depression	1. Sedation 2. Insomnia (similar to placebo)	1. Sedation 2. Headache 3. Fatigue

Abbreviation: HD, Huntington disease.

Boston State Hospital began with a 4-week baseline period in which medications were not changed (14 patients were taking DRBAs) followed by 4 weeks on placebo where all DRBAs were discontinued; then, a 6-week treatment period with TBZ starting at 50 mg/d titrated to 100 mg/d to 150 mg/d. It ended with a 2-week TBZ washout period on placebo. The primary outcome measure was mean frequency of dyskinetic movements per minute as reported by a blinded rater; 8 patients (33%) had complete resolution of TD, 6 (25%) had marked improvement; another 6 had little or no change; and 4 patients did not complete the study (2 developed severe malaise, 1 withdrew due to exacerbation of psychosis, and 1 was lost to follow-up).[50] Compared with placebo, TBZ was found to significantly reduce TD by 64%. Ondo and colleagues[51] reported a prospective, single-blind study of 20 patients with TD (mean duration 43.7 months) who were videotaped before and after treatment with TBZ. One patient withdrew from the study due to sedation. Videotapes were randomized and scored using the motor subset of the AIMS by a blinded rater. The average improvement on the AIMS score was 54.2% (from 17.9 to 8.2; $P<.0001$) after an average treatment period of 20.3 weeks on a mean daily dose of 57.9 mg/d, 11 patients rated themselves as markedly improved, 6 as moderately improved, and 2 as moderately improved.[51]

Two large, retrospective reports of TBZ in hyperkinetic movement disorders have supported its beneficial role in TD.[52,53] Combined, they report greater than 84% of TD patients (a total of 242 patients) that rated their improvement as either moderate or marked. These 2 studies also shed light on the most common AEs of TBZ, which included sedation (25.0%–36.5%), parkinsonism (15.4%–28.5%), depression (7.6%–15.0%), insomnia (4.9%–11.0%), anxiety (5.1%–10.3%), and akathisia (7.6%–9.5%).[52,53] Essentially, all TBZ-related AEs have been shown to be dose related and decrease with dose reduction. They also can be managed with antidepressants, stimulants, and other pharmacologic strategies if patients otherwise benefit from TBZ. Both the 2013 American Academy of Neurology (AAN) guideline and a recently published systematic review gave TBZ a level C (possibly effective) recommendation in the consideration of treatment of TD, based on lack of double-blind, placebo-controlled studies.[54,55]

TBZ is quickly metabolized into α-dihydrotetrabenazine and β-dihydrotetrabenazine (half-life 5–7 h) via hepatic isoenzyme CYP2D6. Because of its short half-life, TBZ typically is dosed 3 times a day.[56] TBZ should be started at low doses (12.5–25 mg/d) with careful titration (typical therapeutic dose, 50–75 mg/d) and monitoring for AEs. It is recommended by the FDA that patients receiving more than 50 mg of TBZ per day be genotyped for CYP2D6, but the various genotypes do not reliably predict the frequency of AEs.[56] With this need for frequent dosing and a side-effect profile restricting its use, a strong interest grew in the development of novel VMAT2 inhibitors. Although TBZ has been approved for the treatment of chorea associated with Huntington disease, it has not been approved for the treatment of TD.

Deutetrabenazine

DTBZ is a deuterated version of TBZ, incorporating 6 atoms of the naturally occurring and nontoxic isotope deuterium or heavy hydrogen in its molecule.[47] Deuterium-carbon bonds are stronger than hydrogen-carbon bonds, thus more resistant to metabolizing cytochrome P450 enzymes like CYP2D6.[57] This provides significant pharmacokinetic advantage (ie, longer half-life) over TBZ without altering target pharmacology. DTBZ is dosed twice a day versus 3 times daily (half-life 9–10 h), with a lower dose per administration to achieve similar clinical effect (6 mg of DTBZ is approximately the equivalent of 12.5 mg TBZ).[58] DTBZ first obtained FDA approval for the treatment of Huntington chorea in April 2017 after the pivotal First-HD trial demonstrated safety and efficacy.[59,60] This was followed by approval for the treatment of TD in August 2017 based on the results of 2 pivotal trials, Aim to Reduce Movements in Tardive Dyskinesia (ARM-TD) and Addressing Involuntary Movements in Tardive Dyskinesia (AIM-TD).[61,62]

ARM-TD was a phase 3, double-blind, multicenter trial of 177 patients with moderate to severe TD (AIMS $\geq$6) that were randomized 1:1 to either placebo or DTBZ.[61] Patients were allowed to continue DRBAs provided there was no recent change in medications. The DTBZ group was started at 12 mg/d, with weekly titration of 6 mg/d until either adequate TD control was achieved, a significant AE occurred, or the maximal allowable dose of 48 mg/d was reached. This was followed by a 6-week maintenance period and 1-week washout. The primary endpoint was the change in AIMS score from baseline to week 12 as assessed by 2 blinded video raters who were movement disorder specialists. Secondary endpoints included treatment success at week 12 on the Clinical Global Impression of Change (CGIC) and Patient Global Impression of Change (PGIC). The mean daily dose was 38.8 mg at the end of the study period. There was a mean 3.0-point reduction in AIMS score for DTBZ versus 1.6 in the placebo group ($P = .019$), a treatment difference of 1.4. Although the percentage of patients who achieved treatment success on the CGIC (48.2% vs 40.4%) and PGIC (42.9% vs 29.8%) favored DTBZ, these differences did not reach statistical significance. Most common AEs for DTBZ versus placebo were somnolence (13.8% vs 10.2%), insomnia (6.9% vs 1.7%), and akathisia (5.2% vs 0%). Discontinuation rates because of AEs were 1.7% versus 3.4%, respectively. Neither DTBZ nor placebo group experienced any worsening in parkinsonism and rates of psychiatric AEs were low: anxiety (3.4% vs 6.8%), depressed mood/depression (1.7% vs 1.7%), and suicidal ideation (0% vs 1.7%).

AIM-TD was a second-phase 3, double-blind, multicenter trial of 298 patients randomized 1:1:1:1 to receive fixed doses of DTBZ 12 mg/d, 24 mg/d, 36 mg/d, or matching placebo for 8 weeks after a 4-week titration period.[62] The primary endpoint was change in AIMS score from baseline to week 12 based on blinded video assessments. From baseline to week 12, change in least squares mean AIMS score improved by −3.3 points in the DTBZ 36 mg/d group, −3.24 in the 24 mg/d group, and −2.1 points in the 12 mg/d group, with a significant treatment difference of −1.9 points ($P = .001$), −1.8 points ($P = .003$), and −0.7 points ($P = .217$), respectively, compared with placebo.[62] The investigators defined treatment success as "much improved" or "very much improved" on the CGIC, which was accomplished in 49% of patients receiving 24 mg/d ($P = .014$) and 44% of those receiving 36 mg/d ($P = .059$) compared with 28% with 12 mg/d and 26% with placebo. There was no significant difference in PGIC outcomes between DTBZ and placebo. The most common AE was headache (5%). There were no other single AEs for DTBZ (all doses pooled) with incidence greater than or equal to 5% or greater than that observed for placebo. Discontinuation rates because of AEs were 4.1% for DTBZ (all doses pooled) versus 2.8% for placebo. 2 patients (1%) died, 1 each in the 24 mg/d and 36 mg/d groups; neither death was deemed related to study drug.[62]

Pooling the data across both trials,[63] the number needed to treat (NNT) for greater than 50% reduction of the AIMS score at the therapeutic doses of DTBZ versus placebo was 7 (95% CI, 4–18). DTBZ was well tolerated, with low rates of AEs in both ARM-TD and AIM-TD. AE-related discontinuation occurred among 3.6% of patients randomized to DTBZ (at any dose) versus 3.1% for placebo, yielding a number needed to harm of 189 (not significant). A recently published open-label extension study, analyzing 331 patients treated for a mean of 352.9 days, confirmed safety outcomes of both trials, demonstrating that DTBZ is well tolerated for long-term use in TD patients.[64] DTBZ has received a level A (established as effective) recommendation for the treatment of TD.[55]

Valbenazine

The metabolites of TBZ possess several chiral centers that generate isomers with different VMAT2 binding affinity.[65] Once characterized, VBZ was developed as a purified parent drug of TBZ that metabolizes into an isomer of α-dihydrotetrabenazine with a combined half-life of 15 hours to 22 hours.[66] This allowed for a convenient once-daily dosing. VBZ also was designed to metabolize slowly, minimizing high peak plasma concentrations thereby improving tolerability.[66] Its limited range of metabolites reduces the likelihood of off-target effects that can occur with TBZ metabolites.[47,66] These pharmacokinetic and pharmacodynamic advantages made VBZ an attractive agent for further study in TD.

KINECT 2 was a phase 2, 6-week, double-blind, placebo-controlled dose-titration study that randomized 102 patients with moderate or severe TD to placebo or VBZ, 25 mg/d, with titration to a maximum of 75 mg/d; 76% of the VBZ group reached this maximum allowed dose.[67] The primary efficacy endpoint was change in AIMS from baseline at week 6 scored by 2 blinded video raters. Secondary efficacy endpoint was CGIC. At week 6, least squares mean AIMS scores were reduced by −2.6 points for the VBZ group compared with −0.2 for placebo ($P = .0005$).[67] CGIC and PGIC results also favored VBZ versus placebo as a rating of "much improved" or "very much improved" occurred in 66.7% versus 15.9% ($P<.0001$) and 57.8% versus 31.8% ($P = .001$), respectively. Treatment-emergent AE rates were 49% in the VBZ and 33% in the placebo subjects. The most common AE (VBZ vs placebo) were fatigue and headache (9.8% vs 4.1%) and constipation and urinary tract infection (3.9% vs 6.1%). These results supported further study in a phase 3 trial.

KINECT 3 was a phase 3, randomized, double-blind, placebo-controlled trial of VBZ in TD.[68] It was designed similarly KINECT to 2. This 6-week study randomized 234 patients (of whom 86% received concomitant DRBAs) 1:1:1 to once-daily placebo or VBZ (40 or 80 mg/d). Least squares mean AIMS scores improved by −1.9 points for VBZ, 40 mg/d ($P = .002$); −3.2 for VBZ, 80 mg/d ($P<.001$); and only −0.1 for placebo. In a pooled analysis of both trials, 36.5% of patients receiving VBZ (both doses) versus 12.4% receiving placebo had a greater than 50% reduction of AIMS scores, yielding an NNT of 5 (95% CI, 3–7).[69] The most common AEs reported (VBZ vs placebo) were somnolence (5.4 vs 3.2%), headache (4.5 vs 3.2%), fatigue (4.0 vs 2.4%), dry mouth (4.0 vs 0.8%), vomiting (3.0 vs 0%), and urinary tract infection (2.5 vs 4.8%).[69] KINECT 3 did note that 4.2% of VBZ patients reported akathisia and suicidal ideation versus 1.3% and 5.3% in placebo, respectively.[68] The 1-year KINECT 3 extension study of 198 patients supported long-term efficacy, safety, and tolerability of VBZ in TD.[70] The recently published data from KINECT 4 (clinicaltrials.gov, NCT02405091), which included 48 weeks of open-label treatment with VBZ followed by a 4-week washout, demonstrated sustained and clinically meaningful improvement of TD, and VBZ generally was well tolerated without notable changes in the psychiatric status of patients.[71]

Based on these data, VBZ received FDA approval for the treatment of TD in April 2017. VBZ has a level A recommendation for the treatment of TD.[55]

Non–vesicular Monoamine Transporter Type 2 Pharmacologic Agents

Benzodiazepines

The γ-aminobutyric acid (GABA)ergic system has been implicated in the pathophysiology of TD.[72] Benzodiazepines are allosteric GABA$_A$ agonists that hyperpolarize neurons by increasing Cl$^-$ influx and frequently are used in the treatment of TD.[73]

Clonazepam was evaluated in a 12-week, double-blind, randomized, crossover trial of 19 chronically ill patients with TD taking DRBAs.[74] Overall, a 37.1% reduction (P<.001) in dyskinesia was noted from baseline after 12 weeks using the Maryland Psychiatric Research Center movement disorders scale. Patients with dystonic symptoms (n = 6) showed greater benefit (41.5% reduction) than the remainder with choreoathetoid dyskinesia (n = 13; 26.5% reduction).[74] The investigators followed 5 patients for an additional 9 months and noted they developed tolerance to clonazepam; however, an antidyskinetic effect was recaptured after a 2-week drug holiday. Clonazepam has a level B recommendation (probably effective) for the treatment of TD.[55]

Diazepam and alprazolam are shorter-acting benzodiazepines for which the effectiveness in TD remains unclear. An open-label study of 21 patients with TD demonstrated improvement in AIMS scores with diazepam.[75] A 24-week, randomized, placebo-controlled, crossover study of 13 patients using blinded rating did not find improvement with diazepam.[76] A small study comparing alprazolam, diazepam, and placebo showed no benefit for TD.[77] Alprazolam has not been studied in a randomized trials; only case reports have been described.[78]

Ginkgo biloba

Ginkgo biloba extract (EGb-761) is obtained from the fan-shaped leaves and seeds of the Ginkgo biloba tree (or maidenhair tree) and has antioxidative properties.[79] It is among the most sold medicinal plants in the world and commonly used in traditional Chinese medicine. In a 12-week, double-blind, randomized, placebo-controlled trial of 157 patients with schizophrenia and TD, EGb-761 reduced AIMS scores by an average of 2.13 (P<.001) compared with 0.1 for placebo[80]; 51.3% of patients in the EGb-761 group experienced greater than 30% reduction in AIMS score compared with just 5.1% of placebo (P<.001). Although additional studies are needed to confirm these data, Gingko biloba has been given a level B recommendation for the treatment of TD.[55]

Amantadine

Amantadine, initially developed as an antiviral agent, is a noncompetitive N-methyl-$_D$-aspartate antagonist with antiglutamatergic properties, now commonly used in the management of levodopa-induced dyskinesias.[81] It was first reported to improve TD in 1971 after 2 small case series.[82,83] The investigators subsequently performed 2 double-blind, crossover studies of amantadine 100 mg 3 times and twice daily versus matching placebo for 10 days (14 patients and 10 patients, respectively) that were negative.[84] More recently, 2 small studies evaluated amantadine in TD patients taking DRBAs and noted positive results.[85,86] Angus and colleagues[85] reported a double-blind, randomized, placebo-controlled, 7-week-per-arm, crossover trial of amantadine initiated at 100 mg/d and titrated to 300 mg/d maintained for 3 weeks. The mean AIMS score was significantly lower in the amantadine group than placebo (7.312 vs 8.188; P<.05). Pappa and colleagues[86] reported a double-blind, randomized, placebo-controlled, 2-week-per-arm, crossover trial of amantadine up to 400 mg/d. Patients receiving amantadine exhibited a reduced mean AIMS score (13.5–10.5; P = .000) whereas the placebo group showed no reduction. These studies supported the short-term use of amantadine; however, given the mixed results and small study sizes, amantadine has a level C recommendation for the treatment of TD.[55]

Other Pharmacologic Treatments

There are several other oral agents for which there is insufficient evidence to support their use in TD.[54,55] These include cholinergic agents (eg, donepezil, physostigmine, choline, and galantamine),[87,88] anticholinergics (eg, benztropine),[37] antioxidants other than Ginkgo biloba (eg, vitamin B_6 and vitamin E), baclofen, buspirone, eicosapentaenoic acid, calcium channel blockers, acetazolamide, melatonin, zonisamide, and propranolol.[55]

Trihexyphenidyl, an anticholinergic, showed improvement in TD from data of 2 retrospective studies using 10 mg/d to 32 mg/d in 3 of 8 patients[89] and 6 mg/d to 12 mg/d in 8 of 21 patients.[90] This is consistent with the observation that anticholinergics are useful in primary dystonia.[91] The risk of cognitive AEs and worsening of OBL stereotypies, however, limit their use and it is generally discouraged in TD.[92,93]

Zolpidem, a nonbenzodiazepine hypnotic, has been reported to be effective for the treatment of TD and tardive akathisia in a small series of 3 patients.[94] Placebo-controlled study is needed to further document effectiveness of zolpidem in TD.

Levetiracetam is an antiepileptic that targets synaptic vesicle glycoprotein 2A and may modulate vesicle release.[95] Two small open-label trials[96,97] and a small randomized trial[98] demonstrated reduced severity of TD. The latter was a 12-week, double-blind study of 50 patients receiving levetiracetam (500–3000 mg/d) versus placebo. AIMS scores declined 43.5% from baseline in the levetiracetam group compared with 18.7% for placebo ($P = .022$); however, there was a high dropout rate because of psychiatric disorientation, nonadherence, loss to follow-up, and unrelated stressors.[98] Although the results were somewhat promising, further studies have not been done and levetiracetam has been given a has been given a level U (inadequate evidence) recommendation for the treatment of TD.[55]

Lastly, although there is some evidence that initiating or switching to atypical antipsychotics can help reduce TD,[99,100] based on the knowledge that all atypical antipsychotics (with the possible exception of clozapine) can cause TD, both the 2013 AAN guidelines and a recent systematic review do not recommend the use of these agents to treat TD.[54,55]

DEEP BRAIN STIMULATION

Deep brain stimulation (DBS) is a well-recognized and widely used treatment option for many movement disorders, including Parkinson disease, essential tremor, and dystonia.[101] DBS in TD typically is reserved for severe, disabling, medically refractory cases (level C recommendation).[55] A recent systematic review and metanalysis found that the majority of DBS studies in TD to date are open-label case reports or part of open-label case series of dystonia of various etiologies.[102] All cases were related to use of neuroleptics, except those of 2 patients, which were a result of metoclopramide exposure.[103,104] A majority of cases target bilateral posteroventral globus pallidus internus (GPi), although a few cases of subthalamic nucleus DBS also have been successfully reported with long-term follow-up.[105,106] Across 51 cases of DBS in classical TD, in which the outcome measure was change in AIMS score, the mean percentage of AIMS score improvement was 62 ± 15% after DBS surgery (median 58%; range 33%–90%).[102] In cases of TD, the Burke-Fahn-Marsden (BFM) scale has been most widely used. The BFM motor score improvement across 67 cases was 76 ± 21% after DBS (median 82%; range 7%–100%).[102] The limitations of these data are the differences across case reports, including phenomenology, severity, clinical assessments, frequency of follow-up, and the lack of prospective, controlled trial.

OTHER TREATMENT OPTIONS
Botulinum Toxin

Botulinum neurotoxin (BoNT) is derived from *Clostridium* bacteria and acts on presynaptic vesicular release complex proteins to reduce neurotransmission.[107] It has emerged as one the most versatile therapeutic options in medicine. Within movement disorders, BoNT type A (onabotulinumtoxinA) is approved for the treatment of blepharospasm, craniocervical dystonia, and limb spasticity.[107] There have been no controlled trials studying the effects of BoNT in the treatment of TD. Several case reports, case series, and open-label reports, however, have shown promising results.[108–110] A majority of reports include patients with focal symptoms, such as OBL stereotypies or TD that had failed other pharmacologic treatments. Slotema and colleagues[111] performed a single-blind (raters only) 33-week study of 12 patients with orofacial TD receiving BoNT every 3 months for 3 treatments. Although there was a nonsignificant ($P = .15$) reduction in TD severity overall, in the patients with no change in their antipsychotic medication (ie, stable doses; n = 8), the reduction was significant (AIMS score 4.81–3.0; $P = .035$). After the study, 50% of the patients preferred to continue treatment with BoNT. Notable limitations of BoNT in the treatment of TD are the need for technical expertise (which can vary significantly between injectors), need for reinjection, and the potential for perioral, lingual, or neck injections to cause dysarthria and dysphagia. In the absence of controlled trials, BoNT currently has a level U recommendation for the treatment of TD.[55]

Electroconvulsive Therapy

Electroconvulsive therapy (ECT) uses a small electric current to produce a generalized cerebral seizure under general anesthesia, primarily used for the management of severe, treatment-resistant psychiatric conditions.[112] Multiple case reports have described improvement of TD after ECT in patients treated for depression or schizophrenia.[113–115] Yasui-Furukori and colleagues[116] reported a retrospective series of 18 patients receiving ECT that demonstrated a mean AIMS score improvement from 19.1 ± 4.7 to 9.6 ± 4.2. These findings contrast with reports (albeit quite dated) of worsening TD,[117] emergence of TD,[118] or no change in TD[119] with ECT. Overall, the 2013 AAN guidelines concluded that there is insufficient evidence (level U) for the efficacy of ECT in treating TD.[54]

SUMMARY

The aim of this review is to provide a summary of the current treatment options for TD with emphasis on recent developments; 2017 was a pivotal year for TD with the approval of 2 new drugs, VBZ and DTBZ, bringing with them renewed interest and attention to the condition. The management of TD remains challenging, however, given the heterogeneity of cases and limited treatment options. There are many important areas of research specifically addressing those patients who remain refractory to treatment despite recent developments. As discussed previously, many other agents with different mechanisms and tolerance profiles have shown promise but need to be studied in large, controlled, multicenter trials. In an era of precision medicine, better understanding the pathophysiology and underlying genetics of TD will lead to new, targeted treatments. The development of patient registries to provide long-term data will be essential for such endeavors. Conceivably, the development of newer antipsychotics that do not cause TD may reduce disease burden significantly. Physician education, however, regarding the judicious use of current DRBAs remains central to the prevention and management of TD.

DISCLOSURE

Dr H.H. Bashir has nothing to disclose. Dr J. Jankovic has received research/training funding from Allergan; CHDI Foundation; Dystonia Coalition; F. Hoffmann-La Roche Ltd; Huntington Study Group; Medtronic Neuromodulation; Merz

Pharmaceuticals; Michael J Fox Foundation for Parkinson Research; National Institutes of Health; Neurocrine Biosciences; Parkinson's Foundation; Parkinson Study Group; Revance Therapeutics, Inc; and Teva Pharmaceutical Industries. He has served as a consultant/advisory board member for Abide; Aeon BioPharma; Nuvelution; Retrophin; and Teva Pharmaceutical Industries Ltd. He has served on editorial boards of *Expert Review of Neurotherapeutics*; *Journal of Parkinson's Disease*; Medlink; *Neurology in Clinical Practice*; *The Botulinum Journal*; PeerJ; *Therapeutic Advances in Neurologic Disorders*; *Neurotherapeutics*; *Tremor and Other Hyperkinetic Movements*; *Toxins*; and UpToDate. He has received royalties from Cambridge; Elsevier; Future Science Group; Hodder Arnold; Medlink: Neurology; Lippincott Williams and Wilkins; and Wiley-Blackwell.

REFERENCES

1. Faurbye A, Rasch PJ, Petersen PB, et al. Neurological symptoms in pharmacotherapy of psychoses. Acta Psychiatr Scand 1964;40(1):10–27.
2. Uhrbrand L, Faurbye A. Reversible and irreversible dyskinesia after treatment with perphenazine, chlorpromazine, reserpine and electroconvulsive therapy. Psychopharmacologia 1960;1(5):408–18.
3. Waln O, Jankovic J. An update on tardive dyskinesia: from phenomenology to treatment. Tremor Other Hyperkinet Mov (N Y) 2013;3:1–11.
4. Macaluso M, Flynn A, Preskorn SH. Tardive dyskinesia: a historical perspective. J Psychiatr Pract 2017;23(2):121–9.
5. Savitt D, Jankovic J. Tardive syndromes. J Neurol Sci 2018;389:35–42.
6. Frei K, Truong DD, Fahn S, et al. The nosology of tardive syndromes. J Neurol Sci 2018;389:10–6.
7. Obeso JA. The Movement Disorders journal 2016 and onward. Mov Disord 2016;31(1):1–2.
8. McEvoy J, Carroll B, Gandhi S, et al. Effect of tardive dyskinesia on quality of life: patient-reported symptom severity is associated with deficits in physical, mental, and social functioning (P4.077). Neurology 2018;90(15 Supplement): P4.077.
9. Kovacs N, Balas I, Janszky J, et al. Status dystonicus in tardive dystonia successfully treated by bilateral deep brain stimulation. Clin Neurol Neurosurg 2011;113(9):808–9.
10. Rohani M, Munhoz RP, Shahidi G, et al. Fatal status dystonicus in tardive dystonia due to depletion of deep brain stimulation's pulse generator. Brain Stimul 2017;10(1):160–1.
11. Pileggi DJ, Cook AM. Neuroleptic malignant syndrome. Ann Pharmacother 2016;50(11):973–81.
12. Ballesteros J, González-Pinto A, Bulbena A. Tardive dyskinesia associated with higher mortality in psychiatric patients: results of a meta-analysis of seven independent studies. J Clin Psychopharmacol 2000;20(2):188–94.
13. Niemann N, Jankovic J. Treatment of tardive dyskinesia: a general overview with focus on the vesicular monoamine transporter 2 inhibitors. Drugs 2018;78(5): 525–41.
14. Tepper SJ, Haas JF. Prevalence of tardive dyskinesia. J Clin Psychiatry 1979; 40(12):508–16.
15. Kane JM, Woerner M, Lieberman J. Tardive dyskinesia: prevalence, incidence, and risk factors. J Clin Psychopharmacol 1988;8(4 Suppl):52S–6S.

16. Gardos G, Casey DE, Cole JO, et al. Ten-year outcome of tardive dyskinesia. Am J Psychiatry 1994;151(6):836–41.
17. Glazer WM, Morgenstern H, Doucette JT. Predicting the long-term risk of tardive dyskinesia in outpatients maintained on neuroleptic medications. J Clin Psychiatry 1993;54(4):133–9.
18. Correll CU, Schenk EM. Tardive dyskinesia and new antipsychotics. Curr Opin Psychiatry 2008;21(2):151–6.
19. Woods SW, Morgenstern H, Saksa JR, et al. Incidence of tardive dyskinesia with atypical versus conventional antipsychotic medications: a prospective cohort study. J Clin Psychiatry 2010;71(4):463–74.
20. Miller DD, Caroff SN, Davis SM, et al. Extrapyramidal side-effects of antipsychotics in a randomised trial. Br J Psychiatry 2008;193(4):279–88.
21. Carbon M, Kane JM, Leucht S, et al. Tardive dyskinesia risk with first- and second-generation antipsychotics in comparative randomized controlled trials: a meta-analysis. World Psychiatry 2018;17(3):330–40.
22. Hálfdánarson Ó, Zoëga H, Aagaard L, et al. International trends in antipsychotic use: a study in 16 countries, 2005-2014. Eur Neuropsychopharmacol 2017; 27(10):1064–76.
23. Domino ME, Swartz MS. Who are the new users of antipsychotic medications? Psychiatr Serv 2008;59(5):507–14.
24. Mulder R, Hamilton A, Irwin L, et al. Treating depression with adjunctive antipsychotics. Bipolar Disord 2018;20(Suppl 2):17–24.
25. D'Abreu A, Akbar U, Friedman JH. Tardive dyskinesia: epidemiology. J Neurol Sci 2018;389:17–20.
26. D'Abreu A, Friedman JH. Tardive dyskinesia-like syndrome due to drugs that do not block dopamine receptors: rare or non-existent: literature review. Tremor Other Hyperkinet Mov (N Y) 2018;8:570.
27. Frei K. Tardive dyskinesia: who gets it and why. Parkinsonism Relat Disord 2019; 59:151–4.
28. Lo Y-C, Peng Y-C. Amisulpride withdrawal dyskinesia: a case report. Ann Gen Psychiatry 2017;16:25.
29. Thomson AM, Wallace J, Kobylecki C. Tardive dyskinesia after drug withdrawal in two older adults: clinical features, complications and management. Geriatr Gerontol Int 2019;19(6):563–4.
30. Pugin D, Bally J, Horvath J, et al. Life-threatening neuroleptic withdrawal emergent syndrome resembling status dystonicus. Parkinsonism Relat Disord 2017; 35:96–7.
31. Cerovecki A, Musil R, Klimke A, et al. Withdrawal symptoms and rebound syndromes associated with switching and discontinuing atypical antipsychotics: theoretical background and practical recommendations. CNS Drugs 2013; 27(7):545–72.
32. Mejia NI, Jankovic J. Tardive dyskinesia and withdrawal emergent syndrome in children. Expert Rev Neurother 2010;10(6):893–901.
33. Solmi M, Pigato G, Kane JM, et al. Clinical risk factors for the development of tardive dyskinesia. J Neurol Sci 2018;389:21–7.
34. Patterson-Lomba O, Ayyagari R, Carroll B. 62 predictors of tardive dyskinesia in psychiatric patients taking concomitant antipsychotics. CNS Spectr 2019;24(1): 207–8.
35. Wijegunaratne H, Qazi H, Koola MM. Chronic and bedtime use of benztropine with antipsychotics: is it necessary? Schizophr Res 2014;153(1–3):248–9.

36. Miller DD, McEvoy JP, Davis SM, et al. Clinical correlates of tardive dyskinesia in schizophrenia: baseline data from the CATIE schizophrenia trial. Schizophr Res 2005;80(1):33–43.
37. Bergman H, Soares-Weiser K. Anticholinergic medication for antipsychotic-induced tardive dyskinesia. Cochrane Database Syst Rev 2018;(1):CD000204.
38. Hauser RA, Truong D. Tardive dyskinesia: out of the shadows. J Neurol Sci 2018; 389:1–3.
39. Vijayakumar D, Jankovic J. Drug-induced dyskinesia, part 2: treatment of tardive dyskinesia. Drugs 2016;76(7):779–87.
40. Viguera AC, Baldessarini RJ, Hegarty JD, et al. Clinical risk following abrupt and gradual withdrawal of maintenance neuroleptic treatment. Arch Gen Psychiatry 1997;54(1):49–55.
41. Mentzel TQ, van der Snoek R, Lieverse R, et al. Clozapine monotherapy as a treatment for antipsychotic-induced tardive dyskinesia: a meta-analysis. J Clin Psychiatry 2018;79(6).
42. Ricciardi L, Pringsheim T, Barnes TRE, et al. Treatment recommendations for tardive dyskinesia. Can J Psychiatry 2019;64(6):388–99.
43. Hawkins T, Berman BD. Pimavanserin: a novel therapeutic option for Parkinson disease psychosis. Neurol Clin Pract 2017;7(2):157–62.
44. Nasrallah HA, Fedora R, Morton R. Successful treatment of clozapine-nonresponsive refractory hallucinations and delusions with pimavanserin, a serotonin 5HT-2A receptor inverse agonist. Schizophr Res 2019;208:217–20.
45. Zutshi D, Cloud LJ, Factor SA. Tardive syndromes are rarely reversible after discontinuing dopamine receptor blocking agents: experience from a university-based movement disorder clinic. Tremor Other Hyperkinet Mov (N Y) 2014; 4:266.
46. Yaffe D, Forrest LR, Schuldiner S. The ins and outs of vesicular monoamine transporters. J Gen Physiol 2018;150(5):671–82.
47. Jankovic J. Dopamine depleters in the treatment of hyperkinetic movement disorders. Expert Opin Pharmacother 2016;17(18):2461–70.
48. Chen JJ, Ondo WG, Dashtipour K, et al. Tetrabenazine for the treatment of hyperkinetic movement disorders: a review of the literature. Clin Ther 2012;34(7): 1487–504.
49. Niemann N, Jankovic J. Real-world experience with VMAT2 inhibitors. Clin Neuropharmacol 2019;42(2):37–41.
50. Kazamatsuri H, Chien C, Cole JO. Treatment of tardive dyskinesia. I. Clinical efficacy of a dopamine-depleting agent, tetrabenazine. Arch Gen Psychiatry 1972;27(1):95–9.
51. Ondo WG, Hanna PA, Jankovic J. Tetrabenazine treatment for tardive dyskinesia: assessment by randomized videotape protocol. Am J Psychiatry 1999; 156(8):1279–81.
52. Jankovic J, Beach J. Long-term effects of tetrabenazine in hyperkinetic movement disorders. Neurology 1997;48(2):358–62.
53. Kenney C, Hunter C, Jankovic J. Long-term tolerability of tetrabenazine in the treatment of hyperkinetic movement disorders. Mov Disord 2007;22(2):193–7.
54. Bhidayasiri R, Fahn S, Weiner WJ, et al. Evidence-based guideline: treatment of tardive syndromes: report of the Guideline Development Subcommittee of the American Academy of Neurology. Neurology 2013;81(5):463–9.
55. Bhidayasiri R, Jitkritsadakul O, Friedman JH, et al. Updating the recommendations for treatment of tardive syndromes: a systematic review of new evidence and practical treatment algorithm. J Neurol Sci 2018;389:67–75.

56. Mehanna R, Hunter C, Davidson A, et al. Analysis of CYP2D6 genotype and response to tetrabenazine. Mov Disord 2013;28(2):210–5.
57. Mullard A. Deuterated drugs draw heavier backing. Nat Rev Drug Discov 2016; 15(4):219–21.
58. Teva Pharmaceuticals USA Inc. AUSTEDO (deutetrabenazine): US prescribing information. Available at: http://www.fda.gov.2017. Accessed July 1, 2019.
59. Huntington Study Group, Frank S, Testa CM, Stamler D, et al. Effect of deutetrabenazine on chorea among patients with huntington disease: a randomized clinical trial. JAMA 2016;316(1):40–50.
60. Bashir H, Jankovic J. Deutetrabenazine for the treatment of Huntington's chorea. Expert Rev Neurother 2018;18(8):625–31.
61. Fernandez HH, Factor SA, Hauser RA, et al. Randomized controlled trial of deutetrabenazine for tardive dyskinesia: the ARM-TD study. Neurology 2017;88(21): 2003–10.
62. Anderson KE, Stamler D, Davis MD, et al. Deutetrabenazine for treatment of involuntary movements in patients with tardive dyskinesia (AIM-TD): a double-blind, randomised, placebo-controlled, phase 3 trial. Lancet Psychiatry 2017; 4(8):595–604.
63. Citrome L. Deutetrabenazine for tardive dyskinesia: a systematic review of the efficacy and safety profile for this newly approved novel medication-What is the number needed to treat, number needed to harm and likelihood to be helped or harmed? Int J Clin Pract 2017;71(11). https://doi.org/10.1111/ijcp. 13030.
64. Fernandez HH, Stamler D, Davis MD, et al. Long-term safety and efficacy of deutetrabenazine for the treatment of tardive dyskinesia. J Neurol Neurosurg Psychiatry 2019;90(12):1317–23.
65. Yao Z, Wei X, Wu X, et al. Preparation and evaluation of tetrabenazine enantiomers and all eight stereoisomers of dihydrotetrabenazine as VMAT2 inhibitors. Eur J Med Chem 2011;46(5):1841–8.
66. Müller T. Valbenazine granted breakthrough drug status for treating tardive dyskinesia. Expert Opin Investig Drugs 2015;24(6):737–42.
67. O'Brien CF, Jimenez R, Hauser RA, et al. NBI-98854, a selective monoamine transport inhibitor for the treatment of tardive dyskinesia: a randomized, double-blind, placebo-controlled study. Mov Disord 2015;30(12):1681–7.
68. Hauser RA, Factor SA, Marder SR, et al. KINECT 3: a phase 3 randomized, double-blind, placebo-controlled trial of valbenazine for tardive dyskinesia. Am J Psychiatry 2017;174(5):476–84.
69. Citrome L. Valbenazine for tardive dyskinesia: a systematic review of the efficacy and safety profile for this newly approved novel medication-What is the number needed to treat, number needed to harm and likelihood to be helped or harmed? Int J Clin Pract 2017;71(7). https://doi.org/10.1111/ijcp.12964.
70. Factor SA, Remington G, Comella CL, et al. The effects of valbenazine in participants with tardive dyskinesia: results of the 1-year KINECT 3 extension study. J Clin Psychiatry 2017;78(9):1344–50.
71. Lindenmayer J-P, Marder SR, Singer C, et al. 77 long-term valbenazine treatment in patients with schizophrenia/schizoaffective disorder or mood disorder and tardive dyskinesia. CNS Spectr 2019;24(1):214–5.
72. Teo JT, Edwards MJ, Bhatia K. Tardive dyskinesia is caused by maladaptive synaptic plasticity: a hypothesis. Mov Disord 2012;27(10):1205–15.
73. Lin C-C, Ondo WG. Non-VMAT2 inhibitor treatments for the treatment of tardive dyskinesia. J Neurol Sci 2018;389:48–54.

74. Thaker GK, Nguyen JA, Strauss ME, et al. Clonazepam treatment of tardive dyskinesia: a practical GABAmimetic strategy. Am J Psychiatry 1990;147(4): 445–51.

75. Singh MM, Becker RE, Pitman RK, et al. Diazepam-induced changes in tardive dyskinesia: suggestions for a new conceptual model. Biol Psychiatry 1982; 17(6):729–42.

76. Weber SS, Dufresne RL, Becker RE, et al. Diazepam in tardive dyskinesia. Drug Intell Clin Pharm 1983;17(7–8):523–7.

77. Csernansky JG, Tacke U, Rusen D, et al. The effect of benzodiazepines on tardive dyskinesia symptoms. J Clin Psychopharmacol 1988;8(2):154–5.

78. Jordan HW, Williams BC. Tardive dyskinesia successfully treated with alprazolam. J Natl Med Assoc 1990;82(9):673–5.

79. Singh B, Kaur P, Gopichand, et al. Biology and chemistry of Ginkgo biloba. Fitoterapia 2008;79(6):401–18.

80. Zhang W-F, Tan Y-L, Zhang X-Y, et al. Extract of Ginkgo biloba treatment for tardive dyskinesia in schizophrenia: a randomized, double-blind, placebo-controlled trial. J Clin Psychiatry 2011;72(5):615–21.

81. Vijayakumar D, Jankovic J. Drug-induced dyskinesia, part 1: treatment of levodopa-induced dyskinesia. Drugs 2016;76(7):759–77.

82. Vale S, Espejel MA. Amantadine for dyskinesia tarda. N Engl J Med 1971; 284(12):673.

83. Decker BL, Davis JM, Jonowsky DS, et al. Amantadine hydrochloride treatment of tardive dyskinesia. N Engl J Med 1971;285(15):860. Available at: http://www.ncbi.nlm.nih.gov/pubmed/5570853.

84. Janowsky DS, El-Yousef MK, Davis JM, et al. Effects of amantadine on tardive dyskinesia and pseudo-parkinsonism. N Engl J Med 1972;286(14):785.

85. Angus S, Sugars J, Boltezar R, et al. A controlled trial of amantadine hydrochloride and neuroleptics in the treatment of tardive dyskinesia. J Clin Psychopharmacol 1997;17(2):88–91.

86. Pappa S, Tsouli S, Apostolou G, et al. Effects of amantadine on tardive dyskinesia: a randomized, double-blind, placebo-controlled study. Clin Neuropharmacol 2010;33(6):271–5.

87. Tammenmaa IA, Sailas E, McGrath JJ, et al. Systematic review of cholinergic drugs for neuroleptic-induced tardive dyskinesia: a meta-analysis of randomized controlled trials. Prog Neuropsychopharmacol Biol Psychiatry 2004;28(7): 1099–107.

88. Tammenmaa-Aho I, Asher R, Soares-Weiser K, et al. Cholinergic medication for antipsychotic-induced tardive dyskinesia. Cochrane Database Syst Rev 2018;(3):CD000207.

89. Kang UJ, Burke RE, Fahn S. Natural history and treatment of tardive dystonia. Mov Disord 1986;1(3):193–208.

90. Suzuki T, Hori T, Baba A, et al. Effectiveness of anticholinergics and neuroleptic dose reduction on neuroleptic-induced pleurothotonus (the Pisa syndrome). J Clin Psychopharmacol 1999;19(3):277–80.

91. Burke RE, Fahn S, Marsden CD. Torsion dystonia: a double-blind, prospective trial of high-dosage trihexyphenidyl. Neurology 1986;36(2):160–4.

92. Desmarais JE, Beauclair L, Annable L, et al. Effects of discontinuing anticholinergic treatment on movement disorders, cognition and psychopathology in patients with schizophrenia. Ther Adv Psychopharmacol 2014;4(6):257–67.

93. Vinogradov S, Fisher M, Warm H, et al. The cognitive cost of anticholinergic burden: decreased response to cognitive training in schizophrenia. Am J Psychiatry 2009;166(9):1055–62.

94. Waln O, Jankovic J. Zolpidem improves tardive dyskinesia and akathisia. Mov Disord 2013;28(12):1748–9.

95. Abou-Khalil BW. Antiepileptic drugs. Continuum (Minneap Minn) 2016;22(1 Epilepsy):132–56.

96. Konitsiotis S, Pappa S, Mantas C, et al. Levetiracetam in tardive dyskinesia: an open label study. Mov Disord 2006;21(8):1219–21.

97. Bona JR. Treatment of neuroleptic-induced tardive dyskinesia with levetiracetam: a case series. J Clin Psychopharmacol 2006;26(2):215–6.

98. Woods SW, Saksa JR, Baker CB, et al. Effects of levetiracetam on tardive dyskinesia: a randomized, double-blind, placebo-controlled study. J Clin Psychiatry 2008;69(4):546–54.

99. Grover S, Hazari N, Kate N, et al. Management of tardive syndromes with clozapine: a case series. Asian J Psychiatr 2014;8:111–4.

100. Chan H-Y, Chiang S-C, Chang C-J, et al. A randomized controlled trial of risperidone and olanzapine for schizophrenic patients with neuroleptic-induced tardive dyskinesia. J Clin Psychiatry 2010;71(9):1226–33.

101. Lozano AM, Lipsman N, Bergman H, et al. Deep brain stimulation: current challenges and future directions. Nat Rev Neurol 2019;15(3):148–60.

102. Macerollo A, Deuschl G. Deep brain stimulation for tardive syndromes: systematic review and meta-analysis. J Neurol Sci 2018;389:55–60.

103. Pouclet-Courtemanche H, Rouaud T, Thobois S, et al. Long-term efficacy and tolerability of bilateral pallidal stimulation to treat tardive dyskinesia. Neurology 2016;86(7):651–9.

104. Gruber D, Trottenberg T, Kivi A, et al. Long-term effects of pallidal deep brain stimulation in tardive dystonia. Neurology 2009;73(1):53–8.

105. Meng D-W, Liu H-G, Yang A-C, et al. Long-term effects of subthalamic nucleus deep brain stimulation in tardive dystonia. Chin Med J (Engl) 2016;129(10):1257–8.

106. Deng Z-D, Li D-Y, Zhang C-C, et al. Long-term follow-up of bilateral subthalamic deep brain stimulation for refractory tardive dystonia. Parkinsonism Relat Disord 2017;41:58–65.

107. Jankovic J. Botulinum toxin: state of the art. Mov Disord 2017;32(8):1131–8.

108. Hennings JMH, Krause E, Bötzel K, et al. Successful treatment of tardive lingual dystonia with botulinum toxin: case report and review of the literature. Prog Neuropsychopharmacol Biol Psychiatry 2008;32(5):1167–71.

109. Kasravi N, Jog MS. Botulinum toxin in the treatment of lingual movement disorders. Mov Disord 2009;24(15):2199–202.

110. Jankovic J. An update on new and unique uses of botulinum toxin in movement disorders. Toxicon 2018;147:84–8.

111. Slotema CW, van Harten PN, Bruggeman R, et al. Botulinum toxin in the treatment of orofacial tardive dyskinesia: a single blind study. Prog Neuropsychopharmacol Biol Psychiatry 2008;32(2):507–9.

112. Weiner RD, Reti IM. Key updates in the clinical application of electroconvulsive therapy. Int Rev Psychiatry 2017;29(2):54–62.

113. Chacko RC, Root L. ECT and tardive dyskinesia: two cases and a review. J Clin Psychiatry 1983;44(7):265–6.

114. Nobuhara K, Matsuda S, Okugawa G, et al. Successful electroconvulsive treatment of depression associated with a marked reduction in the symptoms of tardive dyskinesia. J ECT 2004;20(4):262–3.

115. Peng L-Y, Lee Y, Lin P-Y. Electroconvulsive therapy for a patient with persistent tardive dyskinesia. J ECT 2013;29(3):e52–4.

116. Yasui-Furukori N, Nakamura K, Katagai H, et al. The effects of electroconvulsive therapy on tardive dystonia or dyskinesia induced by psychotropic medication: a retrospective study. Neuropsychiatr Dis Treat 2014;10:1209.

117. Holcomb HH, Sternberg DE, Heninger GR. Effects of electroconvulsive therapy on mood, parkinsonism, and tardive dyskinesia in a depressed patient: ECT and dopamine systems. Biol Psychiatry 1983;18(8):865–73.

118. Roth SD, Mukherjee S, Sackeim HA. Electroconvulsive therapy in a patient with mania, parkinsonism, and tardive dyskinesia. Convuls Ther 1988;4(1):92–7.

119. Asnis GM, Leopold MA. A single-blind study of ECT in patients with tardive dyskinesia. Am J Psychiatry 1978;135(10):1235–7.

Principles of Medical and Surgical Treatment of Cerebral Palsy

Eric M. Chin, MD[a],*, Hilary E. Gwynn, MD[a],
Shenandoah Robinson, MD[b], Alexander H. Hoon Jr, MD, MPH[a]

KEYWORDS

- Cerebral palsy • Movement disorders • Management principles • Complex care

KEY POINTS

- In cases of cerebral palsy, early brain injury or dysgenesis results in a wide variety of movement disorders as well as associated nonmotor impairments.
- Successful management to optimize independence, participation, and quality of life requires individualized multidisciplinary care throughout the lifespan.
- Many symptomatic treatments of specific manifestations are available and widely used, including physical therapy, medications, and neurosurgical and orthopedic interventions. Most lack strong evidence of efficacy. For any intervention, open dialogue between patients, families, and providers regarding therapeutic options and expected benefits and potential side effects is essential.
- Modern imaging and genetic investigations have significantly advanced understanding of the causes and can improve treatment in some individual cases.
- It is important to identify comorbid medical, cognitive, and mental health disorders as these can contribute significantly to outcome.

OVERVIEW: NATURE OF THE PROBLEM

Cerebral palsy (CP) describes "a group of disorders of the development of movement and posture, causing activity limitation, that are attributed to non-progressive disturbances that occurred in the developing fetal or infant brain. The motor disorders of CP are often accompanied by disturbances of sensation, cognition, communication, perception, and/or behavior, and/or by a seizure disorder."[1] CP is the most common cause of physical disability in children (2–3/1000 live births worldwide).[2] After decades of variability in prevalence rates of CP, advances in prenatal and neonatal care,

[a] Department of Neurology and Developmental Medicine, Kennedy Krieger Institute, 707 North Broadway, Baltimore, MD 21205, USA; [b] Department of Neurosurgery, Johns Hopkins University School of Medicine, Phipps Building Rm 101, 600 North Wolfe Street, Baltimore, MD 21287, USA
* Corresponding author.
E-mail address: chine@kennedykrieger.org

Neurol Clin 38 (2020) 397–416
https://doi.org/10.1016/j.ncl.2020.01.009
0733-8619/20/© 2020 Elsevier Inc. All rights reserved.
neurologic.theclinics.com

including therapeutic hypothermia for perinatal hypoxic-ischemic encephalopathy[3] and antenatal magnesium for preterm delivery[4] finally appear to be improving rates in developed countries.[5]

The underlying causes of CP range from brain malformations to preterm white matter injury, hypoxic-ischemic injury, prenatal, perinatal, or postnatal stroke, genetic disorders, central nervous system infection, or early traumatic brain injury. In developed countries, only 2% to 10% of cases are attributable to perinatal hypoxia-ischemia.[6] Most cases are associated with periventricular white matter injury[7] attributable to hypoxic-ischemic and neuroinflammatory preterm insults. Although the initial brain insult is considered "static," the manifestations over the lifetime are dynamic processes that require lifelong management. Causes of motor deficits that instead follow a progressive course with continuing central nervous system injury are known as "masqueraders"[8] or "mimics"[9] of CP, and include a variety of genetic and metabolic disorders.

As the diagnosis of CP permits widely heterogeneous etiologies and anatomic patterns of brain abnormality, motor phenotypes in individuals with CP are often equally complex. Qualitatively, recognizable movement disorders range from spasticity to dystonia, choreoathetosis, tremor, and myoclonus (and often combinations of the above). Although spasticity is the most commonly recognized movement disorder in CP, roughly one-quarter of individuals demonstrate a clinically significant additional or alternative movement disorder.[10] In currently accepted nomenclature, motor phenotypes of CP are classified by the dominant movement abnormality into spastic, dyskinetic, ataxic, and mixed subtypes. However, even within a physiologic CP subtype (eg, "spastic" or "dyskinetic"), there can be wide variation in severity, coexisting movement disorders, and treatment response.

None of the etiologies of CP impact motor pathways in isolation, and coexisting diagnoses are common. The primary insult/malformation itself frequently (but variably) impacts many additional neurologic and neurocognitive domains:

- Epilepsy: 22% to 40% of children with CP develop epilepsy; children with hemiplegic or quadriplegic motor impairment are at particular risk.[11]
- Cognition: Approximately half of individuals with CP also have intellectual disability.[11] Many others have communication difficulties,[12] attentional difficulties,[13] or specific learning disabilities.[14]
- Somatosensation: Cortical sensory deficits are ubiquitous,[15] and measurable hypoesthesia and hyperalgesia are prevalent.[16]
- Chronic pain is also prevalent but poorly characterized to date.[17]
- Other sensory deficits: Most individuals with CP have visual impairment, and 12% to 25% have hearing impairment.[11]
- Oromotor dysfunction: 80% of individuals with CP (particularly individuals with dyskinetic components) require nonoral feeding at some point in their lifetime.[11]

Additional complications of CP arise not from the initial brain injury but from resulting physiologic or psychological stressors:

- Orthopedic deformity: Children with CP are at high risk for hip deformity or scoliosis. Both are rare in children with mild motor impairment but prominent in most severely affected individuals by adulthood.[18,19]
- Disuse-related complications: Decreased mobility itself is linked to complications spanning many organ systems ranging from muscle atrophy to cardiometabolic disorders (including obesity, diabetes mellitus, hypertension, and hyperlipidemia), restrictive lung disease, skin breakdown, a decrease in gut motility, and a systemic hypercoagulable, proinflammatory state.[20]

- Mental health: Diagnosed prevalence of anxiety and mood disorders in individuals with CP each reach 20% to 30% in adulthood.[21]

There is no cure for CP, and treatments used are largely symptomatic with a focus on quality of life and participation in society.[22] As described above, individual needs vary widely along a number of dimensions. Therefore, individual management plans must be equally diverse and versatile. In this brief review, we summarize general principles of treatment of CP and refer elsewhere for more comprehensive discussion of individual topics.

MANAGEMENT GOALS AND PATIENT EVALUATION

Defining achievable and meaningful goals of care should represent the beginning of any management discussion. Although goal selection is highly individualized, current and developmentally predicted level of gross motor functioning can help shape discussion (**Table 1**).

Following careful assessment, specific motor phenotypes may be established and targeted. Caveats include:

- In individuals with mixed CP, the "dominant" movement disorder may not cause the most impairment.
- Movement disorders may be positional, intermittent, or stimulus or activity induced, and so tailored examination with careful observation is beneficial.
- Movement quality evolves over development both in neurotypical people as well as in individuals with CP. Changes over time may be particularly pronounced in individuals with dyskinetic CP.[24]
- Superimposed epileptiform movements can vary in semiology and can be complex, and the clinician must maintain a high degree of suspicion for seizure-related movements.

Identification of specific etiologies is essential for early diagnosis (including ruling out masqueraders) and for guiding treatment selection. Brain MRI is the accepted

Table 1 Common treatment goals	
Gross Motor Functional Classification System, Extended and Revised (GMFCS E&R; from Palisano et al,[23] 2008)	**Spectrum of Treatment Goals**
I	Walks without limitations	**From less motor impairment**
II	Walks with limitations	Increased motor precision (eg, in writing, driving)
		Improved gait efficiency/community ambulation
III	Walks using a hand-held mobility device	Improved gait stability/household ambulation
		More independent self-care (eg, dressing, bathing)
IV	Self-mobility with limitations; may use powered mobility	Improved standing/exercise ambulation
		More stable sitting
V	Transported in a manual wheelchair	Prevention of orthopedic deformity
		Ease of care
		Comfort
		To more motor impairment

Treatment goals are highly personal but are often constrained by an individual's current level of gross motor functioning. The GMFCS E&R is a commonly used classification framework for individuals with CP. Note that goals should reflect thoughtful individualized discussion and do not neatly fall on a rigid spectrum—for example, chronic pain is common for individuals with CP across the spectrum of motor impairment (GMFCS E&R I-V; [17]).

standard screening evaluation for all individuals with CP[25] and is the first step in the etiologic evaluation. Macroscopic sequelae of brain injury/malformations are apparent in 83% to 86% of individuals with CP.[26]

Genetic and metabolic testing are not currently routinely recommended for individuals with CP, but suspicion of a masquerader or a discordance between clinical and imaging findings should prompt further investigation.[27] Currently available whole-exome sequencing now shows a 14% yield for clear pathogenic variants even without case preselection when obtained by a specialty clinic.[28] Increasing clinical utility for genetic/metabolic testing may lead to more common use in the future. Early identification of masqueraders is particularly important as prompt treatment can mitigate or prevent symptoms in selected disorders (eg, dietary modification in glutaric aciduria type 1, supplementation for cerebral folate deficiency, or enzyme cofactor replacement for molybdenum cofactor deficiency type A; reviewed in Jinnah and colleagues[29]).

Appropriate identification of coexisting medical and developmental diagnoses is equally imperative to successful management—both via selection of appropriate therapeutic goals and identification of barriers to care implementation.

- Medical complexity in CP can span multiple organ systems, and physiologic stability is essential for any successful treatment program.
- Neurocognitive impairments can affect patient and family ability to understand or implement a management plan. Therefore, formal evaluation of cognitive and communicative strengths and weaknesses is important.[30] Of note, verbal clarity does not necessarily reflect cognitive ability, and up to one-quarter of children with severe dysarthria have normal or borderline cognition.[12]
- Mental health diagnoses and environmental stressors (affecting the patient and/ or caregivers) are also important determinants of participation in society, quality of life, and ability to carry out a demanding treatment program.[31]

Therefore, successful treatment frequently requires consideration of cognition, language, learning, and behavior with interdisciplinary support from families, medical providers, therapists, educators, and other members of the community.

PHARMACOLOGIC TREATMENT OPTIONS

Systemic medications remain a mainstay of medical treatment of individuals with CP. At present, treatment selection remains largely symptom-driven and directed at specific movement disorders (**Table 2**), although hints at targeted, pathogenesis-based treatments are beginning to emerge. Systemic medications are commonly used for generalized hypertonia (eg, oral baclofen, diazepam, and tizanadine for spasticity), but efficacy may be limited by side effects. Furthermore, normalization of tone does not necessarily normalize motor control.[39] Medical management of dystonia and choreoathetosis seen in dyskinetic CP is particularly challenging—mechanisms are not well understood, and medications used have little supporting evidence and variable efficacy.[40]

Pathogenesis-targeted treatments offer a possible road to personalized medicine. Evidence toward targeted treatments is building along 2 directions: (1) correction of the underlying genetic/metabolic disorder and (2) identification of idiosyncratic (either positive or negative) treatment responses to specific modalities for particular etiologies. Gene-modifying and metabolic therapies are rapidly evolving and beginning to show the capacity to modify the natural history of specific genetic movement disorders (see Pearson and colleagues[9] and Mohammad and colleagues[41] for further

Table 2
Commonly used medications for the treatment of specific movement disorders in cerebral palsy

Medication	Dose	Frequency	Spasticity	Dystonia	Choreoathetosis	Myoclonus	Tremor	Notes
Oral baclofen[33]	Start at 2.5 mg TID; usual target 2 mg/kg/d (maximum 80mg/d)[102]	BID-TID	■	■				
Benzodiazepines								
Oral diazepam[34]	Adults: 2–10 mg divided 2–4 times/day. Children: 0.05–0.1 mg/kg divided 2–4 times/day (maximum of 0.8 mg/kg/d)[38]	2–4× daily PRN	■	■				Beneficial perioperative orthopedic surgery and for nighttime spasms
Oral clonazepam	0.01–0.3 mg/kg/d divided 2–3 times/day[38]	BID	■				■	Beneficial for exaggerated startle
Other antiepileptics								
Valproic acid	Initial: 5–10 mg/kg/d divided 2–4 times/day. Maintenance: 15–60 mg/kg/d up to 4000 mg/d divided 2–4 times/day[38]	BID-TID	■			■		Requires lab monitoring
Levetiracetam	20–60 mg/kg/d[32]	BID				■		
Gabapentin[35]	Initial: 5 mg/kg/d. Maintenance: 15–90 mg/kg/d divided 3 times daily[32]	BID-TID		■		■		Also helpful for neuropathic pain
Dopaminergic medications								

(continued on next page)

Table 2
(continued)

Medication	Dose	Frequency	Spasticity	Dystonia	Choreoathetosis	Myoclonus	Tremor	Notes
Levodopa/carbidopa	Initial: 0.5–1 mg/kg/day levodopa. Typical maintenance dose: 1–5 mg/kg levodopa[32]	BID-TID						Dosage for dopa-responsive dystonia; less evidence for other dystonias[32]
Other oral medications								
Tizanidine hydrochloride	Adult: Initial: 1 mg PO q8h prn. Maximum 36 mg/d. Child < age 10: Initial: 1mg nightly. Child age >10 yr: Initial: 2 mg nightly. Maintenance: 0.3–0.5 mg/kg/d divided 4 times daily[38]	TID						
Dantrolene sodium	Adult: Typically 100 mg/d divided 4 times daily (maximum 400 mg/d). Children > age 5: 0.5 mg/kg/d divided twice daily. Maximum 12 mg/kg divided 4 times daily[38]	BID						May worsen weakness; requires lab monitoring[38]
Tetrabenazine	Initial: 12.5 mg daily. Maintenance: 25–150 mg/d[32]	BID-TID						
Trihexyphenidyl	Initial: 1–2 mg/d. Maintenance: 2–60 mg/d[32]	BID-TID						Monitor intraocular pressure

Primidone	10–25 mg/kg/d or 25–125 mg/d (Maximum 250 mg/d)[32,38]		Requires lab monitors
Propranolol	1–2 mg/kg[32]		
Cannabinoids (eg, CBD, THC)	Not established		Insufficient data for tone management[36]
Injected/infused medications			
Botulinum toxin A and B[37]	Variable	q3–6 mo as required	Local/segmental treatment
Intrathecal baclofen pump	50–1600 µg/d	Higher doses for dystonia	

Green squares indicate first-line medications for specific movement disorders. Yellow squares indicate additional medications that may be considered for the movement disorder shown.

Recommendations reflect existing evidence[38] as well as the authors' clinical experience.

Abbreviations: BID, twice daily; TID, 3 times daily; CBD, cannabidiol; THC, tetrahydrocannabinol.

discussion). Currently detailed phenotypic descriptions, including response to treatment are available for many genetic etiologies (**Table 3**), which can be helpful for "tailoring" treatment regimens.

Targeted injections/infusions also warrant discussion. For example, for severe refractory spasticity or dystonia, intrathecal baclofen is often beneficial, especially when goals include improved comfort and ease of care. For focal/segmental spasticity, local botulinum toxin injection is a widely used approach.[54] Botulinum injections reliably decrease tone and strength in the targeted muscle and when used judiciously can help support gait and function in children without fixed contractures. However, efficacy declines with age, and muscle atrophy accumulates with repeated doses— limiting long-term use.[55] Phenol injections can also be considered for treatment-refractory lower-extremity spasticity.[56]

NONPHARMACOLOGIC THERAPY-BASED, SURGICAL, AND COMBINATION MANAGEMENT

Physical therapy and other nonpharmacologic treatments have long been cornerstones of habilitative and rehabilitative care in CP. A wide range of nonpharmacologic treatments are available, and treatment approaches are constantly evolving. Again, heterogeneity in populations and in techniques used has received limited high-quality study, and there is little consensus on optimal treatment paradigms. That said, large therapeutic trials now offer convincing evidence for or against some specific therapies (**Table 4**), and useful principles are beginning to emerge (**Box 1**).[37]

Selective dorsal rhizotomy is a widely used neurosurgical procedure, which reduces spasticity primarily in the legs by interrupting the sensory component of the deep tendon reflex. It is most often beneficial in selected children with spastic diplegia without dystonia—i.e. those with relatively preserved strength and selective motor control; those able to participate in prolonged rehabilitation; and those for whom less-invasive interventions have not been beneficial.[71] Transient short-term side effects may include sensory or bowel/bladder symptoms, but long-term complications are rare.[72]

Deep brain stimulation (DBS) involves implanting electrodes within deep gray structures including the globus pallidus. Stimulation is controlled by a generator placed subcutaneously in the upper chest. DBS has been very successful for patients with *DYT-1*-related genetic dystonia; more generally, outcome data in patients with dyskinetic CP are limited and heterogeneous.[73] Genetic diagnosis (see **Table 3**) and movement disorder characteristics (dystonia versus chorea and/or athetosis) likely contribute to this variability.[74]

Surgical orthopedic interventions are commonly used for maladaptive musculoskeletal conditions that develop over time in many children with CP. Surgical procedures include tendon lengthening to correct contractures, tendon transfers to reestablish muscle balance, rotational osteotomies for torsional deformities, and spine, hip, and/or foot stabilization. Careful preoperative planning (including optimization of nutritional status and tone) improves outcomes,[75] including optimization of nutritional status and tone. Controlled trials of specific orthopedic surgical interventions, including single-event multilevel surgery (in which multiple joints are operated on in 1 procedure to reduce burden of hospitalization/recovery) are needed to fully demonstrate efficacy.[76] With regard to scoliosis surgery, although full consensus has not been reached,[77] the recommendation leans toward operating at curves less than 90°.[78,79]

Table 3
Treatment considerations for selected childhood-onset movement disorders

Gene and Corresponding Condition	Description of Movement Disorder	Treatment Considerations
TOR1A: Early-onset isolated dystonia (DYT1)	Isolated dystonia typically beginning distally in middle childhood frequently progressing over months to years sparing the larynx and neck[42]	Oral/injected medication is similar to that in dystonia more broadly. Internal globus pallidus (GPi) DBS often produces sustained efficacy for refractory cases[43]
GCH1: Autosomal dominant dopa-responsive dystonia (DYT5a)[44]	Classically with diurnally varying childhood-onset dystonia beginning distally with gradual progression to generalized dystonia with pyramidal symptoms although an expanding recognized phenotypic spectrum	Typically dramatic and sustained response to relatively low doses of orally administered levodopa (20–30 mg/kg/d)
SGCE: Myoclonus-dystonia (DYT11)	Myoclonus frequently with focal/segmental dystonia beginning in childhood with clinical course ranging from spontaneous remission to gradual progression[45]	Response to many therapies has been reported including benzodiazepines, antiepileptic drugs, L-dopa, zolpidem, and ventral intermedius nucleus or GPi DBS[46]
GNAO1-related movement disorder	Episodic choreoathetotic movement disorder. Early hypotonia with later dystonia is common. Frequently progressive motor and cognitive deficits[47]	Hyperkinetic movements can be very treatment resistant[48]. Topiramate has been suggested as first-line for chorea[48], cases have also reported response to tetrabenazine, GPi DBS,[47] or intrathecal baclofen[49]
GCDH: Glutaric aciduria type 1[50]	Stepwise motor decline during early childhood (before 3 years) with development of dystonia, axial hypotonia, and later rigid parkinsonism	Frequently preventable with oral carnitine supplementation early in life. However, symptoms that do arise can be very refractory with little evidence of benefit for treatments beyond baclofen (oral or intrathecal) and benzodiazepines.[51] Response to DBS has been discouraging to date[52]
DDC: Aromatic L-amino acid decarboxylase deficiency[53]	Variable degrees of (typically nonprogressive) axial hypotonia with limb hypertonia; typical movement disorders include oculogyric crises, dystonia, or hypokinesia	Response to dopaminergic agents and pyridoxine have been reported, and trials are recommended, but data on efficacy is limited

As cohorts of individuals with monogenic movement disorders are increasingly well described in the literature, descriptions emerge of the extent of the neurologic phenotype as well as response to specific interventions. It should be noted that most evidence along these lines is at the case series level with a few small randomized controlled trials.

Table 4
Selected nonpharmacologic therapies used for symptomatic treatment of cerebral palsy[37]

Treatment	Major Effects and Level of Evidence (Evidence alert traffic light system: Green light: "Effective, therefore do it"; Yellow light: "Measure: Uncertain effect"; Red light: "Ineffective, therefore don't do it")	Contraindications for Use
Noninvasive treatments		
Serial casting	Improves range of motion at the ankles. Effects may be short-lived but may be functionally helpful in selected partially ambulatory individuals. Other indications (eg, use at knees) lack adequate evidence. Not physiologically plausible as a means of directly impacting spasticity	Heterotopic ossification; Bone fracture/dislocation, occlusive venous/arterial disease[57]
Orthotics (eg, ankle-foot orthotics)	Low-to-very low quality of evidence for/against benefit on gait parameters, limb function, or prevention of contracture	Insufficient voluntary dorsiflexion control; Fixed equinus deformity; Insufficient heel strike; Hypertonic reflex foot activity; Lack of ambulation[58]
Surgical treatments		
Selective dorsal rhizotomy	Effective for reducing spasticity and improving gait kinematics; Evidence for improved gross motor functioning but no evidence regarding translation to improved participation in activities	Dystonia; Ataxia; Fixed contractures[59]
Single-event multilevel surgery with associated therapy	Low-quality supporting evidence of improved long-term functional mobility	Severe weakness; Uncontrolled spasticity or dystonia; Progressive neurologic disorder; Inability to perform postoperative rehabilitation[60]

Four commonly used treatments are outlined here with summaries of evidence for specific indications as well as typical contraindications. Evidence is derived from a systematic review[37] and, as in that reference, uses the evidence alert traffic light system: green light, effective, therefore do it; yellow light: measure has uncertain effect; red light, ineffective therefore don't do it.

Box 1
Principles of therapy in cerebral palsy

Types of therapy used in management of CP are too numerous and varied to list. The following principles reflect existing evidence as well as the authors' approach when prescribing courses of therapy.

Dose of therapy

The "dose" may be more important than the method used for some therapies. As an example, constraint-induced movement therapy (CIMT) is a form of intensive therapy for individuals with hemiplegic CP in which the less-impaired hand is restrained for (typically) 14 days during which focused repetitive tasks and shaping activities are performed for 6 hours per day to overcome "learned [or] developmental non-use."[61] Comparisons between studies suggest that more therapy (up to 90 hours over 15 days) yields more and longer-lasting benefits for individuals with hemiplegic CP. However, for both CIMT and bimanual therapy (in which coordinated use of both hands together), dose/response relationships are seen.[62,63] Combination with adjuncts ranging from functional electrical stimulation[64] to transcranial magnetic stimulation[65] or virtual reality programs[66] also shows promise. There remains marked variability in individual outcomes.

In practice, the authors assume that there arfe diminishing returns for ever higher doses of therapy, but optimal doses, durations, and intensities (high-intensity "bursts" versus distributed over time) are generally not known.[61] Therefore, we recommend setting realistic, measurable, individualized goals to be accomplished over defined time periods with periodic assessment of therapeutic gains versus burden of increased care.

Types of therapy

Evidence is building to support use of specific therapies for specific indications and against efficacy for others.[37] Again using the example of hemiplegic CP, intensive CIMT, and bimanual therapy both have evidence supporting efficacy,[62,63] and neurodevelopmental therapy has evidence against its efficacy. However, evidence for many treatments is limited and inadequate to make strong recommendations for or against them.

One emerging principle is that "top/down" task-oriented therapy goals may be more effective than "bottom-up" goals focused on basic functions or prerequisite skills.[62]

Timing of therapy

Transition points: Permanent (eg, surgery) and long-lasting (eg, botulinum toxin therapy) procedures alter biomechanics (eg, decreased muscle strength in the period after multilevel orthopedic surgery[67]). Therefore, guidelines emphasize the importance of intensive postsurgical (and postbotulinum[62]) therapy[68] throughout the recovery period, but specific evidence-based protocols are only beginning to emerge.[67]

Early intervention: Much current policy and medical practice prioritizes early detection of CP and early initiation of therapy. Evidence has emerged to support benefits of some early interventions.[69] However, early childhood brain plasticity is likely better considered a dynamic period of rapid change than an open-and-shut critical period.[70] Although early diagnosis and therapy may represent an opportunity, submaximal early intervention should not be seen as a reason to lose hope.

ADJUSTING TREATMENT AND EVALUATION OF OUTCOME

As most treatment is symptomatic and marked by variable efficacy and side effect profiles (as well as possible rebound effects), the authors use the following principles (with guidance from Koy and colleagues[32]):

- Acknowledge uncertainty about benefit and potential side effects when initiating treatment. Safety and efficacy studies have not been formally evaluated for many medications (particularly for children). Furthermore, even routine therapy sessions may not be well tolerated by some people. Most children and young adults report pain during physical or occupational therapy, and parents of children with CP report that stretching is the most frequent routinely painful activity.[80] Therapeutic standing, assisted walking, assisted sitting, and splint use have also been reported as painful.[81]
- Identify clear, measurable goals *before* initiating titration. If goals are not reachable with tolerable side effects, all involved should be willing to consider discontinuing a therapeutic trial if side effects outweigh benefits.
- Start with a low dose (with the initial dose at a time and place with careful observation to monitor for idiosyncratic reactions), increase slowly, and avoid abrupt discontinuation.
- Objective outcome measures (**Table 5**) remain somewhat limited at present. Although subjective, patients and parents report an important measure of efficacy. Therapists are important allies in this regard—depending on the situation, their functional measurements may be best used either as blinded observations of treatment effects or an integrated component of multidisciplinary assessment.
- Providers must be thoughtful when treatment plans do not produce the expected results (**Table 6**). Unexpected treatment failure should prompt reexamination of clinical status, benefit/risk profiles of applicable treatments, and diagnoses.
- A broad spectrum of neurorestorative therapies are under preclinical investigation but are currently unproven.[94] Despite biologic plausibility, many clinical trials have suffered from a lack of a standardized, systematic approach—making comparison difficult.[95] However, patients and families often turn to experimental complementary, alternative, or integrative medical therapies when conventional therapies do not provide the results desired—and enthusiasm has outpaced effective regulation. For example, cell-based (stem cell) clinics have arisen promising dramatic benefits beyond those suggested by current evidence. Treatments are generally very costly to families, and there have been several reports of serious adverse effects (including death) after treatments.[96] Therefore,

Table 5
Examples of assessments in cerebral palsy

Assessment Type	Examples	Uses
Overall functioning	Gross Motor Function Measure[82] (gross motor) WeeFIM[83] (self-care, mobility, cognition)	Global assessment of motor functioning
Segmental	Medical Research Council (muscle strength)[84] Modified Ashworth Scale (spasticity)[85] Tardieu (spasticity)[86]	Phenotyping, longitudinal monitoring, assessing treatment response
Movement disorder specific	Hypertonia Assessment Tool[87] Barry-Albright Dystonia Scale[88] Scale for the Assessment and Rating of Ataxia[89]	
Infant evaluation	Prechtl's Assessment of General Movements[90] Hammersmith Infant Neurological Exam[91] Alberta Infant Motor Scale[92]	Early identification/ diagnosis/risk stratification

Many instruments are used to measure and quantify various aspects of motor functioning in CP. This table is not exhaustive but illustrates types of assessments that may be used. In most cases, multiple types of assessments are used in a complementary manner (eg, to comment on single-joint function, qualities of movement disorders present, and on effects on functional status).

Table 6	
Why treatment plans can fail	
Reason	**Comments/Examples**
Incorrect/incomplete diagnosis	Neuromuscular and neurometabolic disorders may initially appear similar to individuals with CP and only later demonstrate clear progressive decline. Within a diagnosis of CP, dystonia can easily be overshadowed by spasticity, which can lead to suboptimal medical management[93]
Insufficient treatment	There may be limitations from an insurance or psychosocial perspective
Inappropriate treatment	Children with dystonia are not good candidates for selective dorsal rhizotomy[59]
Limited effective treatment options	Hyperkinetic movements are notoriously difficult to treat
Overlooked comorbidity: pain, anxiety or mood	Patient/family motivation is critical for the therapies that are required to complement and make medical or surgical interventions successful
Patient expectations differ from provider goals	Benefit from intervention is typically limited. Realistic, concrete goals should be set jointly between providers and families, communicated clearly, and reevaluated regularly
Side effects > benefits	Some surgical interventions, both orthopedic and neurosurgical, can produce unwanted reduction in motor strength. Paradoxically, spasticity can be useful in some situations for scaffolding postures[93]

Treatment plans, even when well planned and well coordinated, may fail to achieve expected results. Potential pitfalls are outlined here.

patients, families and clinicians should discuss evidence of benefits/risks (as well as, often, lack of evidence) when considering using unproven treatments.[97]

TREATMENT OVER THE LIFESPAN

Functional status and adaptive needs change over the lifespan for individuals with CP. During childhood, the primary focus is placed on optimizing developmental gains in motor and cognitive ability. Motor abilities for children unable to ambulate independently can peak at age 7 to 8 years and may decline during adolescence.[98] The transition to adulthood is also a particularly challenging period, and establishing independence and maintaining health/quality of life are key goals for adolescents and adults with CP.

Surveillance guidelines reflect these changing needs. Although some considerations, such as pain, should be evaluated at every visit,[99] other surveillance (such as screening for orthopedic deformity) requires a more complex schedule[100] based on age and functional status. Motor, cognitive, language, and academic development, as well as vision, hearing, and mental health, should be closely monitored in all children with CP.[30]

Community participation remains a significant challenge for adolescents and adults with CP. In 1 cohort, 79% of respondents aged 18 to 30 years finished 12 or more years of school, but only 23% held a driver's license or were competitively employed (although continued schooling and lack of available work were included in reasons for unemployment). Only 5% were married, although 74% reported having friends. Roughly one-third of respondents regularly strolled around the neighborhood or engaged in sports.[101] That said, 1 study reported that over 90% of children and adults with CP reported overall life satisfaction, and even more predicted overall life satisfaction 5 years in the future.[101]

SUMMARY

CP is a complex, heterogeneous disorder. Successful management requires timely, accurate assessment and treatment of both motor and nonmotor manifestations. Prenatal and perinatal neuroprotective strategies offer the promise of decreasing prevalence and severity of CP, but neurorestorative strategies remain experimental. Advanced imaging modalities and genetic testing frequently provide etiologic clarity and are proving increasingly helpful for guiding management plans.

In the setting of interindividual heterogeneity, individualized treatment plans with close monitoring of effects and tolerability represent the gold standard of care. Well-designed, controlled studies are beginning to build evidence for and against specific therapies to achieve specific goals. At present, evidence for medical and surgical treatments (eg, selective dorsal rhizotomy) largely relates to body structure-level endpoints (eg, tone reduction), whereas therapy trials have largely targeted functional (activity level-based) outcomes. Therefore, no treatment to date has high-quality evidence on both the body structure level and on the functional level.[37] Bridging this divide should be a priority for therapeutic trials to maximize individual participation at home, in the community, and in the workplace.

ACKNOWLEDGMENTS

EMC was supported by Eunice Kennedy Shriver National Institute of Child Health and Human Development (2 T32 HD7414-26) during the writing of this manuscript. Topics discussed in this review also relate to ongoing work (EMC, SR, and AHH) supported by the Cerebral Palsy Alliance Research Foundation (PG16617), the Johns Hopkins Neurosurgery Pain Research Institute, and the Johns Hopkins Blaustein Pain Research and Education Endowment. We also acknowledge Bruce Shapiro, Elaine Stashinko, and Mary Leppert for feedback on this manuscript.

REFERENCES

1. Rosenbaum P, Paneth N, Leviton A, et al. A report: the definition and classification of cerebral palsy April 2006. Dev Med Child Neurol Suppl 2007;109:8–14.
2. Himmelmann K, Uvebrant P. The panorama of cerebral palsy in Sweden part XII shows that patterns changed in the birth years 2007–2010. Acta Paediatr 2018; 107(3):462–8.
3. Jacobs SE, Berg M, Hunt R, et al. Cooling for newborns with hypoxic ischaemic encephalopathy. Cochrane Database Syst Rev 2013;(1):CD003311.
4. Berger R, Söder S. Neuroprotection in preterm infants. Biomed Res Int 2015; 2015:257139.
5. Sellier E, Platt MJ, Andersen GL, et al. Decreasing prevalence in cerebral palsy: a multi-site European population-based study, 1980 to 2003. Dev Med Child Neurol 2016;58(1):85–92.
6. Eunson P. Aetiology and epidemiology of cerebral palsy. Paediatr Child Health 2012;22(9):361–6.
7. Krägeloh-Mann I, Horber V. The role of magnetic resonance imaging in elucidating the pathogenesis of cerebral palsy: a systematic review. Dev Med Child Neurol 2007;49(2):144–51.

8. Lee RW, Poretti A, Cohen JS, et al. A diagnostic approach for cerebral palsy in the genomic era. Neuromolecular Med 2014;16(4):821–44.
9. Pearson TS, Pons R, Ghaoui R, et al. Genetic mimics of cerebral palsy. Mov Disord 2019;34(5):625–36.
10. Westbom L, Hagglund G, Nordmark E. Cerebral palsy in a total population of 4-11 year olds in southern Sweden. Prevalence and distribution according to different CP classification systems. BMC Pediatr 2007;7:41.
11. Odding E, Roebroeck ME, Stam HJ. The epidemiology of cerebral palsy: incidence, impairments and risk factors. Disabil Rehabil 2006;28(4):183–91.
12. Sigurdardottir S, Vik T. Speech, expressive language, and verbal cognition of preschool children with cerebral palsy in Iceland. Dev Med Child Neurol 2010;53(1):74–80.
13. Bottcher L. Children with spastic cerebral palsy, their cognitive functioning, and social participation: a review. Child Neuropsychol 2010;16(3):209–28.
14. Schenker R, Coster WJ, Parush S. Neuroimpairments, activity performance, and participation in children with cerebral palsy mainstreamed in elementary schools. Dev Med Child Neurol 2005;47(12):808–14.
15. Wingert JR, Burton H, Sinclair RJ, et al. Tactile sensory abilities in cerebral palsy: deficits in roughness and object discrimination. Dev Med Child Neurol 2008; 50(11):832–8.
16. Blankenburg M, Junker J, Hirschfeld G, et al. Quantitative sensory testing profiles in children, adolescents and young adults (6-20 years) with cerebral palsy: hints for a neuropathic genesis of pain syndromes. Eur J Paediatr Neurol 2018; 22(3):470–81.
17. Penner M, Xie WY, Binepal N, et al. Characteristics of pain in children and youth with cerebral palsy. Pediatrics 2013;132(2):e407–13.
18. Hägglund G, Pettersson K, Czuba T, et al. Incidence of scoliosis in cerebral palsy. Acta Orthop 2018;89(4):443–7.
19. Soo B, Howard JJ, Boyd RN, et al. Hip displacement in cerebral palsy. J Bone Joint Surg Am 2006;88(1):121–9.
20. Peterson MD, Gordon PM, Hurvitz EA, et al. Secondary muscle pathology and metabolic dysregulation in adults with cerebral palsy. Am J Physiol Endocrinol Metab 2012;303(9):E1085–93.
21. Whitney DG, Warschausky SA, Ng S, et al. Prevalence of mental health disorders among adults with cerebral palsy. Ann Intern Med 2019. https://doi.org/10.7326/m18-3420.
22. Schiariti V, Selb M, Cieza A, et al. International Classification of Functioning, Disability and Health Core Sets for children and youth with cerebral palsy: a consensus meeting. Developmental Medicine & Child Neurology 2015;57(2):149–58.
23. Palisano RJ, Rosenbaum P, Bartlett D, et al. Content validity of the expanded and revised Gross Motor Function Classification System. Dev Med Child Neurol 2008;50(10):744–50.
24. Lesný I. The development of athetosis. Dev Med Child Neurol 1968;10(4):441–6.
25. Mink JW, Jenkins ME, Whelan MA, et al. Practice parameter: diagnostic assessment of the child with cerebral palsy: report of the Quality Standards Subcommittee of the American Academy of Neurology and the Practice Committee of the Child Neurology Society. Neurology 2004;63(10):1985–6.
26. Scheck SM, Boyd RN, Rose SE. New insights into the pathology of white matter tracts in cerebral palsy from diffusion magnetic resonance imaging: a systematic review. Dev Med Child Neurol 2012;54(8):684–96.

27. Springer A, Dyck Holzinger S, Andersen J, et al. Profile of children with cerebral palsy spectrum disorder and a normal MRI study. Neurology 2019;93(1): e88–96.

28. McMichael G, Bainbridge MN, Haan E, et al. Whole-exome sequencing points to considerable genetic heterogeneity of cerebral palsy. Mol Psychiatry 2015; 20(2):176–82.

29. Jinnah HA, Albanese A, Bhatia KP, et al. Treatable inherited rare movement disorders. Mov Disord 2018;33(1):21–35.

30. Bøttcher L, Stadskleiv K, Berntsen T, et al. Systematic cognitive monitoring of children with cerebral palsy – the development of an assessment and follow-up protocol. Scand J Disabil Res 2015;18(4):304–15.

31. Downs J, Blackmore AM, Epstein A, et al. The prevalence of mental health disorders and symptoms in children and adolescents with cerebral palsy: a systematic review and meta-analysis. Dev Med Child Neurol 2018;60(1):30–8.

32. Koy A, Lin J-P, Sanger TD, et al. Advances in management of movement disorders in children. Lancet Neurol 2016;15(7):719–35.

33. Milla PJ, Jackson AD. A controlled trial of baclofen in children with cerebral palsy. J Int Med Res 1977;5(6):398–404.

34. Whelan MA, Delgado MR. Practice parameter: pharmacologic treatment of spasticity in children and adolescents with cerebral palsy (an evidence-based review): report of the quality standards subcommittee of the American Academy of Neurology and the practice committee of the child neurology society. Neurology 2010;75(7):669.

35. Liow NY-K, Gimeno H, Lumsden DE, et al. Gabapentin can significantly improve dystonia severity and quality of life in children. Eur J Paediatr Neurol 2016;20(1): 100–7.

36. Libzon S, Schleider LB-L, Saban N, et al. Medical cannabis for pediatric moderate to severe complex motor disorders. J Child Neurol 2018;33(9):565–71.

37. Novak I, McIntyre S, Morgan C, et al. A systematic review of interventions for children with cerebral palsy: state of the evidence. Dev Med Child Neurol 2013;55(10):885–910.

38. Edgar TS. Oral pharmacotherapy of childhood movement disorders. J Child Neurol 2003;18(1_suppl):S40–9.

39. Sahrmann SA, Norton BJ. The relationship of voluntary movement of spasticity in the upper motor neuron syndrome. Ann Neurol 1977;2(6):460–5.

40. Monbaliu E, Himmelmann K, Lin J-P, et al. Clinical presentation and management of dyskinetic cerebral palsy. Lancet Neurol 2017;16(9):741–9.

41. Mohammad SS, Paget SP, Dale RC. Current therapies and therapeutic decision making for childhood-onset movement disorders. Mov Disord 2019;34(5): 637–56.

42. Balint B, Bhatia KP. Isolated and combined dystonia syndromes - an update on new genes and their phenotypes. Eur J Neurol 2015;22(4):610–7.

43. Panov F, Gologorsky Y, Connors G, et al. Deep brain stimulation in DYT1 dystonia: a 10-year experience. Neurosurgery 2013;73(1):86–93 [discussion: 93].

44. Furukawa Y. GTP Cyclohydrolase 1-deficient dopa-responsive dystonia. In: Adam MP, Ardinger HH, Pagon RA, et al, editors. GeneReviews. Seattle (WA): University of Washington, Seattle; 2002. p. 1993–2020. Available at: https://www.ncbi.nlm.nih.gov/books/NBK1508/.

45. Peall KJ, Kurian MA, Wardle M, et al. SGCE and myoclonus dystonia: motor characteristics, diagnostic criteria and clinical predictors of genotype. J Neurol 2014;261(12):2296–304.

46. Raymond D, Saunders-Pullman R, Ozelius L. SGCE Myoclonus-Dystonia. In: Adam MP, Ardinger HH, Pagon RA, et al, editors. GeneReviews® [Internet]. Seattle: University of Washington; 2003. p. 1993–2020. Available from: https://www.ncbi.nlm.nih.gov/books/NBK1414/.

47. Danti FR, Galosi S, Romani M, et al. Encephalopathy: broadening the phenotype and evaluating treatment and outcome. Neurol Genet 2017;3(2):e143.

48. Sakamoto S, Monden Y, Fukai R, et al. A case of severe movement disorder with GNAO1 mutation responsive to topiramate. Brain Dev 2017;39(5):439–43.

49. Waak M, Mohammad SS, Coman D, et al. GNAO1-related movement disorder with life-threatening exacerbations: movement phenomenology and response to DBS. J Neurol Neurosurg Psychiatry 2018;89(2):221–2.

50. Kölker S, Christensen E, Leonard JV, et al. Diagnosis and management of glutaric aciduria type I--revised recommendations. J Inherit Metab Dis 2011;34(3):677–94.

51. Kyllerman M, Skjeldal O, Christensen E, et al. Long-term follow-up, neurological outcome and survival rate in 28 Nordic patients with glutaric aciduria type 1. Eur J Paediatr Neurol 2004;8(3):121–9.

52. Elkaim LM, Alotaibi NM, Sigal A, et al. Deep brain stimulation for pediatric dystonia: a meta-analysis with individual participant data. Dev Med Child Neurol 2019;61(1):49–56.

53. Wassenberg T, Molero-Luis M, Jeltsch K, et al. Consensus guideline for the diagnosis and treatment of aromatic L-amino acid decarboxylase (AADC) deficiency. Orphanet J Rare Dis 2017;12(1). https://doi.org/10.1186/s13023-016-0522-z.

54. Valentine J, Davidson S-A, Bear N, et al. Botulinum toxin and surgical intervention in children and adolescents with cerebral palsy: who, when and why do we treat? Disabil Rehabil 2019. https://doi.org/10.1080/09638288.2019.1644381.

55. Multani I, Manji J, Hastings-Ison T, et al. Botulinum toxin in the management of children with cerebral palsy. Paediatr Drugs 2019;21(4):261–81.

56. Chang EY, Ghosh N, Yanni D, et al. A review of spasticity treatments: pharmacological and interventional approaches. Critical Reviews™ in Physical and Rehabilitation Medicine 2013;25(1–2).

57. McNee AE, Will E, Lin J-P, et al. The effect of serial casting on gait in children with cerebral palsy: preliminary results from a crossover trial. Gait Posture 2007;25(3):463–8.

58. Ofluoglu D. Orthotic management in cerebral palsy. Acta Orthop Traumatol Turc 2009;43(2):165–72 [in Turkish].

59. Nordmark E, Josenby AL, Lagergren J, et al. Long-term outcomes five years after selective dorsal rhizotomy. BMC Pediatr 2008;8:54.

60. Rutz E, Baker R, Tirosh O, et al. Are results after single-event multilevel surgery in cerebral palsy durable? Clin Orthop Relat Res 2013;471(3):1028–38.

61. Sakzewski L, Gordon A, Eliasson A-C. The state of the evidence for intensive upper limb therapy approaches for children with unilateral cerebral palsy. J Child Neurol 2014;29(8):1077–90.

62. Novak I, Honan I. Effectiveness of paediatric occupational therapy for children with disabilities: a systematic review. Aust Occup Ther J 2019. https://doi.org/10.1111/1440-1630.12573.

63. Hoare BJ, Wallen MA, Thorley MN, et al. Constraint-induced movement therapy in children with unilateral cerebral palsy. Cochrane Database Syst Rev 2019;(4):CD004149.

64. Xu K, Wang L, Mai J, et al. Efficacy of constraint-induced movement therapy and electrical stimulation on hand function of children with hemiplegic cerebral palsy: a controlled clinical trial. Disabil Rehabil 2012;34(4):337–46.

65. Kirton A, Andersen J, Herrero M, et al. Brain stimulation and constraint for perinatal stroke hemiparesis: The PLASTIC CHAMPS Trial. Neurology 2016;86(18): 1659–67.

66. Rostami HR, Arastoo AA, Nejad SJ, et al. Effects of modified constraint-induced movement therapy in virtual environment on upper-limb function in children with spastic hemiparetic cerebral palsy: a randomised controlled trial. NeuroRehabilitation 2012;31(4):357–65.

67. van Bommel EEH, Arts MME, Jongerius PH, et al. Physical therapy treatment in children with cerebral palsy after single-event multilevel surgery: a qualitative systematic review. A first step towards a clinical guideline for physical therapy after single-event multilevel surgery. Ther Adv Chronic Dis 2019;10. 2040622319854241.

68. Bromham N, Dworzynski K, Eunson P, et al, Guideline Committee. Cerebral palsy in adults: summary of NICE guidance. BMJ 2019;364:l806.

69. Novak I, Morgan C, Adde L, et al. Early, accurate diagnosis and early intervention in cerebral palsy: advances in diagnosis and treatment. JAMA Pediatr 2017; 171(9):897–907.

70. Bruer J. The myth of the first three years: a new understanding of early brain development and lifelong learning. New York: Simon and Schuster; 2010.

71. Enslin JMN, Langerak NG, Fieggen AG. The evolution of selective dorsal rhizotomy for the management of spasticity. Neurotherapeutics 2019;16(1):3–8.

72. Jeffery SMT, Markia B, Pople IK, et al. Surgical outcomes of single-level bilateral selective dorsal rhizotomy for spastic diplegia in 150 consecutive patients. World Neurosurg 2019. https://doi.org/10.1016/j.wneu.2018.12.187.

73. Koy A, Timmermann L. Deep brain stimulation in cerebral palsy: challenges and opportunities. Eur J Paediatr Neurol 2017;21(1):118–21.

74. Elia AE, Bagella CF, Ferré F, et al. Deep brain stimulation for dystonia due to cerebral palsy: a review. Eur J Paediatr Neurol 2018;22(2):308–15.

75. Berry JG, Glaspy T, Eagan B, et al. Pediatric complex care and surgery comanagement: preparation for spinal fusion. J Child Health Care 2019. https://doi.org/10.1177/1367493519864741.

76. Jea A, Dormans J. Single-event multilevel surgery: contender or pretender. Pediatrics 2019;143(4). https://doi.org/10.1542/peds.2019-0102.

77. Miller DJ, Flynn JJM, Pasha S, et al. Improving health-related quality of life for patients with nonambulatory cerebral palsy: who stands to gain from scoliosis surgery? J Pediatr Orthop 2019. https://doi.org/10.1097/BPO.0000000000001424.

78. Hollenbeck SM, Yaszay B, Sponseller PD, et al. The pros and cons of operating early versus late in the progression of cerebral palsy scoliosis. Spine Deform 2019;7(3):489–93.

79. Brooks JT, Sponseller PD. What's new in the management of neuromuscular scoliosis. J Pediatr Orthop 2016;36(6):627–33.

80. McKearnan KA, Kieckhefer GM, Engel JM, et al. Pain in children with cerebral palsy: a review. J Neurosci Nurs 2004;36(5):252–9.

81. Hadden KL, von Baeyer CL. Pain in children with cerebral palsy: common triggers and expressive behaviors. Pain 2002;99(1–2):281–8.

82. Michaelis U. Gross Motor Function Measure (GMFM-66 & GMFM 88) user's manual 2nd edition clinics in developmental medicine edited by D.J. Russell,

P.L Rosenbaum, M. Wright, L.M Avery London, UK: Mac Keith Press, 2013 £70.00 (Spiral Binding), pp 290 ISBN. Dev Med Child Neurol 2015;57(12):1188.

83. Uniform Data System for Medical Rehabilitation. 2016. The WeeFIM II® Clinical Guide, Version 6.4. Buffalo: UDSMR.

84. Compston A. Aids to the investigation of peripheral nerve injuries. Medical Research Council: Nerve Injuries Research Committee. His Majesty's Stationery Office: 1942; pp. 48 (iii) and 74 figures and 7 diagrams; with aids to the examination of the peripheral nervous system. By Michael O'Brien for the Guarantors of Brain. Saunders Elsevier: 2010; pp. [8] 64 and 94 Figures. Brain 2010; 133(10):2838–44.

85. Bohannon RW, Smith MB. Interrater reliability of a modified Ashworth scale of muscle spasticity. Phys Ther 1987;67(2):206–7.

86. Haugh AB, Pandyan AD, Johnson GR. A systematic review of the Tardieu Scale for the measurement of spasticity. Disabil Rehabil 2006;28(15):899–907.

87. Jethwa A, Mink J, Macarthur C, et al. Development of the hypertonia assessment tool (HAT): a discriminative tool for hypertonia in children. Dev Med Child Neurol 2010;52(5):e83–7.

88. Barry MJ, VanSwearingen JM, Albright AL. Reliability and responsiveness of the Barry-Albright Dystonia Scale. Dev Med Child Neurol 1999;41(6):404–11.

89. Schmitz-Hübsch T, du Montcel ST, Baliko L, et al. Development and validation of a new ataxia rating scale: scale for the assessment and rating of Ataxia (SARA). Akt Neurol 2005;32(S4). https://doi.org/10.1055/s-2005-919541.

90. Einspieler C, Prechtl HFR. Prechtl's assessment of general movements: a diagnostic tool for the functional assessment of the young nervous system. Ment Retard Dev Disabil Res Rev 2005;11(1):61–7.

91. Romeo DM, Ricci D, Brogna C, et al. Use of the hammersmith infant neurological examination in infants with cerebral palsy: a critical review of the literature. Dev Med Child Neurol 2016;58(3):240–5.

92. Darrah J, Bartlett D, Maguire TO, et al. Have infant gross motor abilities changed in 20 years? A re-evaluation of the Alberta Infant Motor Scale normative values. Dev Med Child Neurol 2014;56(9):877–81.

93. Pranzatelli MR. Oral pharmacotherapy for the movement disorders of cerebral palsy. J Child Neurol 1996;11(1_suppl):S13–22.

94. Finch-Edmondson M, Morgan C, Hunt RW, et al. Emergent prophylactic, reparative and restorative brain interventions for infants born preterm with cerebral palsy. Front Physiol 2019;10:15.

95. Jantzie LL, Scafidi J, Robinson S. Stem cells and cell-based therapies for cerebral palsy: a call for rigor. Pediatr Res 2018;83(1–2):345–55.

96. Novak I, Walker K, Hunt RW, et al. Concise review: stem cell interventions for people with cerebral palsy: systematic review with meta-analysis. Stem Cells Transl Med 2016;5(8):1014–25.

97. Oppenheim WL. Complementary and alternative methods in cerebral palsy. Dev Med Child Neurol 2009;51(Suppl 4):122–9.

98. Hanna SE, Rosenbaum PL, Bartlett DJ, et al. Stability and decline in gross motor function among children and youth with cerebral palsy aged 2 to 21 years. Dev Med Child Neurol 2009;51(4):295–302.

99. Fehlings D. Pain in cerebral palsy: a neglected comorbidity. Dev Med Child Neurol 2017;59(8):782–3.

100. Wynter M, Gibson N, Willoughby KL, et al. Australian hip surveillance guidelines for children with cerebral palsy: 5-year review. Dev Med Child Neurol 2015; 57(9):808–20.

101. Mesterman R, Leitner Y, Yifat R, et al. Cerebral palsy—long-term medical, functional, educational, and psychosocial outcomes. J Child Neurol 2009;25(1): 36–42.
102. He Y, Brunstrom-Hernandez JE, Thio LL, et al. Population pharmacokinetics of oral baclofen in pediatric patients with cerebral palsy. The Journal of pediatrics 2014;164(5):1181–8.

Wilson Disease
An Overview and Approach to Management

Caitlin Mulligan, MD[a], Jeff M. Bronstein, MD, PhD[b],*

KEYWORDS

- Wilson disease • Copper • Movement disorder • Chelation

KEY POINTS

- Wilson disease is a treatable genetic disorder of copper metabolism leading to excess copper deposition, and it affects function in multiple organ systems, most commonly the liver and the brain.
- Screening laboratory investigations for Wilson disease should include serum copper, serum ceruloplasmin, and 24-hour urinary copper. Other tests, such as brain MRI and liver biopsy, can be helpful, although genetic testing can provide definitive diagnosis.
- Serum copper level is low in Wilson disease.
- Current treatment involves limiting copper intake in the diet, reducing copper absorption with zinc, chelation therapy to remove copper from the tissues, and treating the symptoms. Early recognition of Wilson disease portends a better prognosis for recovery with therapy.

INTRODUCTION

Wilson disease is one of the few movement disorders in which there are therapies that modify disease progression. This disease is caused by copper overload primarily in the liver and brain caused by reduced copper excretion secondary to genetic mutations in the ATP7B gene. Excessive copper leads to a variety of clinical presentations, including neurologic symptoms, acute or chronic liver failure, and/or psychiatric manifestations. Because it is a rare autosomal recessive disorder presenting with such diverse manifestations, there is often a delay in the diagnosis and treatment, which is unfortunate because it is treatable. This article reviews the clinical presentation, epidemiology, genetics, pathophysiology, diagnosis, and management of Wilson disease. Given that there is no universally agreed-on algorithm for treatment, we also offer an approach to Wilson disease management based on our experience.

[a] Department of Neurosciences, University of California, San Diego, 9500 Gilman Drive #0886, La Jolla, CA 92092, USA; [b] Department of Neurology, David Geffen School of Medicine at UCLA, 710 Westwood Plaza, Los Angeles, CA 90095, USA
* Corresponding author.
E-mail address: jbronste@mednet.ucla.edu

Neurol Clin 38 (2020) 417–432
https://doi.org/10.1016/j.ncl.2020.01.005
0733-8619/20/© 2020 Elsevier Inc. All rights reserved.

CLINICAL PRESENTATION

Wilson disease was first described in 1912 by Dr Samuel Alexander Kinnier Wilson.[1] In his article published in Brain, he described several cases of progressive neurologic dysfunction associated with cirrhosis of the liver that ended in death. He proposed the disease may be called "progressive lenticular degeneration," although ultimately it was known as Wilson disease, named after him. Many of the core features of Wilson disease were described in his initial article, with the most prominent symptoms of neurologic dysfunction, cirrhosis, and psychiatric features, although it is now known that there are other systems involved as well. There is great variability in the symptoms that patients with Wilson disease present with, and for that reason it is sometimes referred to as the great masquerader.[2] It must be kept in mind that there is likely a large referral bias to many of the case series, so the frequency of neurologic, psychiatric, and hepatic presentations varies considerably. One study of 282 patients with Wilson disease in India found that 15% of patients presented with hepatic symptoms only, 69% with neurologic symptoms, 4% with hepatic and neurologic symptoms, and 2% with psychiatric symptoms only.[3] Other studies have varied in the estimation, with hepatologists reporting hepatic presentation in up to 68%.[4] Psychiatric problems are often underappreciated early in the disease.

AGE AT PRESENTATION

Wilson disease generally presents in childhood and young adulthood. The most common age of presentation is 10 to 20 years,[3,5,6] but patients can present before the age of 5 years[7,8] and after the age of 70 years.[9] In 1 study, 3.8% of 1223 patients with genetically confirmed Wilson disease became symptomatic at 40 years of age or later.[10] Thus, although most patients present early in life, Wilson disease could still be considered in the differential diagnosis for patients presenting in middle age. Several studies have suggested that patients with primarily hepatic presentations tend to be younger than those with neurologic presentations, although both can occur early and late in life.[11]

NEUROLOGIC SYMPTOMS

The neurologic symptoms of Wilson disease are varied, but most refer to dysfunction in the extrapyramidal system. Wilson[1] originally described the neurologic symptoms as being purely extrapyramidal, with symptoms of involuntary movements, tremor, dystonic smile, dysphagia, and dysarthria. This description still holds true, and neurologic symptoms of Wilson disease include dysarthria, dystonia, gait abnormalities, tremor, parkinsonism, chorea, and (more rarely) seizures. Depending on the study, there have been a range of reported frequencies of these symptoms. A review of several independent case series suggests that dysarthria is the most common neurologic symptom at presentation, followed by gait abnormality/ataxia/cerebellar, dystonia, parkinsonism, and others as summarized in **Table 1**.[2,3,12,13] The dystonia in Wilson disease can be focal, segmental, or generalized,[14] although the focal dystonia of facial expression causing involuntary smiling is known as risus sardonicus and is fairly common in Wilson disease.[12] Classically, a rubral wing-beating tremor has been described in Wilson disease, although tremor can also be present at rest, with posture, or with action.

HEPATIC DYSFUNCTION

There is a spectrum of symptoms from hepatic dysfunction in Wilson disease, ranging from asymptomatic increase in liver enzyme levels to fulminant liver failure.

Table 1
Summary of neurologic symptoms at presentation based on 4 independent case series

Neurologic Manifestations at Onset	Patients (%)
Dysarthria	46–97
Gait abnormality/ataxia/cerebellar	28–75
Dystonia	38–69
Parkinsonism	12–58
Postural tremor	55
Dysphagia	50
Chorea/athetosis	6–30
Seizures	6–28
Rest tremor	4

Data from Refs.[2,3,12,13]

Typically, early in the disease there is mild increase in transaminitis, which progresses to chronic active hepatitis, followed by fibrosis and then cirrhosis.[15] Cirrhosis may begin compensated and progress to decompensated cirrhosis with ascites, coagulopathy, varices, and encephalopathy. The most common symptoms at presentation are jaundice, anorexia, and emesis, occurring in 37% to 44%, followed by ascites in about 23% to 36%, and hepatosplenomegaly in 16% to 29%.[15] The presence of cirrhosis at presentation portends an increased risk of mortality.[16] Interestingly, there seems to be a low risk of hepatocellular carcinoma in patients with Wilson disease.[17,18]

PSYCHIATRIC MANIFESTATIONS

Psychiatric manifestations are often the first symptom of Wilson disease, but these symptoms do not often lead to the diagnosis until neurologic or hepatic symptoms develop. Wilson described "emotionalism" in 8 of the 12 cases in his initial description of the disease.[1] Psychiatric symptoms can be variable, but affective disorders are more common than psychosis,[19] and common psychiatric features include personality changes, depression, cognitive changes, and anxiety.[20] Personality changes can take the form of aggression, disinhibition, or obsessiveness. Two large case series suggest that many patients have psychiatric symptoms at the time of presentation.[20,21] One retrospective case series identified psychiatric manifestations in 64.8% of patients.[20] In another study of 195 patients, 51% had psychiatric symptoms at the time of presentation and 20% had seen psychiatrists before the diagnosis of Wilson disease.[21] The delay in diagnosis in patients with primary psychiatric symptoms, estimated to be about 28 months,[22] is much greater than other presentations of Wilson disease, which averaged 12 months in a separate study.[6] This finding is not surprising because depression is common in this age group and mild neurologic side effects such as tremor can be side effects of medications to treat them.

OPHTHALMOLOGIC DYSFUNCTION

The first description of Kayser-Fleischer rings was in 1902 and 1903, before the initial description of Wilson disease. There was initially debate about its association with Wilson disease, but several studies have established that Kayser-Fleischer rings are present in 90% to 99% of cases with neurologic symptoms.[5,23] However, only a little more than half of patients with hepatic presentations have Kayser-Fleischer rings.[23] The presence of Kayser-Fleischer rings represents copper deposition and is best identified by a slit lamp examination performed by an experienced ophthalmologist. However, a recent study also suggests that some patients with Wilson disease with normal slit lamp examinations were shown to have abnormal anterior segment optical coherence tomography,[24] suggesting that imaging of the corneal membrane may be more sensitive to detecting copper deposition than the traditional slit lamp examination.

OTHER CLINICAL MANIFESTATIONS

Wilson disease can have effects on several other organ systems, including hematologic (anemia and thrombocytopenia), renal, endocrine, and cardiac systems. Coombs-negative hemolytic anemia and episodes of jaundice caused by hemolysis can occur independent of liver disease, although it is rarely the presenting symptom.[11] The kidneys can be involved in Wilson disease, again independent of liver disease, and there are reports of renal tubular acidosis and aminoaciduria. Effects on the bone and joints can present as arthralgias, and some patients have been misdiagnosed with rheumatoid arthritis.[11] There are various endocrinological effects, including growth and puberty disorders, hypoparathyroidism, dysmenorrhea, and infertility.[25] In addition, patients with Wilson disease have also been found to have mild changes in electrocardiography and diastolic dysfunction.[26,27]

GENETICS AND EPIDEMIOLOGY

Wilson disease is an autosomal recessive condition, although it was not until 1985 that it was linked to chromosome 13.[28] In 1993, 2 separate groups described mutations in the ATP7B gene in patients with Wilson disease.[29,30] Subsequently, there have been more than 500 mutations in the ATP7B described[31]; however, there is still much to learn. Individual gene mutations have not been reliably associated with different presentations of Wilson disease,[32] although there is some evidence that truncating mutations may be associated with earlier onset than missense mutations[33] and patients with frameshift mutations may be more likely to develop neurologic symptoms.[34] Interestingly, there are case reports of monozygotic twins who are phenotypically discordant for Wilson disease.[35–37] This finding strongly suggests there must be at least some contribution of environmental and epigenetic factors contributing to Wilson disease. However, there has been limited success in identifying other genetic loci that may modify the Wilson disease phenotype, with several genes implicated, including genes involved in triglyceride metabolism, lipid metabolism, and antioxidant pathways.[38] Environmental factors thought to make a difference include gender,[32] iron,[39] and dietary factors.[39]

Wilson disease is a rare disorder, although the prevalence has varied depending on the study, with the most widely cited prevalence of 1 in 30,000.[40] More recent studies in China[41] and France[42] suggest a lower prevalence of 1 in 56,000 to 1 in 66,000, respectively. The frequency of individuals carrying pathogenic mutations is higher than expected. This finding has been confirmed in multiple populations in France,[43] the United Kingdom,[44] and China.[45] In addition, 1 study showed a higher than expected frequency of Wilson disease in the offspring of patients with Wilson disease.[46] Thus, there is some debate about the true prevalence of Wilson disease and whether there are patients with Wilson disease that have not been diagnosed and are not being picked up in the epidemiologic studies. In addition, there may be incomplete penetrance, and there is at least 1 case in the literature of a patient carrying 2 mutations in the ATP7B gene presenting with hepatitis but without any evidence of alteration in copper metabolism.[47]

PATHOPHYSIOLOGY

Copper is a cofactor in many enzymes and is necessary for normal metabolism. One example is cytochrome c oxidase, which is involved in the final step of the electron transport chain and uses copper as a cofactor to perform this function. People consume approximately 1 mg/d of copper in their diets and excrete 90% of the unused copper in bile, which is eventually eliminated in stool and the remainder in the urine. In Wilson disease, patients cannot excrete copper efficiently in the bile and therefore it accumulates in the liver and brain.

Wilson disease is caused by a defect in the ATP7B gene, which encodes a P-type adenosine triphosphatase. The function of this protein is to load copper onto apoceruloplasmin in the Golgi apparatus to become ceruloplasmin in hepatocytes. Normally, the ceruloplasmin would then be excreted into bile with copper bound to it, functioning as the major pathway to remove excess copper from the body. In Wilson disease, the malfunction of the ATP7B protein leads to an inability to load copper onto ceruloplasmin in the Golgi apparatus, and therefore an inability to appropriately excrete copper into bile (**Fig. 1**). As a result, copper builds up in the hepatocyte and subsequently leaks into the blood. Copper exists in 2 pools in the blood: ceruloplasmin bound (85%–95%) and non–ceruloplasmin bound or free copper (5%–15%), which is loosely bound to albumin and available for uptake by cells or to participate in metabolism.[48] Apoceruloplamin is ceruloplasmin unbound to copper and is quickly degraded in the blood stream, leading to a low serum ceruloplasmin levels in Wilson disease. Because most serum copper is normally bound to ceruloplasmin and ceruloplasmin levels are low in Wilson disease, total serum copper level is low in the disease and free unbound copper level is increased. Copper toxicity is thought to be mediated by oxidative stress and creation of free radicals, mediated by free copper participating in metabolic reactions.[5] Ultimately, it is this copper toxicity

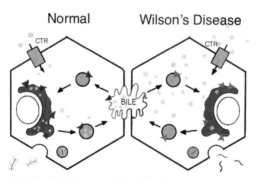

Fig. 1. In normal metabolism (*left*), copper (*gold dots*) enters hepatocyte cytoplasm via the copper transporter (CTR) and into the Golgi apparatus (*brown*) by an ATPase (*blue*) coded by the ATP7B gene. Copper is then transported via vesicles and secreted into bile in the free state or into the plasma protein bound (ceruloplasmin). A defective Wilson ATPase (*red*) results in impaired copper transport into the Golgi and vesicles and decreased secretion into bile. Intracellular copper level increases, leading to hepatocyte cell death and copper leakage into the plasma. A greater portion of apoceruloplasmin remains unbound to copper in Wilson disease and is secreted into the plasma. It is then rapidly degraded, which results in lower ceruloplasmin level.

that leads to the hepatic and neurologic dysfunction. The pathophysiology of the skeletal and hematologic problems seen in some patients with Wilson is poorly understood.

DIAGNOSIS
Laboratory Tests

Several laboratory investigations are helpful in establishing the diagnosis of Wilson disease, and these are summarized here, followed by the diagnostic criteria.

Ceruloplasmin
Serum ceruloplasmin level is low in most patients with Wilson disease. It is known that other conditions may also cause ceruloplasmin level to be low, including individuals heterozygous for ATP7B mutations, as well as other disease affecting the loss of protein (eg, nephrotic system) or synthesis of protein (eg, end-stage liver disease, malnutrition). In addition, increases in ceruloplasmin level may occur as an acute phase reactant[49] and with other hormonal conditions such as pregnancy and while taking oral contraceptives.[50] Studies have suggested that the sensitivity of low ceruloplasmin level (<20 mg/dL) for Wilson disease range from 80% to 99%,[3,5,51] although the specificity is lower. A large study of serum ceruloplasmin in China found that the sensitivity of ceruloplasmin level less than 20 mg/dL for Wilson disease was 99% and the specificity was 80.9%, but less than 15 mg/dL had a lower sensitivity of 95% and higher specificity of 95%.[51] In addition, with patients with hepatic presentations, low ceruloplasmin level may be less predictive of Wilson disease, and 1 study found that low ceruloplasmin level in the setting of liver disease had a positive predictive value of 5.9%.[52] Thus, the other factors, such as clinical presentation and other laboratory tests, are needed to make the diagnosis of Wilson disease.

Serum copper and free copper
Serum copper level is a measure of the total copper in the serum, regardless of whether it is bound to protein (ceruloplasmin or albumin) or unbound (free). Because ceruloplasmin level is low in Wilson disease, and copper is mostly carried by ceruloplasmin in the serum, the total serum copper level is typically low in patients with Wilson disease despite the disease being caused by copper overload. The serum copper is not indicative or useful on its own, but free copper is a marker of disease. Although some specialized laboratory tests are able to measure free copper level directly, this is not widely available and thus free copper level is typically calculated by subtracting ceruloplasmin level (mg/dL) times 3 from total serum copper level (μg/dL) to estimate the level of non–ceruloplasmin-bound copper. Normal free copper level is less than 10 μg/dL, and in Wilson disease it is typically higher than this. However, because free copper level is an indirect value, it can be negative and is not always reliable.

Urinary copper
The urinary excretion of copper is an important measure of copper excretion. As mentioned earlier, normally copper is excreted mainly through bile; in Wilson disease, the biliary copper excretion is reduced and there is increased urinary copper excretion as a result. For accurate interpretation of the urinary copper, patients must take home a copper-free container to collect urine for a full 24 hours. This requirement can be challenging in pediatric patients and, if urine is not collected correctly, there can be a falsely low value. In Wilson disease, 24-hour urinary copper level is typically more than 100 μg in 24 hours in adults. If urinary copper level is mildly increased and there is a question of Wilson disease, urinary copper can be measured before and after penicillamine to evaluate whether urinary copper level increases after penicillamine

(500 mg every 12 hours), which would be expected if there is an excess of copper stored in tissues.

Additional blood tests

Liver function tests, including aspartate aminotransferase (AST), alanine amino-transferase (ALT), gamma-glutamyl transferase, bilirubin, alkaline phosphatase, and prothrombin time, can be helpful measures of liver function. A complete blood count can show Coombs-negative hemolytic anemia, thrombocytopenia, and so forth.

MRI Brain

For those patients with neurologic symptoms, MRI of the brain can be helpful to establish any stereotypical findings consistent with Wilson disease, as well as to rule out other causes of neurologic symptoms. Although the so-called face of the giant panda sign, which consists of increased T2 signal in the midbrain, has been thought to be pathognomonic for Wilson disease, there are multiple MRI changes that can occur in Wilson disease. An excellent retrospective study of 100 patients with early-onset extrapyramidal disorders compared them with 56 patients with Wilson and found that the face of the giant panda sign was present in only 14% of patients with Wilson disease and 0% of patients with other pediatric extrapyramidal disorders, and thus it is fairly specific but not sensitive.[53] Other MRI findings include signal changes in the basal ganglia, thalami, pons, and white matter, as well as atrophy.[53] MRI lesions are reversible in most patients with treatment, and were correlated with clinical improvement in 1 study, although patients with extensive changes were less likely to improve.[54]

Liver Biopsy

Liver biopsy is sometimes obtained as part of the diagnostic work-up for Wilson disease, especially in patients with hepatic presentations. Total hepatic copper is the most useful diagnostic from the liver biopsy, and has a sensitivity estimated to be 83% when liver copper level is greater than 250 μg/g.[55] Stains such as rhodanine detect the abnormal presence of lysosomal copper but are not sensitive for the diagnosis.[56] False-negatives caused by sampling error remain a significant problem in using liver biopsies for the diagnosis of Wilson disease.[55,57]

Genetic Testing

Genetic testing of the ATP7B gene is considered the gold standard for diagnosis of Wilson disease. However, because of the variability in genetic mutations that have been described, looking for common polymorphisms misses possible pathogenic mutations, and direct sequencing of the entire gene is recommended.[58]

DIAGNOSTIC CRITERIA

In 2003, the Leipzig criteria for the diagnosis of Wilson disease were put forth by the European Association for the Study of the Liver (EASL).[50] These criteria consider both clinical and laboratory data to establish the diagnosis and are summarized in **Table 2**. The criteria use a combination of clinical examination and laboratory findings, with a diagnosis established after achieving at least 4 points. These criteria are used in research settings; however, they also can be helpful for practicing physicians who are trying to establish the diagnosis of Wilson disease, especially in settings in which genetic testing is difficult to obtain.

Table 2
Diagnostic criteria for Wilson disease according to Leipzig criteria

Clinical or Laboratory Finding		Points
Kayser-Fleischer Rings	Present	2
	Absent	0
Neurologic Symptoms or MRI Findings	Severe	2
	Mild	1
	Absent	0
Serum Ceruloplasmin Level (g/L)	<0.1	2
	0.1–0.2	1
	Normal (>0.2)	0
24-h Urinary Copper	>2× upper limit of normal	2
	1–2× upper limit of normal	1
	Normal	0
	Normal, but >5× upper limit of normal after D-penicillamine	2
Coombs-negative Hemolytic Anemia	Present	1
	Absent	0
Total Liver Copper Level (μmol/g)	>5× upper limit of normal (>4)	2
	Increased (0.8–4)	1
	Normal (<0.8)	−1
	Rhodanine-positive granules present	1
Genetic Mutation	Present on both chromosomes	4
	Present on 1 chromosome	1
	Absent	0
Total Score	Diagnosis established	4
	Diagnosis possible, more tests needed	3
	Diagnosis unlikely	2 or less

Adapted from Liver EA for the S of the. EASL Clinical Practice Guidelines: Wilson's disease. *J Hepatol.* 2012;56(3):671-685; with permission.

MANAGEMENT

The overall goal of therapy is to establish normal copper homeostasis by balancing copper intake and excretion. In patients with copper overload, the goal of therapy is net negative copper balance, which can be achieved by increasing excretion via chelation therapy, as well as reducing copper absorption with zinc and reducing dietary intake. Once proper balance is established, maintenance can often be achieved using zinc and low-copper diet alone, but it sometimes requires ongoing chelation.

MEDICATIONS

Multiple medications are approved for the treatment of Wilson disease, with 1 medication currently under study in a phase III clinical trial for Wilson disease. The medications vary in mechanism, side effects, and potency, which is summarized in **Table 3**. D-Penicillamine and trientine both work as chelating agents by binding with copper, which is then eliminated in the urine and therefore promotes copper excretion. In contrast, zinc salts inhibit the absorption of copper from the diet by inducing expression of the endogenous copper chelator metallothionine in the gut and liver. Bischoline-tetrathiomolybdate is currently under study, but has a novel mechanism of action and it works by complexing free copper to albumin, sequestering free copper

Table 3
Medications for Wilson disease

Drug	Mechanism	Dosing	Side Effects	Potency
D-Penicillamine	Chelates copper and promotes urinary excretion	Titrated up to 1 g/d, divided into 2–4 doses Must be taken 30 min before meals or 2 h after meals	Fever, rash, anemia, bone marrow suppression, lymphadenopathy, lupuslike syndrome, worsening neurologic symptoms	Very effective at attaining negative copper balance, 5–10 mg/d in early therapy[60]
Trientine	Chelates copper and promotes urinary excretion	Titrated up to 1 g/d, divided into 2–4 doses Must be taken 30 min before meals or 2 h after meals	Proteinuria, bone marrow suppression, autoimmune reactions, worsening neurologic symptoms	Less effective attaining negative copper balance, 2–3 mg/d in early therapy[60]
Zinc salts	Induces metallothionine in gastrointestinal epithelium and inhibits copper absorption	50 mg TID Must be taken at least 1 h before or after meals	Gastrointestinal upset	Weak, <1 mg/d[60]
Bis-choline-tetrathiomolybdate (under phase III clinical trial)	Complexes free copper with albumin	15 mg/d	Transaminitis, bone marrow suppression	To be determined

Abbreviation: TID, 3 times a day.

from participating in metabolic reactions.[48] A similar drug, ammonium tetrathiomolybdate, was previously studied with beneficial anticopper effects, but it was too unstable for practical use.[59] The drugs also differ in effectiveness in reducing total body copper level, with D-penicillamine being the most potent at copper efflux, and zinc salts being least potent.[60] A large retrospective study of patients receiving trientine and D-penicillamine supports the 2 drugs having similar effectiveness, but with increased side effects in the D-penicillamine group.[61] However, the quality of studies comparing the efficacy of anticopper medications has been limited to smaller, unrandomized trials.[62] A meta-analyses does support the superiority of D-penicillamine to placebo, but there was mixed evidence comparing zinc with D-penicillamine.[62] When chelation therapy is indicated, the authors generally prefer starting with trientine rather than D-penicillamine because it has fewer side effects.

The potential for neurologic worsening is another important consideration in selecting a treatment of Wilson disease. The frequency of worsening neurologic symptoms early after starting chelation therapy has been described in many studies, occurring between less than 10% and 50% of patients.[61,63–65] It remains unclear whether there is a difference in the frequency of neurologic worsening between chelating agents.[62] Increase of serum free copper level precedes neurologic worsening in patients treated with trientine, [48] and it has been suggested that chelation increases the free copper, which is available to create free radicals and contributes to further damage. For this reason, chelation therapy should be started at low dose if the patient has neurologic symptoms and needs to be closely monitored. If neurologic decline does occur, the dose of the chelator should be reduced or even stopped and zinc therapy should be used. This situation can often be a conundrum because the goal is to reduce copper levels in brain and the liver as fast as possible to limit permanent damage, but chelating too fast with traditional chelators can cause additional damage. Thus, the novel mechanism of tetrathiomolybdate as complexing free copper is attractive theoretically, and the recent phase II trial supports the low rate of neurologic worsening,[59] although larger studies are needed and underway.

LIVER TRANSPLANT

Liver transplant is an effective therapy for patients with liver disease. Transplant of a normally functioning liver into a patient with Wilson disease essentially restores normal copper excretion, as well as normal liver function. However, liver transplant is a complex procedure requiring lifelong immunosuppression and is typically reserved for patients with acute liver failure or decompensated cirrhosis.[56,66]

DIET

Following a low-copper diet is a commonsense lifestyle modification that should work to reduce the overall copper load to the body. In general, it is recommended that patients should try to consume less than 1 mg/d of total copper, which is not difficult to achieve by avoiding the highest copper content foods (ie, shellfish and liver) and eating other foods rich in copper (ie, chocolate, nuts, dried fruits, beans, and mushrooms) in moderation. Water can contain high concentrations of copper if it comes from copper piping. Most water filters do not remove copper, although running the water to flush the pipes greatly reduces the levels. Purified or distilled water contain almost no copper. Avoid using copper cooking pots as well.

There is little direct evidence of the effectiveness of a low-copper diet in treating Wilson disease,[67] but it is logical to reduce the intake within reason.

SYMPTOM MANAGEMENT

Although much of the focus is on anticopper therapies, symptom management is also an important component of medical therapy. Hepatic complications such as esophageal varices and ascites are treated symptomatically similar to advanced liver disease of other causes. For neurologic symptoms, medications to treat parkinsonism, such as carbidopa/levodopa, can be tried but are not necessarily effective.[12] Treatments for dystonia can be tried, including anticholinergic medications such as trihexiphenidyl or local muscle relaxants with botulinum toxin injections for focal dystonia. Deep brain stimulation targeting ventral intermediate nucleus of thalamus for tremor and the globus pallidus interna for dystonia have been tried, but with variable success in a limited number of patients.[68] In addition, taking a multidisciplinary approach and involving speech therapy for dysarthria and dysphagia, as well as physical therapy and occupational therapy, may be helpful as well. Psychiatric manifestations can be managed with serotonin reuptake inhibitors or neuroleptics, although there is some evidence that patients with Wilson disease are more sensitive to neuroleptics.[19]

PREVENTION

Once a patient is diagnosed with Wilson disease, siblings at risk should be screened. Because Wilson disease is an autosomal recessive disease, siblings of affected patients are at a 25% risk of having the disease. Siblings, whether or not they are symptomatic, should be screened with liver function tests, neurologic examination, ophthalmologic examination, and functional tests of copper metabolism (ceruloplasmin, 24-hour urinary copper), or genetic testing. If the specific genetic mutations are known, siblings can be tested for those polymorphisms or with haplotype analysis of polymorphisms in genes flanking ATP7B.[58] In addition, there have been efforts to develop population screening tests for newborns to detect presymptomatic Wilson disease. Although initial studies of ceruloplasmin were unsuccessful, a new test quantifying the amount of ATP7B protein in serum is promising for an appropriate screening tool.[69]

PROGNOSIS

Before the development of medical therapies, Wilson disease was inevitably a fatal disease.[1] Early diagnosis is important and has been shown to be associated with reduced mortality and need for liver transplant,[16,50,70] and the life expectancy is estimated to be near that of the general population.[71] In addition, health-related quality of life in treated patients with Wilson disease is similar to that of the general population.[72] However, compliance is an important factor for prognosis,[71] and there are reports of death in patients who were previously well controlled on medications who became noncompliant.[73] With regard to reversibility of symptoms, most evidence suggests that both neurologic and hepatic symptoms improve with appropriate therapy in most patients,[5,16,74,75] although dystonia may be the least likely of the neurologic symptoms to respond to treatment.[75] Psychiatric symptoms are also expected to improve with anticopper treatment, although there may a plateau in response after 2 years of treatment.[20] Despite a favorable response to treatment in most patients, there are also reports of patients who have died despite early diagnosis and treatment, and there is a concept that some patients do not respond conventionally to copper-reducing agents.[70,76]

APPROACH TO MANAGEMENT

There is no consensus on treating patients with Wilson disease, but there is some general agreement on overall approach. The authors would like to share our treatment approach at Wilson disease center of excellence.

When starting anticopper therapy on a newly diagnosed patient, the goal of therapy is to achieve a net negative copper balance. However, the urgency of copper level reduction should be evaluated depending on the clinical scenario. When symptoms are already present, there is a more urgent need to reduce copper level for the best chance of symptom reversal and to prevent further disease progression, and thus the more potent chelating medications are indicated. In asymptomatic patients, there is less urgency to reduce copper levels and it may be possible to use zinc and a low-copper diet alone.

For asymptomatic patients, the authors typically start with zinc 50 mg 3 times per day on an empty stomach along with a low-copper diet. The authors monitor neurologic symptoms and liver function tests as well as urinary copper excretion every 3 months. If the patient develops symptoms at any time, we add a chelating agent. If the urinary copper level increases from baseline, we also consider adding a chelating agent at that time.

For symptomatic patients, we typically use trientine if available through the patient health insurance because of the preferable side effect profile, but D-penicillamine is an appropriate alternative if trientine is not available. For both medications, we typically start with a dosage of 250 mg/d on an empty stomach and increase by 250-mg increments every 7 to 14 days to a maximum of 1000 to 1500 mg daily divided into 2 to 3 doses. For children and adults who weigh less than 45 kg (100 lb), we recommend starting with 250 mg daily with a maximum total daily dose of 20 mg/kg in 2 or 3 divided doses. We monitor the neurologic status closely and reduce the dose if there is evidence of decline at any point. Liver function tests, complete blood count with platelets, serum copper and ceruloplasmin, and 24-hour urine copper are monitored approximately every 3 months during chelation. We find the 24-hour urine copper to be more accurate than spot serum free copper levels (indirectly measured) for monitoring copper status. Urine copper level increases once chelation is initiated but eventually come down as copper stores are depleted. Once the 24-hour urine copper level decreases to 100-200 μg/d, which often can take 6 to 12 months, the patient enters the maintenance phase of therapy.

In the maintenance phase of therapy, the goal is to maintain a net even copper balance. After chelation therapy, many patients are able to achieve this with zinc and low-copper diet alone, although some patients remain on low-dose chelation therapy. As discussed earlier, we use urinary copper as a marker of copper status, which is monitored every 6 months in the maintenance phase along with serum copper, ceruloplasmin, blood counts, and liver function tests. An increase in the urinary copper to more than 100 μg/d suggests an increase in systemic copper stores, which reflects noncompliance or insufficient anticopper therapy. This condition should be addressed by stressing compliance, adding back chelating drug, or increasing the dose of chelator therapy until urinary copper level decreases to less than 100 μg/d again. Because of the chronic nature of Wilson disease and the potential for worsening with noncompliance, we continue to monitor laboratory tests every 6 months indefinitely for patients with Wilson.

DISCLOSURE

C. Mulligan: none. J.M. Bronstein: site principal investigator of the phase 2 and 3 trials of tetrathiomolybdate in Wilson disease run by Alexion and has received funds only to complete these studies.

REFERENCES

1. Wilson SAK. Progressive lenticular degeneration: A familial nervous disease associated with cirrhosis of the liver. Brain 1912;34(4):295–507.
2. Soltanzadeh A, Soltanzadeh P, Nafissi S, et al. Wilson's disease: A great masquerader. Eur Neurol 2007;57(2):80–5.
3. Taly AB, Meenakshi-Sundaram S, Sinha S, et al. Wilson disease: Description of 282 patients evaluated over 3 decades. Medicine (Baltimore) 2007;86(2):112–21.
4. Weiss KH, Gotthardt DN, Klemm D, et al. Zinc Monotherapy Is Not as Effective as Chelating Agents in Treatment of Wilson Disease. Gastroenterology 2011;140(4):1189–98.e1.
5. Brewer GJ, Yuzbasiyan-Gurkan V. Wilson disease. Medicine (Baltimore) 1992;71(3):139–64.
6. Walshe JM, Yealland M. Wilson's disease: The problem of delayed diagnosis. J Neurol Neurosurg Psychiatry 1992;55(8):692–6.
7. Kim JW, Kim JH, Seo JK, et al. Genetically confirmed Wilson disease in a 9-month old boy with elevations of aminotransferases. World J Hepatol 2013;5(3):156.
8. Beyersdorff A, Findeisen A. Morbus Wilson: Case report of a two-year-old child as first manifestation. Scand J Gastroenterol 2006;41(4):496–7.
9. Ala A, Borjigin J, Rochwarger A, et al. Wilson disease in septuagenarian siblings: Raising the bar for diagnosis. Hepatology 2005;41(3):668–70.
10. Ferenci P, Członkowska A, Merle U, et al. Late-Onset Wilson's Disease. Gastroenterology 2007;132(4):1294–8.
11. Saito T. Presenting symptoms and natural history of Wilson disease. Eur J Pediatr 1987;146(3):261–5.
12. Machado A, Chien HF, Deguti MM, et al. Neurological manifestations in Wilson's disease: Report of 119 cases. Mov Disord 2006;21(12):2192–6.
13. Starosta-Rubinstein S, Young AB, Kluin K, et al. Clinical Assessment of 31 Patients With Wilson's Disease: Correlations With Structural Changes on Magnetic Resonance Imaging. Arch Neurol 1987;44(4):365–70.
14. Svetel M, Kozić D, Stefanova E, et al. Dystonia in Wilson's disease. Mov Disord 2001;16(4):719–23.
15. Boga S, Ala A, Schilsky ML. Hepatic features of Wilson disease. In: Członkowska A, Schilsky ML, editors. Handbook of clinical neurology, vol. 142. Amsterdam: Elsevier; 2017. p. 91–9. https://doi.org/10.1016/B978-0-444-63625-6.00009-4.
16. Beinhardt S, Leiss W, Stättermayer AF, et al. Long-term Outcomes of Patients With Wilson Disease in a Large Austrian Cohort. Clin Gastroenterol Hepatol 2014;12(4):683–9.
17. van Meer S, de Man RA, van den Berg AP, et al. No increased risk of hepatocellular carcinoma in cirrhosis due to Wilson disease during long-term follow-up. J Gastroenterol Hepatol 2015;30(3):535–9.
18. Pfeiffenberger J, Mogler C, Gotthardt DN, et al. Hepatobiliary malignancies in Wilson disease. Liver Int 2015;35(5):1615–22.
19. Srinivas K, Sinha S, Taly AB, et al. Dominant psychiatric manifestations in Wilson's disease: A diagnostic and therapeutic challenge! J Neurol Sci 2008;266(1–2):104–8.
20. Akil M, Schwartz J, Dutchak D, et al. The psychiatric presentations of Wilson's disease. J Neuropsychiatry Clin Neurosci 1991;3(4):377–82.
21. Dening TR, Berrios GE. Wilson's Disease: Psychiatric Symptoms in 195 Cases. Arch Gen Psychiatry 1989;46(12):1126–34.

22. Zimbrean PC, Schilsky ML. Psychiatric aspects of Wilson disease: a review. Gen Hosp Psychiatry 2014;36(1):53–62.
23. Steindl P, Ferenci P, Dienes HP, et al. Wilson's disease in patients presenting with liver disease: A diagnostic challenge. Gastroenterology 1997;113(1):212–8.
24. Broniek-Kowalik K, Dzieżyc K, Litwin T, et al. Anterior segment optical coherence tomography (AS-OCT) as a new method of detecting copper deposits forming the Kayser–Fleischer ring in patients with Wilson disease. Acta Ophthalmol 2019. https://doi.org/10.1111/aos.14009.
25. Kapoor N, Shetty S, Thomas N, et al. Wilson's disease: An endocrine revelation. Indian J Endocrinol Metab 2014;18(6):855–7.
26. Buksińska-Lisik M, Litwin T, Pasierski T, et al. Cardiac assessment in Wilson's disease patients based on electrocardiography and echocardiography examination. Arch Med Sci 2017;15(4):857–64.
27. Quick S, Reuner U, Weidauer M, et al. Cardiac and autonomic function in patients with Wilson's disease. Orphanet J Rare Dis 2019;14(1):22.
28. Frydman M, Bonne-Tamir B, Farrer LA, et al. Assignment of the gene for Wilson disease to chromosome 13: linkage to the esterase D locus. Proc Natl Acad Sci U S A 2006;82(6):1819–21.
29. Tanzi RE, Petrukhin K, Chernov I, et al. The Wilson disease gene is a copper transporting ATPase with homology to the menkes disease gene. Nat Genet 1993;5(4):344–50.
30. Bull PC, Thomas GR, Rommens JM, et al. The Wilson disease gene is a putative copper transporting P-type ATPase similar to the menkes gene. Nat Genet 1993;5(4):327–37.
31. Kenney SM, Cox DW. Sequence variation database for the Wilson disease copper transporter, ATP7B. Hum Mutat 2007;28(12):1171–7.
32. Ferenci P, Stremmel W, Członkowska A, et al. Age and Sex but Not ATP7B Genotype Effectively Influence the Clinical Phenotype of Wilson Disease. Hepatology 2019;69(4):1464–76.
33. Merle U, Weiss KH, Eisenbach C, et al. Truncating mutations in the Wilson disease gene ATP7B are associated with very low serum ceruloplasmin oxidase activity and an early onset of Wilson disease. BMC Gastroenterol 2010;10:8.
34. Kluska A, Kulecka M, Litwin T, et al. Whole-exome sequencing identifies novel pathogenic variants across the ATP7B gene and some modifiers of Wilson's disease phenotype. Liver Int 2019;39(1):177–86.
35. Członkowska A, Gromadzka G, Chabik G. Monozygotic female twins discordant for phenotype of Wilson's disease. Mov Disord 2009;24(7):1066–9.
36. Kegley KM, Sellers MA, Ferber MJ, et al. Fulminant wilson's disease requiring liver transplantation in one monozygotic twin despite identical genetic mutation: Case report. Am J Transplant 2010;10(5):1325–9.
37. Takeshita Y, Shimizu N, Yamaguchi Y, et al. Two families with Wilson disease in which siblings showed different phenotypes. J Hum Genet 2002;47(10):543–7.
38. Czlonkowska A, Litwin T, Dusek P, et al. Wilson disease. Nat Rev Dis Prim 2018;4(1):21.
39. Medici V, Weiss KH. Genetic and environmental modifiers of Wilson disease. In: Członkowska A, Schilsky ML, editors. Handbook of clinical neurology, vol. 142. Amsterdam: Elsevier; 2017. p. 35–41. https://doi.org/10.1016/B978-0-444-63625-6.00004-5.
40. Kulkarni A, Sharma VK. Wilson's disease. In: Quah SR, editor. International encyclopedia of public health, vol. 369. Amsterdam: Elsevier; 2016. p. 424–33. https://doi.org/10.1016/B978-0-12-803678-5.00495-1.

41. Cheung KS, Seto WK, Fung J, et al. Epidemiology and natural history of Wilson's disease in the Chinese: A territory-based study in Hong Kong between 2000 and 2016. World J Gastroenterol 2017;23(43):7716–26.
42. Poujois A, Woimant F, Samson S, et al. Characteristics and prevalence of Wilson's disease: A 2013 observational population-based study in France. Clin Res Hepatol Gastroenterol 2018;42(1):57–63.
43. Collet C, Laplanche JL, Page J, et al. High genetic carrier frequency of Wilson's disease in France: Discrepancies with clinical prevalence. BMC Med Genet 2018;19(1):143.
44. Coffey AJ, Durkie M, Hague S, et al. A genetic study of Wilson's disease in the United Kingdom. Brain 2013;136(5):1476–87.
45. Jang JH, Lee T, Bang S, et al. Carrier frequency of Wilson's disease in the Korean population: A DNA-based approach. J Hum Genet 2017;62(9):815–8.
46. Dzieżyc K, Litwin T, Chabik G, et al. Families with Wilson's disease in subsequent generations: Clinical and genetic analysis. Mov Disord 2014;29(14):1828–32.
47. Stättermayer AF, Entenmann A, Gschwantler M, et al. The dilemma to diagnose Wilson disease by genetic testing alone. Eur J Clin Invest 2019;e13147. https://doi.org/10.1111/eci.13147.
48. Brewer GJ, Askari F, Dick RB, et al. Treatment of Wilson's disease with tetrathiomolybdate: V. control of free copper by tetrathiomolybdate and a comparison with trientine. Transl Res 2009;154(2):70–7.
49. Gitlin JD. Transcriptional regulation of ceruloplasmin gene expression during inflammation. J Biol Chem 1988;263(13):6281–7.
50. Ferenci P, Caca K, Loudianos G, et al. Diagnosis and phenotypic classification of Wilson disease. Liver Int 2003;23(3):139–42.
51. Xu R, Jiang YF, Zhang YH, et al. The optimal threshold of serum ceruloplasmin in the diagnosis of Wilson's disease: A large hospital-based study. PLoS One 2018;13(1):e0190887.
52. Cauza E, Maier-Dobersberger T, Polli C, et al. Screening for Wilson's disease in patients with liver diseases by serum ceruloplasmin. J Hepatol 1997;27(2):358–62.
53. Prashanth LK, Sinha S, Taly AB, et al. Do MRI features distinguish Wilson's disease from other early onset extrapyramidal disorders? An analysis of 100 cases. Mov Disord 2010;25(6):672–8.
54. Sinha S, Taly AB, Prashanth LK, et al. Sequential MRI changes in Wilson's disease with de-coppering therapy: a study of 50 patients. Br J Radiol 2007;80(957):744–9.
55. Ferenci P, Steindl-Munda P, Vogel W, et al. Diagnostic value of quantitative hepatic copper determination in patients with Wilson's disease. Clin Gastroenterol Hepatol 2005;3(8):811–8.
56. European Association for Study of Liver. EASL Clinical Practice Guidelines: Wilson's disease. J Hepatol 2012;56(3):671–85.
57. Song Y-M, Chen M-D. A single determination of liver copper concentration may misdiagnose Wilson's disease. Clin Biochem 2000;33(7):589–90.
58. Chang IJ, Hahn SH. The genetics of Wilson disease. Handb Clin Neurol 2017;142:19–34.
59. Weiss KH, Askari FK, Czlonkowska A, et al. Bis-choline tetrathiomolybdate in patients with Wilson's disease: an open-label, multicentre, phase 2 study. Lancet Gastroenterol Hepatol 2017;2(12):869–76.
60. Brewer GJ. Novel therapeutic approaches to the treatment of Wilson's disease. Expert Opin Pharmacother 2006;7(3):317–24.

61. Weiss KH, Thurik F, Gotthardt DN, et al. Efficacy and Safety of Oral Chelators in Treatment of Patients With Wilson Disease. Clin Gastroenterol Hepatol 2013; 11(8):1028–35.e2.

62. Appenzeller-Herzog C, Mathes T, Heeres MLS, et al. Comparative effectiveness of common therapies for Wilson disease: A Systematic review and meta-analysis of controlled studies. Liver Int 2019. https://doi.org/10.1111/liv.14179.

63. Litwin T, Dziezyc K, Karliński M, et al. Early neurological worsening in patients with Wilson's disease. J Neurol Sci 2015;355(1–2):162–7.

64. Brewer GJ. Penicillamine should not be used as initial therapy in Wilson's disease. Mov Disord 1999;14(4):551–4.

65. Medici V, Trevisan CP, D'Incà R, et al. Diagnosis and management of Wilson's disease: Results of a single center experience. J Clin Gastroenterol 2006;40(10): 936–41.

66. Roberts EA, Schilsky ML. Diagnosis and treatment of Wilson disease: An update. Hepatology 2008;47(6):2089–111.

67. Russell K, Gillanders LK, Orr DW, et al. Dietary copper restriction in Wilson's disease review-article. Eur J Clin Nutr 2018;72(3):326–31.

68. Hedera P. Treatment of Wilson's disease motor complications with deep brain stimulation. Ann N Y Acad Sci 2014;1315(1):16–23.

69. Jung S, Whiteaker JR, Zhao L, et al. Immuno-SRM as a potential screen for Wilson Disease. J Proteome Res 2017;16(2):862–71.

70. Członkowska A, Tarnacka B, Litwin T, et al. Wilson's disease - Cause of mortality in 164 patients during 1992-2003 observation period. J Neurol 2005;252(6): 698–703.

71. Dzieżyc K, Karliński M, Litwin T, et al. Compliant treatment with anti-copper agents prevents clinically overt Wilson's disease in pre-symptomatic patients. Eur J Neurol 2014;21(2):332–7.

72. Schaefer M, Gotthardt DN, Ganion N, et al. Wilson disease: Health-related quality of life and risk for depression. Clin Res Hepatol Gastroenterol 2016;40(3):349–56.

73. Walshe JM, Dixon AK. Dangers of non-compliance in Wilson's disease. Lancet 1986;327(8485):845–7.

74. Schilsky ML, Scheinberg IH, Sternlieb I. Prognosis of Wilsonian chronic active hepatitis. Gastroenterology 1991;100(3):762–7.

75. Burke JF, Dayalu P, Nan B, et al. Prognostic significance of neurologic examination findings in Wilson disease. Parkinsonism Relat Disord 2011;17(7):551–6.

76. Walshe JM. Cause of death in Wilson disease. Mov Disord 2007;22(15):2216–20.

Treatment of Paroxysmal Dyskinesia

Anna Latorre, MD, PhD, Kailash P. Bhatia, FRCP, MD*

KEYWORDS

- Paroxysmal dyskinesia • PKD • PNKD • PED • PRRT2 • MR-1 • SLC2A1
- Treatment

KEY POINTS

- Paroxysmal dyskinesias are a heterogeneous group of disorders manifesting as recurrent attacks of abnormal moments (dystonic, choreic, ballistic, or a combination of these), without loss of consciousness.
- According to the precipitating factors, they can be classified as paroxysmal kinesigenic dyskinesia (PKD), paroxysmal non-kinesigenic dyskinesia (PNKD), and paroxysmal exercise-induced dystonia (PED).
- Causes can be primary and secondary. Each phenotype can be associated with different gene mutations, most commonly with PRRT2, PNKD (MR-1), and SLC2A1 gene mutations.
- Preventing the attacks by avoiding precipitating factors can be sufficient in controlling the symptoms (especially for PED), but pharmacologic and other nonpharmacologic treatment options are available.
- PKD has an exquisite response to antiepileptic drugs, particularly carbamazepine, whereas benzodiazepine can be effective for PNKD. Refractory paroxysmal dyskinesia may respond to surgical treatment.

OVERVIEW: NATURE OF THE PROBLEM
Definition

Paroxysmal dyskinesias (PxD) are a rare heterogeneous group of disorders manifesting as recurrent attacks of abnormal moments, without loss of consciousness.[1] The abnormal movements may be dystonic, choreic, ballistic, or a combination of these. In medical literature, the terms "paroxysmal" and "dyskinesia" respectively refer to "sudden attack, recurrence or intensification of a disease" and "involuntary jerky or slow writhing movements, often of a fixed pattern, including tics, myoclonus, chorea and dystonia." It is, therefore, clear that the definition is too broad and could

Department of Clinical and Movement Neurosciences, UCL Queen Square Institute of Neurology, University College London, Queen Square, London WC1N 3BG, UK
* Corresponding author.
E-mail address: k.bhatia@ucl.ac.uk

Neurol Clin 38 (2020) 433–447
https://doi.org/10.1016/j.ncl.2020.01.007   **neurologic.theclinics.com**

erroneously include conditions that are not generally considered as PxD by movement disorders experts. The following paragraphs will help in clarifying this aspect.

Historical Aspects

PxD was first described in 1892 by Shuzo Kure[2] in a 23-year-old Japanese man, who had frequent movement-induced paroxysmal attacks from the age of 10. Later in 1901, Gowers[3] reported a child with a similar picture, but he considered the attacks as an epileptic phenomenon. In 1940, Mount and Reback[4] described a 23-year-old man with intermittent choreo-dystonic attacks of the trunk and extremities and labeled this condition "paroxysmal dystonic choreoathetosis." In this case, the attacks were precipitated by alcohol, coffee, or tea intake; fatigue; and smoking, and could last several hours. Over the years, more families with a similar disorder were described, showing a clear autosomal dominant pattern of inheritance. In 1967, Kertesz[5] reported other families with episodic attacks of involuntary movements; but, differently from the previous description, the attacks were very brief in duration and induced by sudden movements. Moreover, they responded well to anticonvulsants, particularly carbamazepine (CBZ). Kerstesz[5] called it "paroxysmal kinesigenic choreoathetosis," to differentiate it from "paroxysmal dystonic choreoathetosis." A third type of PxD was introduced in 1977 by Lance,[6] who used the term paroxysmal exercise-induced dystonia (PED) to describe a family who had attacks lasting between 5 and 30 minutes, provoked by prolonged exercise. It was only in 1995 that Demirkiran and Jankovic[7] merged the many terms adopted, organizing PxD in 3 subtypes: paroxysmal kinesigenic (PKD), paroxysmal non-kinesigenic dyskinesia (PNKD), and PED. A fourth subtype of PxD, characterized by attacks occurring during sleep without detectible trigger, was also proposed (ie, paroxysmal hypnogenic dyskinesias); however, it has been later discovered to be a form of autosomal dominant nocturnal frontal lobe epilepsy in most of the cases, and therefore no longer regarded as a form of PxD.

Classification

The clinical classification of PxD is mostly based on the criteria proposed by Demirkiran and Jankovic (1995),[7] subsequently refined by Bruno and colleagues[8] (2004). This classification relies on the precipitating event, which is considered the best predictor of clinical course and of the underlying genetic cause.[7,9] According to precipitating factors, PxD can be classified as PKD, PNKD, or PED. Secondary categorization is based on duration of the attacks. Finally, a tertiary categorization involves presumed etiology: primary (familial/sporadic) or secondary (**Table 1**). More recently, Erro and colleagues 2014[9] proposed a new classification scheme of primary PxD that includes all of the previously mentioned categorizations as well as the most recent genetic discoveries. This new classification consists of 2 axes: clinical features (axis 1) and genetic determinants (axis 2), as shown in **Box 1**.

Paroxysmal Kinesigenic Dyskinesia

PKD is the most common PxD, and is characterized by brief, self-limiting attacks, precipitated by sudden movements, such as standing up quickly from a chair. A sudden increase in speed, amplitude, or strength, or even the sudden additions of new actions during ongoing steady movements may induce an attack too[7,10]; whereas startle, sound/photo/vestibular stimulation, hyperventilation, or stress can favor them.[10] Usually the attacks last a few seconds up to 1 minute but are multiple during the day.[11] The frequency ranges from less than 1 per month to up to 100 per day. The clinical manifestation exhibited may be dystonia, chorea, ballismus, or a combination thereof, but among these, dystonia is the most common. The attacks may be focal,

Table 1
Clinical features of paroxysmal dyskinesia

	PKD	PNKD	PED
Age at onset	Childhood/teens	Infancy/childhood	Variable
Clinical semiology	Chorea/dystonia	Chorea/dystonia	Dystonia
Precipitating factors	Sudden movement	Coffee, tea, alcohol, stress, fatigue	Prolonged exertion
Duration of attacks	Seconds to minutes	Minutes to hours	Subside with rest (usually 15–40 min)
Frequency of attacks	From 1/mo up to 100/d	From 1/y up to 2–3/d	Dependent on exercise

Abbreviations: PED, paroxysmal exercise-induced dystonia; PKD, paroxysmal kinesigenic dyskinesia; PNKD, paroxysmal non-kinesigenic dyskinesia.

multifocal, or generalized; they most often involve 1 or 2 limbs, but trunk and/or speech (through orofacial involvement) also can be affected.[9,10] Most patients experience "aura" abnormal sensation before the involuntary movements, such as numbness or "pins and needles" in the affected limb or the epigastric region.[11] The "aura" can be used as warning sign to prevent the attacks, for instance by slowing down or "holding tight" the affected limb.[9] There is no pain or loss of consciousness during attacks, and no postictal confusion or drowsiness.[11,12] Onset age in PKD is usually between 7 and 15 years but has been described up to 40 years. There is a higher prevalence in male individuals (4:1, even up to 8:1) in the sporadic form but not in familial cases.[13]

Mutations in the PRRT2 gene are the cause of isolated PKD in approximately 40% to 90% of the cases,[14–18] depending on case ascertainment.[9,19] In PKD, PRRT2 is inherited in an autosomal dominant manner but with variable penetrance ranging from 80% to 90% in familial cases to 30% to 35% in sporadic cases.[20] In PRRT2 carriers, attack frequency peaks during puberty and decreases with age. PRRT2 mutations can cause also 2 related disorders, namely infantile convulsions and

Box 1
Classification of primary paroxysmal dyskinesias according to clinical (Axis I) and genetic (Axis II) characteristics[81]

Axis I: Clinical characteristics
A .Inclusion criteria (1 plus one of 2a, b, or c)
   1. Paroxysmal attacks of dystonia, chorea, ballism (or a mixture of those) with sudden onset and variable duration (seconds to hours).
   2. Paroxysmal dyskinesia are categorized according to the "trigger factor" into one of the following:
      a. Paroxysmal kinesigenic dyskinesia: attacks are triggered by sudden movements, acceleration, or intention to move
      b. Paroxysmal non-kinesigenic dyskinesia: attacks are triggered by coffee, alcohol, and other non-kinesigenic precipitants
      c. Paroxysmal exercise-induced dyskinesia: attacks are triggered by prolonged exercise
B .Exclusion criteria (both 1 and 2)
   1. Symptoms are due to another neurologic condition
   2. Symptoms are psychogenic

Axis II: Genetic characteristics
1. Mutations confirmed in one of the known genes (ie, PRRT2, MR-1, KCNMA1, SLC2A1)
2. No mutations in one of the known genes, or genetic testing has not been performed (undetermined forms)

choreoathetosis (ICCA) and benign familial infantile epilepsy (BFIE), and it has been proposed that ICCA, BFIE, and PKD may represent a spectrum of related disorders.[21] In addition, it is known that PRRT2 mutations can induce additional phenotypes including episodic ataxia and familial hemiplegic migraine.[19,22] When present in a single subject or in the family, these features make the occurrence of PRRT2 mutations more likely. Not all cases of PKD are due to mutations in the PRRT2 gene, and although some cases remain of unknown etiology, others have been attributed to different genes. For instance, mutations in SCN8A can be a cause of the ICCA syndrome,[23] as well as episodic dystonia.[24] Possible PKD cases have also been attributed to mutations in SLC2A1, PNKD (MR-1), KCNMA1, and KCNA1 genes.[25,26] More complex phenotypes, including developmental delays, intellectual disability, and language abnormalities, minor dysmorphic facial features, and/or autism spectrum disorder associated with PKD should raise the suspicion of 16p11.2 (micro) deletions.[27]

Paroxysmal Non-kinesigenic Dyskinesia

The typical PNKD phenotype is characterized by dystonic and/or choreic attacks, lasting from minutes to hours. Precipitating factors include coffee, tea, alcohol, and stress, whereas attacks may be alleviated by sleep. Less frequent triggers comprise change in external temperature, fever, menstruation, and tiredness. The frequency of the attacks is rarely more than 1 a day and most commonly 1 attack per week.[9] The dyskinesias can be generalized or unilateral/focal. They often start in one limb and then spread over the body and become generalized. Speech impairment due to face involvement, with oral dyskinesia or tongue dystonia, can be seen, and occasionally other additional features including oculogyric crises, blepharospasm, risus sardonicus, inability to move, and pain have been reported.[9] Prodromal symptoms, when present, include weakness, shortness of breath, and migraine. Onset is usually in infancy or early childhood.[9] Reliable data on PNKD gender prevalence are not available.

Mutations of the myofibrillogenesis regulator 1 (MR-1) gene were found to be causative of PNKD,[28] and the MR-1 gene was consequently renamed as the PNKD gene. In patients carrying the gene, a general tendency to decreasing attack frequency with aging has been described.

Although PNKD due to MR-1 mutations manifests as isolated PxD, in several gene mutations that have been recently linked to the PNKD spectrum, the involuntary movements are combined with other neurologic features. For instance, in PNKD due to KCNMA1 gene mutations, PxD are combined with a personal or familial history of epilepsy or neurodevelopmental delay.[29] PNKD also can be associated with mutations in SLC2A1,[30,31] ATP1A3,[32–34] ADCY5,[35] or in genes encoding the branched-chain a-ketoacid dehydrogenase complex (maple syrup urine disease).[36,37] Of note, ADCY5 mutations can cause variable phenotypes and may manifest, even within the same patient, with PKD and PNKD,[35,38] whereas ATP1A3, in the context of alternating hemiplegia of childhood, can manifest with hemidystonic attacks resembling PNKD.

Paroxysmal Exercise-Induced Dystonia

The third group of PxD was recognized by Lance (1977),[6] as, differently from PKD, the attacks were not brought on by sudden movements but by physical exhaustion after continuous exertion. Indeed, by definition, PEDs are precipitated by prolonged or sustained exercise. In some cases, fasting, stress, and anxiety could trigger the episodes as well.[9] Most commonly the attacks last from 15 to 40 minutes, and rarely less than 5 minutes.[9] Frequency of attacks ranges from several per day to 1 per month, with most of the patients reporting several attacks per week. The most common presentation is dystonia, but isolated chorea has been also described. It usually has focal/unilateral involvement affecting the lower limbs, and generalization of attacks is rather unusual.[22] Additional features reported during the attacks include oculogyric crises, gait disturbances, clumsiness, weakness, and migraine.[9]

Mutations in SLC2A1 gene are the main cause of PED, which can be isolated or part of a more complex phenotype.[31,39–44] SLC2A1 encodes the glucose transporter type 1 (GLUT1), a membrane-bound protein that facilitates glucose transfer across the blood-brain barrier. Heterozygous mutations in SLC2A1 result in the GLUT1 deficiency syndrome, which is a complex disorder characterized by intellectual impairment, epilepsy, microcephaly, and movement disorders, including paroxysmal forms. PED is considered as a nonclassic variant of the GLUT1 deficiency syndrome,[43] inherited in an autosomal dominant manner, although most cases are de novo.[45]

Pyruvate dehydrogenase complex-E2 (PDC-E2) deficiency and mitochondrial short-chain enoyl-CoA hydratase deficiency (ECHS1) are two potentially treatable neurologic disorders rarely reported to have an initial presentation with only isolated PED.[46,47] Other possible causes of PED are young-onset Parkinson's disease due to Parkin mutation[48] and GCH1 mutations.[9,49]

Summary

PxDs are characterized by recurrent attacks of abnormal movements, typically dystonia, chorea, or a combination of them, without loss of consciousness. According to the precipitating factor, PxDs can be classified into 3 main subtypes: PKD, PNKD, and PED. Each subtype is associated with a causative gene, respectively PRRT2, PNKD (MR-1), and SLC2A1; however, recent genetic findings have extended the spectrum of genes associated with these syndromes, suggesting certain degree of clinical and genetic overlap and refusing the concept that one phenotype is attributable to one single etiology (**Table 2**). Of note, PxD can also be secondary to a variety of acquired, immunologic and neurodegenerative causes[50] (**Table 3**). In this case, the clinical picture might be different from the classic presentation, as they occur later in life compared with the main genetic forms, and manifest with additional signs or symptoms that guide the diagnostic workup.

PATIENT EVALUATION OVERVIEW

It is generally assumed that clinical examination of PxD is normal between the attacks; however, although this might be the case for PRRT2-PKD and for MR-1-PNKD, it is not necessarily true for the other forms, as in many cases they present with additional features. Therefore, the criterion of normal interictal examination should be avoided.

The first relevant step of the diagnostic process is to obtain a detailed personal clinical history. Important features that should be considered comprise the attack's phenomenology, triggers, and duration as well as family history and comorbidities. If possible, the neurologic examination should be performed both during and between the attacks, to identify interictal examination findings that may allow for diagnostic possibilities to be narrowed. When attacks do not occur in the clinical settings, videotapes should be encouraged.

Although the disorder is intermittent in nature, it does not wax and wane over a period of time such as tics. Moreover, considering the phenomenology, it ranges from dystonia to chorea, and rarely involves ballism, but does not encompass tremor or myoclonus. In case of unusual features, such as the lack of specific and consistent

			Other Paroxysmal	
Gene	Subtype	Inheritance	Disorders	Other Features
PRRT2	PKD	AD	Epilepsy, migraine, FHM, ataxia	-
MR-1	PNKD (PKD)	AD	Migraine (rare)	-
SLC2A1	PED (PKD, PNKD)	AD	Ataxia, epilepsy	Anemia, hypotonia, spasticity
KNCMA1	PNKD	AD	Epilepsy	Mental retardation
SCN8A	PKD	AD	Epilepsy	Mental retardation
ECHS1	PED	AR	-	Leigh syndrome
PDC-E2	PED	AR	-	Leigh syndrome
ADCY5	PNKD (PKD, nocturnal)	AD		Axial hypotonia, nonparoxysmal dystonia and chorea
ATP1A3	PNKD (hemidystonic)		Hemiplegia, ataxia	-
GCH1	PED	AD	-	Parkinsonism
Parkin	PED	AR	-	Parkinsonism

Table 2
Most common genetic causes of paroxysmal dyskinesia

In parenthesis, less common subtype.
Abbreviations: AD, autosomal dominant; AR, autosomal recessive; FHM, familial hemiplegic migraine; PDC, pyruvate dehydrogenase complex; PED, paroxysmal exercise-induced dyskinesia; PKD, paroxysmal kinesigenic dyskinesia; PNKD, paroxysmal non-kinesigenic dyskinesias.

triggers, variable durations, and adulthood onset, secondary causes need to be excluded, including functional disorders.

Paroxysmal attacks comprise also epilepsy, tonic spasms, tetany, neuromyotonia, periodic paralyses, and episodic ataxias, which need to be excluded clinically or by additional investigations whenever appropriate.

PED diagnosis can be supported by a low cerebrospinal fluid/serum glucose ratio (<0.60), but as for the other syndrome, it is confirmed by genetic analysis. Some cases could remain unsolved, but treatment is to be pursued empirically.

Summary

The evaluation of patients with PxD is based on ictal and interictal clinical examination, as well as a thorough medical history. The latter should be focused on attack features (such as precipitating triggers, duration, and phenomenology), possible additional symptoms, and detailed family history. The clinical diagnosis can be confirmed by means of appropriate genetic test; however, a definitive cause is not always found. In that event, treatment should be started on an empirical base. When medical history points toward secondary causes, additional investigations might be pursued as appropriate.

MANAGEMENT GOALS

The management of PxD is focused on the reduction of attack frequency and the prevention of secondary complications, such as falls or interference with activities (for instance driving). This goal can be achieved by avoiding precipitating triggers, and/or preventing the attacks by pharmacologic and nonpharmacologic treatments.

Table 3
Secondary causes of paroxysmal dyskinesia

Immune-Mediated Disorders	Vascular	Metabolic Causes	Trauma	Other
Multiple sclerosis and other demyelinating diseases	Stroke	Hypo/hyperglycemia	Central and peripheral	Basal ganglia calcifications
Autoimmune encephalopathy (anti-VGKC, Anti-Caspr2, Hashimoto)	Moyamoya	Hypocalcaemia/ hypoparathyroidism/ pseudohypop-arathyroidism		Central pontine myelinolysis
Systemic autoimmune disorders (SLE-APS-Behcet disease)	Cerebral palsy	Thyrotoxicosis/ hypothyroidism		Kernicterus
Parry-Romberg syndrome		Wilson disease		Encephalitis/ postinfectious
Paraneoplastic limbic encephalitis		Maple syrup urine disease		Brain neoplasm
Celiac disease		Lesch-Nyhan disease		Early-onset Parkinson disease
				Functional disorders

Abbreviations: APS, antiphospholipid syndrome; SLE, systemic lupus erythematosus; VGKC, voltage-gated potassium channel-complex.

If comorbidities, like epilepsy, are present, appropriate treatment should be considered. Importantly, possible side effects of the drugs used should be monitored.

There are no guidelines for the treatment of PxD, which is based on clinical experience and known pathological mechanisms.

In secondary forms of PxD, treatment is mainly focused on the underlying cause, especially when it is reversible.

PHARMACOLOGIC TREATMENT OPTIONS
Paroxysmal Kinesigenic Dyskinesia

PKD is characterized by an exquisite response to antiepileptic drugs (AEDs). The first line of treatment is CBZ, at low dose, but phenytoin is often used too[9,51] (**Table 4**). A dramatic response to AEDs is seen especially in PRRT2-PKD compared with other forms,[52,53] but treatment failure has been reported in homozygous or compound heterozygous PRRT2 mutation carriers.[54,55]

CBZ and oxcarbazepine appear to be equally effective,[56] but other AEDs, such as phenobarbital,[57] levetiracetam,[58] gabapentin,[59] valproic acid,[9] lamotrigine,[60] and topiramate,[61] have been proven to be beneficial to some extent too.

The use of these drugs is based on class IV level of evidence (observational studies without controls).

The biological mechanisms underlying PKD are not entirely clear, therefore the reason why CBZ is the most effective drug is still not known. It has been proposed that the mutant PRRT2 interacts with SNAP-25, a presynaptic Q-SNARE protein involved in the fusion of neurotransmitter vesicles to the cellular membrane, which modulates the kinetics of voltage-gated Ca2+ channels leading to neuronal

Table 4
Most common pharmacologic treatment for paroxysmal dyskinesia

Drug	Daily Dosage	Side Effects	Effective for
CBZ	50–200 mg	Skin rash (particularly in people of Asian descent), aplastic anemia, agranulocytosis, dizziness, drowsiness, nausea, vomiting, dry mouth, edema, loss of balance or coordination	PKD
Oxcarbazepine	75–300 mg	As CBZ	PKD
Phenytoin	100–200 mg	Headache, nausea and vomiting, constipation, dizziness, drowsiness, slurred speech, loss of balance or coordination, insomnia, cardiac arrhythmias, skin reactions	PKD
Lacosamide	50–100 mg	Dizziness, spinning sensation, loss of balance or coordination, blurred vision, nausea and vomiting, drowsiness, tiredness, headache, skin reactions	PKD
Clonazepam	Low dose	Alertness decreased, drowsiness, dysarthria, fatigue, headache, hypotension, mood altered, muscle weakness, nausea, withdrawal syndrome (at low dose)	PNKD
Diazepam	Low dose	As clonazepam	PNKD

Abbreviations: CBZ, carbamazepine; PKD, paroxysmal kinesigenic dyskinesia; PNKD, paroxysmal non-kinesigenic dyskinesia.

hyperexcitability.[62] On this basis, it has been suggested that any voltage-gated sodium channel blockers (such as CBZ, phenytoin, lacosamide) could be potentially therapeutic.

Paroxysmal Non-kinesigenic Dyskinesia

The effect of conventional AEDs is limited in PNKD, but symptoms may respond to benzodiazepines (BDZ), which represent the first-line treatment option. Among them, the most commonly used are clonazepam and diazepam (class IV level of evidence) (see **Table 4**), as either prophylactic or rescue drugs. It has been shown that they are able to reduce both frequency and severity of the attacks in up to 97% of the patients.[8] Other BDZs, including lorazepam, can be effective too. Oxcarbazepine has been recently reported to be beneficial in one case,[63] whereas CBZ is ineffective in most patients.[64] The effect of other drugs on PNKD has been tried with partial success (haloperidol, anticholinergics, gabapentin, levetiracetam, nitric oxide synthetase inhibitors, adenosine agonists/antagonists, acetazolamide, piracetam, and levodopa[65–67]).

ADCY5 patients may have mild functional gain with clonazepam or clobazam, but whether these drugs also improve the paroxysmal episodes is not specifically reported.[68] In ATP1A3, the hemidystonic attacks can be treated by flunarizine, a calcium channel blocker, with dose ranging from 5 to 20 mg/d; however, there are reports of response of hemiplegia/dystonia episodes also to topiramate, ketogenic diet, aripiprazole, steroids, amantadine, and oral ATP.[69]

Paroxysmal Exercise-Induced Dystonia

Compared with other forms of PxD, PED due to GLUT1 mutations respond less to pharmacologic treatment,[64] whereas lifestyle and diet modifications are very important in preventing the attacks. Nevertheless, partial benefit has been reported with levodopa, trihexyphenidyl, and BDZ.[7,13]

If associated with Parkinson's disease or GCH1 mutations, PED improves with levodopa, whereas in ECHS1, the paroxysmal attacks can respectively respond to a mitochondrial cocktail, including thiamine, riboflavin, carnitine, coenzyme Q, vitamin B6, and vitamin C.[70]

NONPHARMACOLOGIC TREATMENT OPTIONS
Paroxysmal Kinesigenic Dyskinesia

Lifestyle: avoidance of established trigger, that is, sudden movements. Stress, sleep deprivation, anxiety, and other triggers can increase the likelihood for PKD episodes, therefore their control can help in preventing attacks.

Paroxysmal Non-kinesigenic Dyskinesia

Lifestyle and diet: avoidance of methylglyoxal-containing food and beverages, such as alcohol, coffee, tea, and chocolate, may benefit these patients, as well as the avoidance of other predisposing factors, such as fatigue. Lifestyle modifications and diet can reduce or almost abolish attacks in up to one-third of patients with MR-1 mutations.[71]

Paroxysmal Exercise-Induced Dystonia

Lifestyle and diet: prolonged continuous exertion in PED may prevent the occurrence of attacks. In case of GLUT1 deficiency, PED can respond to ketogenic diet,[72] but compliance to it can be rather poor, and the modified Atkins diet, with less strict fat-to-nonfat ratio and no restriction of food or fluid intake, has been proposed as an alternative, with good results.[73] More recently, triheptanoin, an odd-chain triglyceride that acts by replenishing metabolic intermediates in the Krebs cycle, has been shown to dramatically reduce the attacks in PED, with the advantage of being better tolerated than the Atkins diet.[74]

The ketogenic diet is successful also for the treatment of PDC-E2 deficiency.[75]

COMBINATION THERAPIES

There are not reports on the use of combination therapies for the treatment of primary PxD, unless the goal is to address both the paroxysmal attacks and comorbidities (such as epilepsy, nonparoxysmal dystonia).

Acetazolamide might be a useful adjunct to CBZ in the treatment of PKD, especially when due to demyelinating lesions.[13]

SURGICAL TREATMENT OPTIONS
Paroxysmal Kinesigenic Dyskinesia

A surgical approach for the treatment of PKD was tried in 4 members of the same family, positive for PRRT2 mutations, with benefit. In 2 members, unilateral stereotactic surgery was performed in 1967, which resulted in complete resolution of the episodes. Based on this result, the other 2 members of the family similarly affected, despite the good response to CBZ, which however reduced but not completely stopped the attacks, decided to undergo the same surgery, consisting of right ventro-oral thalamotomy. Following surgery, the number of attacks reduced significantly in one patient and completely disappeared in the other one.[76]

Paroxysmal Non-kinesigenic Dyskinesia

There are 2 reports on the effective treatment of PNKD with deep brain stimulation (DBS). The first report[77] is about a 26-year-old man with a long history of mental retardation, chorea, and episodes of flexion and jerky movements of the legs, arm, neck, and face. These episodes were classified as PNKD, although his condition remained undiagnosed. He underwent implantation of bilateral DBS in the globus pallidus internus (GPi), with a significant and sustained improvement of the attacks, as well as balance, gross motor function, and walking. In the second report, 2 patients clinically diagnosed with PNKD, refractory to conventional treatment, had a good response to GPi DBS with completely suppression of the PxD.[78]

Bilateral GPi DBS can improve the episodic choreoathetoid and dystonic movements in ADCY5.[68,79]

Paroxysmal Exercise-Induced Dystonia

In a case of PED, of unknown etiology, the dystonic attacks of the right foot ceased completely after left posteroventral medial pallidotomy.[80]

TREATMENT RESISTANCE/COMPLICATIONS/DISEASE RECURRENCE

In most of the patients affected by PKD and PNKD, the symptoms can be easily controlled by the combination of nonpharmacologic and pharmacologic therapies, with low chance of disease recurrence. The response to the pharmacologic treatment seems to be related to the underlying cause, with PRRT2-PKD and MR-1-PNKD being the most successful responders to conventional treatment. In small numbers of refractory cases, surgical approaches have been successful. Treatment of PED largely relies on the avoidance of attack triggers, and a good compliance and response to nonpharmacological treatment has been reported.

The possible side effects are related to the drug used, as detailed in the tables. Worth mentioning, the risk of hypersensitivity reactions to CBZ is increased by the presence of specific human leukocyte antigen (HLA) alleles. The HLA-B*15:02 allele is strongly associated with CBZ-induced Stevens–Johnson syndrome/toxic epidermal necrolysis in populations in which this allele is most common, such as Asian populations. In these populations, the use of CBZ should be avoided and an alternative selected.

EVALUATION OF OUTCOME, ADJUSTMENT OF TREATMENT, AND LONG-TERM RECOMMENDATIONS

Treatment outcome is based on the recurrence of the attacks, and therefore mostly on patient report. In this regard, it might be useful to ask patients to keep a diary of the episodes, specifying the duration and precipitating factors. In case of poor response to the first-line treatment, after adjusting the dose of the recommended drug (keeping in mind that PKD and PNKD usually respond to a low dose of AEDs/BDZ), the other options should be pursued and chosen according to their side-effect profile and patient comorbidities. Differently from PED due to GLUT1 deficiency, the frequency of the episodes in PKD and PNKD decreases with advancing age, and treatment might be unnecessary by that time.

SUMMARY

PxD defines clinical heterogeneous syndromes distinguished by the recurrence of attacks of abnormal movements, triggered by detectable factors, without loss of consciousness. According to the precipitating factors, PxD is classified in PKD, PNKD, and PED; other features, such as duration of the attacks, response to treatment, and etiology, might also help in differentiating them. PxD can be further stratified into primary and secondary disorders. The primary are mostly due to a genetics defect, with PRRT, PNKD (MR-1), and SLC2A1 being the most common gene involved and causing respectively PKD, PNKD, and PED. Nevertheless, the spectrum of genes associated with PxD has been broadened by recent findings, highlighting a clinical and genetic overlap among these syndromes and declining the *one-gene-one-phenotype* notion.

The clinical diagnosis of PxD is based on ictal and interictal neurologic examination, a detailed personal and family medical history, and presence of comorbidities. The clinical diagnosis can be confirmed by means of appropriate genetic test or next generation sequencing approaches. If the clinical evaluation suggest secondary causes, additional investigations should be pursued as appropriate.

The treatment of PxD is based on the combination of nonpharmacologic and pharmacologic approaches. PKD has an excellent response to AEDs (especially CBZ), whereas in many PNKD and PED cases the symptoms can be controlled by avoiding the precipitating factors. Whenever this is not sufficient, the use of drugs, such as BDZ for PNKD, and diet changes, such as ketogenic or Atkins diet for PED due to GLUT1 deficiency, can be effective. Moreover, PKD and PNKD have a benign course, and the recurrence of involuntary movement episodes tends to decrease over the years. Patients with a known genetic cause, such as PRRT2 or PNKD (MR-1), have a better response to conventional treatment compared with the undiagnosed ones; however, in the latter it is recommended to start the appropriate treatment on an empirical basis. Of note, in PxD refractory to conventional treatments, the surgical approach might be considered as an alternative option.

DISCLOSURES

K.P. Bhatia holds research grants from NIHR RfPB, MRC Wellcome Strategic grant (Ref. no.: WT089698), and PD UK (Ref. no.: G-1009) and has received honoraria/financial support to speak/attend meetings from GSK, Boehringer-Ingelheim, Ipsen, Merz, Sun Pharma, Allergan, Teva Lundbeck and Orion pharmaceutical companies. K.P. Bhatia receives royalties from Oxford University Press and a stipend for MDCP editorship. A. Latorre has nothing to disclose.

REFERENCES

1. Bhatia KP. The paroxysmal dyskinesias. J Neurol 1999;246(3):149–55.
2. Kure S. Atypical Thomsen's disease. J Tokyo Med Assoc 1982;(6):505–14.
3. Gowers WR. Epilepsy and other chronic convulsive diseases: Their Causes Symptoms and Treatment. 2nd edition. London: J & A Churchill; 1901.
4. Mount L, Reback S. Familial paroxysmal choreoathetosis. Arch Neuro Psychiatry 1940;44:841–7.
5. Kertesz A. Paroxysmal kinesigenic choreoathetosis. An entity within the paroxysmal choreoathetosis syndrome. Description of 10 cases, including 1 autopsied. Neurology 1967;17(7):680–90.
6. Lance JW. Familial paroxysmal dystonic choreoathetosis and its differentiation from related syndromes. Ann Neurol 1977;2(4):285–93.
7. Demirkiran M, Jankovic J. Paroxysmal dyskinesias: clinical features and classification. Ann Neurol 1995;38(4):571–9.

8. Bruno MK, Hallett M, Gwinn-Hardy K, et al. Clinical evaluation of idiopathic paroxysmal kinesigenic dyskinesia: new diagnostic criteria. Neurology 2004;63(12): 2280–7.

9. Erro R, Sheerin UM, Bhatia KP. Paroxysmal dyskinesias revisited: a review of 500 genetically proven cases and a new classification. Mov Disord 2014;29(9): 1108–16.

10. Bhatia KP. Familial (idiopathic) paroxysmal dyskinesias: an update. Semin Neurol 2001;21(1):69–74.

11. Bruno MK, Hallett M, Gwinn-Hardy K, et al. Clinical evaluation of idiopathic paroxysmal kinesigenic dyskinesia: new diagnostic criteria. Neurology 2004;63(12): 2280–7.

12. Houser MK, Soland VL, Bhatia KP, et al. Paroxysmal kinesigenic choreoathetosis: a report of 26 patients. J Neurol 1999;246(2):120–6.

13. Bhatia KP. Paroxysmal dyskinesias. Mov Disord 2011;26(6):1157–65.

14. Chen WJ, Lin Y, Xiong ZQ, et al. Exome sequencing identifies truncating mutations in PRRT2 that cause paroxysmal kinesigenic dyskinesia. Nat Genet 2011; 43(12):1252–5.

15. Wang JL, Cao L, Li XH, et al. Identification of PRRT2 as the causative gene of paroxysmal kinesigenic dyskinesias. Brain 2011;134(Pt 12):3493–501.

16. Li J, Zhu X, Wang X, et al. Targeted genomic sequencing identifies PRRT2 mutations as a cause of paroxysmal kinesigenic choreoathetosis. J Med Genet 2012; 49(2):76–8.

17. Braak H, Brettschneider J, Ludolph AC, et al. Amyotrophic lateral sclerosis–a model of corticofugal axonal spread. Nat Rev Neurol 2013;9(12):708–14.

18. Lee HY, Huang Y, Bruneau N, et al. Mutations in the gene PRRT2 cause paroxysmal kinesigenic dyskinesia with infantile convulsions. Cell Rep 2012;1(1):2–12.

19. Ebrahimi-Fakhari D, Saffari A, Westenberger A, et al. The evolving spectrum of PRRT2-associated paroxysmal diseases. Brain 2015;138(Pt 12):3476–95.

20. McGovern EM, Roze E, Counihan TJ. The expanding spectrum of paroxysmal movement disorders: update from clinical features to therapeutics. Curr Opin Neurol 2018;31(4):491–7.

21. Heron SE, Grinton BE, Kivity S, et al. PRRT2 mutations cause benign familial infantile epilepsy and infantile convulsions with choreoathetosis syndrome. Am J Hum Genet 2012;90(1):152–60.

22. Gardiner AR, Jaffer F, Dale RC, et al. The clinical and genetic heterogeneity of paroxysmal dyskinesias. Brain 2015;138(Pt 12):3567–80.

23. Gardella E, Becker F, Moller RS, et al. Benign infantile seizures and paroxysmal dyskinesia caused by an SCN8A mutation. Ann Neurol 2016;79(3):428–36.

24. Larsen J, Carvill GL, Gardella E, et al. The phenotypic spectrum of SCN8A encephalopathy. Neurology 2015;84(5):480–9.

25. Tian WT, Huang XJ, Mao X, et al. Proline-rich transmembrane protein 2-negative paroxysmal kinesigenic dyskinesia: clinical and genetic analyses of 163 patients. Mov Disord 2018;33(3):459–67.

26. Yin XM, Lin JH, Cao L, et al. Familial paroxysmal kinesigenic dyskinesia is associated with mutations in the KCNA1 gene. Hum Mol Genet 2018;27(4):757–8.

27. Weber A, Kohler A, Hahn A, et al. Benign infantile convulsions (IC) and subsequent paroxysmal kinesigenic dyskinesia (PKD) in a patient with 16p11.2 microdeletion syndrome. Neurogenetics 2013;14(3–4):251–3.

28. Rainier S, Thomas D, Tokarz D, et al. Myofibrillogenesis regulator 1 gene mutations cause paroxysmal dystonic choreoathetosis. Arch Neurol 2004;61(7): 1025–9.

29. Du W, Bautista JF, Yang H, et al. Calcium-sensitive potassium channelopathy in human epilepsy and paroxysmal movement disorder. Nat Genet 2005;37(7): 733–8.

30. Anheim M, Maillart E, Vuillaumier-Barrot S, et al. Excellent response to acetazolamide in a case of paroxysmal dyskinesias due to GLUT1-deficiency. J Neurol 2011;258(2):316–7.

31. Weber YG, Kamm C, Suls A, et al. Paroxysmal choreoathetosis/spasticity (DYT9) is caused by a GLUT1 defect. Neurology 2011;77(10):959–64.

32. Roubergue A, Roze E, Vuillaumier-Barrot S, et al. The multiple faces of the ATP1A3-related dystonic movement disorder. Mov Disord 2013;28(10):1457–9.

33. Pittock SJ, Joyce C, O'Keane V, et al. Rapid-onset dystonia-parkinsonism: a clinical and genetic analysis of a new kindred. Neurology 2000;55(7):991–5.

34. Rosewich H, Thiele H, Ohlenbusch A, et al. Heterozygous de-novo mutations in ATP1A3 in patients with alternating hemiplegia of childhood: a whole-exome sequencing gene-identification study. Lancet Neurol 2012;11(9):764–73.

35. Friedman JR, Meneret A, Chen DH, et al. ADCY5 mutation carriers display pleiotropic paroxysmal day and nighttime dyskinesias. Mov Disord 2016;31(1):147–8.

36. Carecchio M, Schneider SA, Chan H, et al. Movement disorders in adult surviving patients with maple syrup urine disease. Mov Disord 2011;26(7):1324–8.

37. Temudo T, Martins E, Pocas F, et al. Maple syrup disease presenting as paroxysmal dystonia. Ann Neurol 2004;56(5):749–50.

38. Chen DH, Meneret A, Friedman JR, et al. ADCY5-related dyskinesia: broader spectrum and genotype-phenotype correlations. Neurology 2015;85(23): 2026–35.

39. Zorzi G, Castellotti B, Zibordi F, et al. Paroxysmal movement disorders in GLUT1 deficiency syndrome. Neurology 2008;71(2):146–8.

40. Pons R, Collins A, Rotstein M, et al. The spectrum of movement disorders in Glut-1 deficiency. Mov Disord 2010;25(3):275–81.

41. Schneider SA, Paisan-Ruiz C, Garcia-Gorostiaga I, et al. GLUT1 gene mutations cause sporadic paroxysmal exercise-induced dyskinesias. Mov Disord 2009; 24(11):1684–8.

42. Wang D, Pascual JM, Yang H, et al. Glut-1 deficiency syndrome: clinical, genetic, and therapeutic aspects. Ann Neurol 2005;57(1):111–8.

43. Suls A, Dedeken P, Goffin K, et al. Paroxysmal exercise-induced dyskinesia and epilepsy is due to mutations in SLC2A1, encoding the glucose transporter GLUT1. Brain 2008;131(Pt 7):1831–44.

44. Leen WG, Klepper J, Verbeek MM, et al. Glucose transporter-1 deficiency syndrome: the expanding clinical and genetic spectrum of a treatable disorder. Brain 2010;133(Pt 3):655–70.

45. Weber YG, Storch A, Wuttke TV, et al. GLUT1 mutations are a cause of paroxysmal exertion-induced dyskinesias and induce hemolytic anemia by a cation leak. J Clin Invest 2008;118(6):2157–68.

46. Friedman J, Feigenbaum A, Chuang N, et al. Pyruvate dehydrogenase complex-E2 deficiency causes paroxysmal exercise-induced dyskinesia. Neurology 2017; 89(22):2297–8.

47. Olgiati S, Skorvanek M, Quadri M, et al. Paroxysmal exercise-induced dystonia within the phenotypic spectrum of ECHS1 deficiency. Mov Disord 2016;31(7): 1041–8.

48. Bozi M, Bhatia KP. Paroxysmal exercise-induced dystonia as a presenting feature of young-onset Parkinson's disease. Mov Disord 2003;18(12):1545–7.

49. Dale RC, Melchers A, Fung VS, et al. Familial paroxysmal exercise-induced dystonia: atypical presentation of autosomal dominant GTP-cyclohydrolase 1 deficiency. Dev Med Child Neurol 2010;52(6):583–6.

50. Blakeley J, Jankovic J. Secondary paroxysmal dyskinesias. Mov Disord 2002; 17(4):726–34.

51. Strzelczyk A, Burk K, Oertel WH. Treatment of paroxysmal dyskinesias. Expert Opin Pharmacother 2011;12(1):63–72.

52. Huang XJ, Wang T, Wang JL, et al. Paroxysmal kinesigenic dyskinesia: clinical and genetic analyses of 110 patients. Neurology 2015;85(18):1546–53.

53. Gardiner AR, Bhatia KP, Stamelou M, et al. PRRT2 gene mutations: from paroxysmal dyskinesia to episodic ataxia and hemiplegic migraine. Neurology 2012; 79(21):2115–21.

54. Labate A, Tarantino P, Viri M, et al. Homozygous c.649dupC mutation in PRRT2 worsens the BFIS/PKD phenotype with mental retardation, episodic ataxia, and absences. Epilepsia 2012;53(12):e196–9.

55. Delcourt M, Riant F, Mancini J, et al. Severe phenotypic spectrum of biallelic mutations in PRRT2 gene. J Neurol Neurosurg Psychiatry 2015;86(7):782–5.

56. Yang Y, Su Y, Guo Y, et al. Oxcarbazepine versus carbamazepine in the treatment of paroxysmal kinesigenic dyskinesia. Int J Neurosci 2012;122(12):719–22.

57. Goodenough DJ, Fariello RG, Annis BL, et al. Familial and acquired paroxysmal dyskinesias. A proposed classification with delineation of clinical features. Arch Neurol 1978;35(12):827–31.

58. Chatterjee A, Louis ED, Frucht S. Levetiracetam in the treatment of paroxysmal kinesiogenic choreoathetosis. Mov Disord 2002;17(3):614–5.

59. Chudnow RS, Mimbela RA, Owen DB, et al. Gabapentin for familial paroxysmal dystonic choreoathetosis. Neurology 1997;49(5):1441–2.

60. Uberall MA, Wenzel D. Effectiveness of lamotrigine in children with paroxysmal kinesigenic choreoathetosis. Dev Med Child Neurol 2000;42(10):699–700.

61. Huang YG, Chen YC, Du F, et al. Topiramate therapy for paroxysmal kinesigenic choreoathetosis. Mov Disord 2005;20(1):75–7.

62. Li M, Niu F, Zhu X, et al. PRRT2 mutant leads to dysfunction of glutamate signaling. Int J Mol Sci 2015;16(5):9134–51.

63. Kumar A, Szekely A, Jabbari B. Effective treatment of paroxysmal nonkinesigenic dyskinesia with oxcarbazepine. Clin Neuropharmacol 2016;39(4):201–5.

64. Mink JW. Treatment of paroxysmal dyskinesias in children. Curr Treat Options Neurol 2015;17(6):350.

65. Alemdar M, Iseri P, Selekler M, et al. Levetiracetam-responding paroxysmal nonkinesigenic dyskinesia. Clin Neuropharmacol 2007;30(4):241–4.

66. Coulter DL, Donofrio P. Haloperidol for nonkinesiogenic paroxysmal dyskinesia. Arch Neurol 1980;37(5):325–6.

67. Loscher W, Richter A. Piracetam and levetiracetam, two pyrrolidone derivatives, exert antidystonic activity in a hamster model of paroxysmal dystonia. Eur J Pharmacol 2000;391(3):251–4.

68. Chang FC, Westenberger A, Dale RC, et al. Phenotypic insights into ADCY5-associated disease. Mov Disord 2016;31(7):1033–40.

69. Masoud M, Gordon K, Hall A, et al. Motor function domains in alternating hemiplegia of childhood. Dev Med Child Neurol 2017;59(8):822–8.

70. Mahajan A, Constantinou J, Sidiropoulos C. ECHS1 deficiency-associated paroxysmal exercise-induced dyskinesias: case presentation and initial benefit of intervention. J Neurol 2017;264(1):185–7.

71. Erro R, Bhatia KP. Unravelling of the paroxysmal dyskinesias. J Neurol Neurosurg Psychiatry 2019;90(2):227–34.
72. Ramm-Pettersen A, Nakken KO, Skogseid IM, et al. Good outcome in patients with early dietary treatment of GLUT-1 deficiency syndrome: results from a retrospective Norwegian study. Dev Med Child Neurol 2013;55(5):440–7.
73. Leen WG, Mewasingh L, Verbeek MM, et al. Movement disorders in GLUT1 deficiency syndrome respond to the modified Atkins diet. Mov Disord 2013;28(10): 1439–42.
74. Mochel F, Hainque E, Gras D, et al. Triheptanoin dramatically reduces paroxysmal motor disorder in patients with GLUT1 deficiency. J Neurol Neurosurg Psychiatry 2016;87(5):550–3.
75. McWilliam CA, Ridout CK, Brown RM, et al. Pyruvate dehydrogenase E2 deficiency: a potentially treatable cause of episodic dystonia. Eur J Paediatr Neurol 2010;14(4):349–53.
76. Horisawa S, Sumi M, Akagawa H, et al. Thalamotomy for paroxysmal kinesigenic dyskinesias in a multiplex family. Eur J Neurol 2017;24(10):e71–2.
77. Kaufman CB, Mink JW, Schwalb JM. Bilateral deep brain stimulation for treatment of medically refractory paroxysmal nonkinesigenic dyskinesia. J Neurosurg 2010; 112(4):847–50.
78. van Coller R, Slabbert P, Vaidyanathan J, et al. Successful treatment of disabling paroxysmal nonkinesigenic dyskinesia with deep brain stimulation of the globus pallidus internus. Stereotact Funct Neurosurg 2014;92(6):388–92.
79. Meijer IA, Miravite J, Kopell BH, et al. Deep brain stimulation in an additional patient with ADCY5-related movement disorder. J Child Neurol 2017;32(4):438–9.
80. Bhatia KP, Marsden CD, Thomas DG. Posteroventral pallidotomy can ameliorate attacks of paroxysmal dystonia induced by exercise. J Neurol Neurosurg Psychiatry 1998;65(4):604–5.
81. Erro R, Sheerin UM, Bhatia KP. Paroxysmal dyskinesias revisited: a review of 500 genetically proven cases and a new classification. Mov Disord 2014;29(9): 1108–16.

An Overview of the Current State and the Future of Ataxia Treatments

Kimberly Tsu Kwei, MD, PhD[a], Sheng-Han Kuo, MD[b],*

KEYWORDS

- Cerebellum • Ataxia • Multiple system atrophy • Spinocerebellar ataxia
- Friedreich ataxia • Ataxia treatment

KEY POINTS

- A review paper summarizing current treatments for cerebellar ataxia.
- Review categorizing treatments for cerebellar ataxia by symptomatic treatment and disease-modifying treatments.
- We further separate disease-modifying treatments into those for autosomal dominant, autosomal recessive, and immune-mediated cerebellar ataxias.
- We discuss preclinical and clinical trials currently underway for the treatment of cerebellar ataxia.

INTRODUCTION

The cerebellum is responsible for a multitude of motor functions through the coordination of movements by prediction and is modulated by sensory feedback. Cerebellar ataxia refers to the dysfunction of the cerebellum that leads to problems with gait and balance, eye movements, speech, and hand dexterity.[1] The cerebellum comprises 2 hemispheres separated by the vermis. The 10 lobules of the cerebellum are grouped in 3 lobes; lobules I to V make up the anterior lobe of the cerebellum, lobules VI to IX make up the posterior lobe, and lobule X is the flocculonodular lobe. From functional imaging studies of the cerebellum, the anterior lobe is thought to be

S.-H. Kuo is supported by the NINDS K08 NS083738, R01 NS104423, National Ataxia Foundation, Louis V. Gerstner Jr. Scholarship, Parkinson Foundation, Brain Research Foundation, and International Essential Tremor Foundation; K.T. Kwei is funded by an Edmond J. Safra Fellowship in Movement Disorders through the Michael J. Fox Foundation.
a Division of Movement Disorders, Department of Neurology, Columbia University Medical Center, 610 West 168th Street, Floor 3, New York, NY 10032, USA; b Division of Movement Disorders, Department of Neurology, Columbia University Medical Center, 650 West 168th Street, Room 305, New York, NY 10032, USA
* Corresponding author.
E-mail address: sk3295@columbia.edu

important for motor control, whereas the posterior lobe is more involved in cognitive processing.[2] Thus, patients with cerebellar ataxia may have a variety of motor and nonmotor symptoms affecting their daily activities.

The prevalence of ataxia varies depending on ethnic background and geographic region, because different populations have founder effects for certain types of hereditary ataxias. Most studies have focused on the prevalence of hereditary ataxias. However, some estimates suggest that the prevalence of ataxia ranges from 2.7 to 38.35 per 100,000.[3] A study looking at the global distribution of hereditary ataxias found that the most common autosomal dominant (AD) cerebellar ataxia is spinocerebellar ataxia type 3 (SCA3), and the most common autosomal recessive (AR) ataxia is Friedreich ataxia.[4]

Cerebellar dysfunction can be caused by nutritional deficiencies, immune-mediated cerebellar degeneration, gene defects inherited in AD, AR, or X-linked fashion, as well as neurodegenerative conditions. In the work-up of ataxia, it is important to understand the age of onset and time course of ataxia, family history, and associated medical conditions and signs and symptoms. There are several excellent papers describing the work-up of ataxia,[5–7] and the focus of this paper is not to resummarize an ataxia work-up but instead to highlight current treatments for ataxia as well as those looming on the horizon. **Fig. 1** summarizes current and potential treatments for ataxia.

To understand the development of therapy for ataxia, it is important to know how the severity of ataxia is measured. There are 2 rating scales commonly used to measure ataxia severity. The Scale for the Assessment and Rating of Ataxia (SARA) score is a 40-point scale taking into account gait, stance, and upper and lower extremity motor deficits.[8] It is relatively easy to use in a clinical setting because it is not particularly time consuming. The annual rate of SARA score increase has been found to be 2.11 in SCA1, 1.49 in patients with SCA2, 1.56 in patients with SCA3, and 0.80 in patients with SCA6 in a natural history study in Europe.[9] A US natural history study of SCA also showed comparable disease progression using SARA.[10] Another commonly used scale is the International Cooperative Ataxia Rating Scale (ICARS), which is a 100-point measure of cerebellar dysfunction taking into account eye movement

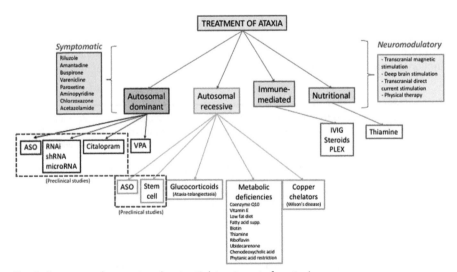

Fig. 1. Summary of current and potential treatments for ataxia.

abnormalities, upper and lower extremity coordination deficits, speech, stance, and gait.[11] A study of 18 patients with static and progressive cerebellar lesions found that the ICARS score can differentiate between the two on certain measures and can detect yearly changes in ataxia in the patients with degenerative cerebellar diseases.[12] Although ICARS was developed earlier than SARA, the latter is now the more commonly used clinical measure for ataxia.

Symptomatic Treatment of Ataxia

Many medications have been examined in an effort to find symptomatic treatment of ataxia by modulating cerebellar function through changes in ion channel function and/or cerebellar physiology. However, most symptomatic treatments have not been tested for an extended period of time, and there is a lack of replicate studies. It is also unknown whether these medications can have additional disease-modifying effects. Nonetheless, the effects of these treatments may provide some symptomatic relief and improve quality of life. **Table 1** summarizes the symptomatic treatments for cerebellar ataxias,[13–19] a few of which we will highlight below. Supplementary Table 1 lists medications that have been tested and were proven noneffective.

Riluzole has been shown to improve function in patients with ataxia as measured by SARA and ICARS scores. It mostly affects axial domains by improving speech and gait. Side effects of riluzole include mild liver enzyme increases and transient vertigo

Table 1
Symptomatic treatment of ataxia

Treatment	Ataxia Type	Evidence	References
Riluzole	SCA, FA	Randomized, double-blind, placebo-controlled trial	Ristori et al,[20] 2010; Romano et al,[21] 2015
Varenicline	SCA3	A randomized, double-blind, placebo-controlled trial	Zesiewicz et al,[22] 2012
Paroxetine	MSA	A randomized, double-blind, placebo-controlled study	Friess et al,[104] 2006
Aminopyridine	EA2	A randomized, double-blind, placebo-controlled, crossover study	Strupp et al,[13] 2011
	SCA6, ADCA	Observational studies	Tsunemi et al,[14] 2010
Amantadine (IV)	MSA	A short-term, open-label study	Youn et al,[15] 2012
Buspirone	MSA-C	Open-label studies	Heo et al,[16] 2008
Acetazolamide	SCA6, EA	Open-label studies and case reports	Baloh and Winder,[24] 1991; Griggs et al,[25] 1978; Harno et al,[26] 2004; Yabe et al,[23] 2001
	PMM2-CDG	A single-blind, randomized withdrawal trial	Martínez-Monseny et al,[27] 2019
Citalopram	FA	Case series (2 patients)	Rohr et al,[17] 1999
Chlorzoxazone	SCA1, SCA2	Rodent studies	Egorova et al,[18] 2016; Bushart et al,[19] 2018

Abbreviations: EA2, episodic ataxia type 2; FA, Friedreich ataxia; MSA, multiple system atrophy; PMM2-CDG, phosphomannomutase congenital disorder of glycosylation; SCA, spinocerebellar ataxia.

but it is generally well tolerated. Although the initial study only observed the effects of riluzole over 8 weeks, a longer study over 12 months demonstrated continued benefits.[20,21] Riluzole is thought to modulate SK channels, which are enriched in Purkinje cells, thereby partially normalizing neuronal firing patterns.

Varenicline is a partial agonist of the alpha-4 beta-2 nicotinic acetylcholine receptor, and was studied in 20 patients with SCA3. A randomized, double-blind, placebo-controlled trial of varenicline demonstrated improved axial symptoms and rapid alternating movements measured by SARA scores. Although relatively well tolerated, varenicline was associated with depression and irritability.[22]

Acetazolamide has been shown to reduce the severity of ataxia in SCA6 patients, who have repeat expansions in the *CACNA1A* gene.[23] The *CACNA1A* gene encodes a voltage-dependent calcium channel, and acetazolamide is thought to be helpful in channelopathies because it lowers the pH and may thus change channel properties. An open-label trial of 6 patients with SCA6 treated with acetazolamide had improvement in ataxia rating scale scores and decreased body sway but the effects were somewhat lessened after 1 year. Similarly, patients with episodic ataxia 2, which is also caused by *CACNA1A* gene mutations, had improvement in cerebellar symptoms with acetazolamide.[24–26] Acetazolamide has also been shown to be effective in treating patients with PMM2 congenital disorder of glycosylation (PMM2-CDG), which causes a cerebellar syndrome that may be mediated by abnormal glycosylation of calcium channels.[27] PMM2-CDG is inherited in an AR manner. Side effects of acetazolamide include low bicarbonate levels and paresthesia.

Neuromodulation of Ataxia

Neuromodulation of the cerebellum has shown promising results for treating cerebellar ataxia.[28] Various studies have used transcranial magnetic stimulation (TMS), transcranial direct current stimulation (tDCS), as well as deep brain stimulation (DBS) to test the effects on cerebellar ataxia. Although DBS involves surgical implantation of electrodes, both TMS and tDCS are noninvasive and all have relatively few side effects. TMS can directly induce action potentials, whereas tDCS can modulate local membrane potentials and neuronal plasticity.[29] Studies of cerebellar neuromodulation are highlighted in **Table 2**,[30–40] but we will focus on a few tDCS studies in more depth here because tDCS is most studied in cerebellar ataxia with a potential for larger-scaled studies in the future.

A case report of 2 patients with SCA2 showed improvement in SARA score, tremor, and upper limb dysmetria immediately after cerebellar tDCS.[41] Nineteen patients with various forms of neurodegenerative ataxias received anodal cerebellar tDCS in a double-blind, sham-controlled crossover study.[35] There was a statistically significant improvement in 1.40 points of SARA score and 4.37 points in ICARS score between the sham and stimulation trials. A drawback of these studies was that the effect was only tested immediately after stimulation, making it unclear the duration of symptomatic improvement in these patients after cessation of tDCS.

A follow-up double-blind, randomized, sham-controlled crossover study looked at cerebellar anodal and spinal cord cathodal tDCS stimulation in 21 patients with degenerative ataxias.[42] This study had a longer stimulation period (2 weeks of stimulation) and had SARA and ICARS performed before the stimulation or sham stimulation, immediately after the 2-week stimulation, and then 1 and 3 months after the stimulation. There was an improvement in SARA and ICARS scores in the stimulation group at all time points after stimulation when compared with prestimulation and also when compared with sham. This study provides evidence of long-duration responses of ataxia with tDCS to the cerebellar region. The ease of use of tDCS and its

Table 2
Neuromodulation and physical exercise for ataxia

Treatment	Ataxia Type	Evidence	References
Physical therapy	SCA7, SCA2, FA	A randomized, open-label study	Ilg et al,[30] 2009; Tercero-Pérez et al,[107] 2019; Velázquez-Pérez et al,[45] 2019
Transcranial magnetic stimulation	SCA1, SCA6, SCA7	A randomized, sham-controlled study and case reports	Kawamura et al,[31] 2018; Shiga et al,[32] 2002; Shimizu et al,[33] 1999
	Posterior circulation stroke	A randomized, double-blind trial	Kim et al,[34] 2014
Transcranial direct current stimulation	SCA, MSA, FA	A randomized, double-blind, sham-controlled study and case report	Benussi et al,[35] 2015; Benussi et al,[42] 2018; Grimaldi and Manto,[36] 2013
Deep brain stimulation	SCA	Case report	Hashimoto et al,[37] 2018
	FXTAS	Case report	dos Santos Ghilardi et al,[38] 2015
	Cerebellar stroke	Case report	Teixeira et al,[39] 2015; Weiss et al,[40] 2015

Abbreviations: FA, Friedreich ataxia; FXTAS, fragile X-associated tremor/ataxia syndrome; MSA, multiple system atrophy; SCA, spinocerebellar ataxia.

relatively longer-lasting effects may be a useful adjunct to symptomatic medical therapy, especially in those patients who do not experience improvement in ataxia from medical therapy.

Exercise as Treatment of Ataxia

Exercise or physical therapy has been a cornerstone in helping patients with cerebellar ataxia. Studies of intensive rehabilitation have shown long-lasting effects physical therapy. A study of 42 patients with degenerative ataxia were separated into 2 groups to receive either 4 weeks of intensive rehabilitation or a delayed start of the same rehabilitation schedule.[43] The immediate rehabilitation group had a greater improvement in SARA scores compared with the delayed start group at 4 weeks after rehabilitation. Although the improvement was attenuated at 12 and 24 weeks after rehabilitation, a significant number of patients still had improvement compared with baseline, which is notable given the progressive worsening of symptoms in degenerative ataxia.

A study of 38 patients with SCA2, randomized into a 24-week neurorehabilitation therapy program or no therapy, showed that there was a significant improvement in SARA scores in those receiving rehabilitation.[44] Notably the improvement in SARA scores between the therapy and no-therapy groups were in the subscores of gait, stance, and sitting, and this improvement occurred in patients across different durations of disease. Another study randomized 30 preclinical patients with SCA2 into either a neurorehabilitation or control group.[45] Although the study did not find differences in SARA scores between the 2 groups after the intervention, there was an improvement in tandem gait, finger-to-nose, and heel-shin tasks in the rehabilitation group only.

Of note, a diverse range of physical activity has been shown to be helpful in improving cerebellar dysfunction. A study showed that intensive cycling in 20 patients with various SCAs led to an improvement in ICARS scores after 4 weeks of cycling.[46] Patients with cerebellar ataxia might be able to engage in diverse exercise and physical therapy, such as rock climbing.[47] Working through rehabilitation on physical functions as basic as swallowing may even be helpful in patients with cerebellar ataxia.[48] These studies highlight the long-lasting effects of exercise and physical therapy in improving ataxia, and may point to a neuromodulatory effect of exercise or to enhance other brain regions.

DISEASE-MODIFYING TREATMENTS OF ATAXIA

The cerebellum has some capacity for cellular and synaptic plasticity in response to injury, and the hope is that this reserve of cerebellar recovery can be accessed in ataxia patients if appropriate treatments are applied in a timely manner.[49] We highlight some current treatments that may be disease modifying as well as hopeful looming prospects in the next few sections. Perhaps the most important message is that identifying the cause of a patient's cerebellar ataxia can be incredibly important as there are a multitude of treatments that can slow down and even halt the progression of ataxia.

Treatment of Nutritional and Immune-Mediated Ataxias

Table 3 lists common causes of nutritional and immune-mediated ataxias, which occur on a time course of weeks to months.[50–52] It is critically important to examine serum B12 and B1 levels and potential autoimmune antibodies in a patient with cerebellar ataxia as these causes could potentially be reversed with the appropriate treatment especially early on in the disease course. The classic triad of Wernicke encephalopathy is altered mental status, ophthalmoplegia, and cerebellar ataxia,[53] and often occurs in the setting of chronic alcoholism. Cancer and gastric bypass surgeries can be causes for Wernicke encephalopathy.[54] Prompt thiamine administration is the treatment of Wernicke encephalopathy.

The most common cause of vitamin B12 deficiency is pernicious anemia, which is an autoimmune atrophic gastritis.[55] Although the gait dysfunction in vitamin B12 deficiency is due to both demyelination of the dorsal columns and central nervous system involvement, there have been cases of vitamin B12 deficiency that cause cerebellar

Table 3
Treatment of immune-mediated and nutritional ataxias

Treatment	Ataxia Type	Evidence	References
IVIG	Opsoclonus myoclonus ataxia syndrome	A randomized, open-label study	de Alarcon et al,[50] 2018
Gluten-free diet, IVIG, steroids	Anti-DGP, antigliadin cerebellar ataxias	Open label	Nanri et al,[51] 2016
IVIG, steroids	Anti-GAD, anti-TPO cerebellar ataxias	Open label	Nanri et al,[51] 2016
Thiamine	Wernicke encephalopathy	Case reports	Chataway and Hardman,[52] 1995; Sinha et al,[53] 2019
Vitamin B12	Pernicious anemia, dietary deficiency	Case reports	Chakrabarty et al,[56] 2014; Stabler,[55] 2013

Abbreviations: Anti-DGP, antideamidated gliadin peptide; anti-GAD, antiglutamic acid decarboxylase antibody; anti-TPO, antithyroperoxidase antibody; IVIG, intravenous immunoglobulin.

degeneration only.[56] Prompt detection of vitamin B12 deficiency in a patient with cerebellar ataxia is critical to prevent clinical worsening and may even reverse the symptoms.

Finally, there are several autoantibodies and paraneoplastic syndromes associated with cerebellar ataxia, and the identification of these causes are important to administer treatment promptly. The most common paraneoplastic autoantibodies are the anti-Yo (associated with breast, uterine, and ovarian cancers), anti-Hu (associated with small-cell lung cancer), anti-Tr (associated with Hodgkin lymphoma), and anti-CV2 (associated with small-cell lung cancer and thymoma) antibodies.[57] Guidelines on the treatment of paraneoplastic ataxias suggest that if treating the underlying cancer does not help, a round of immunotherapy may be helpful. Patients who have autoantibodies detected in the serum may receive a spinal tap to further investigate whether these antibodies are present in the cerebrospinal fluid. These patients with autoantibodies can be treated with either immunoglobulin therapy, steroids, or other immuno-modulatory agents. More randomized controlled trials need to be conducted to examine autoantibody-mediated cerebellar ataxia to determine the optimal immunotherapy tailored to ataxia associated with each individual autoantibody.

Treatment of Autosomal Recessive Ataxias

AR ataxias are a diverse group of progressive ataxias often resulting from dysfunctional metabolic pathways. Most AR ataxias can be categorized in 1 of 3 subgroups: defective mitochondrial metabolism, dysfunctional lipid metabolism, and impaired DNA repair.[58] Some of these AR mutations lead to accumulation of toxic downstream metabolites and reduction of these metabolites can ameliorate the symptoms of the illness and/or modify the disease course.

Wilson disease causes a multitude of neurologic, psychiatric, and ophthalmologic symptoms, including ataxia due to copper accumulation in the brain and liver resulting from a mutation in the *ATP7B* gene that encodes a protein for copper transport. Lifelong treatment with oral copper chelators, such as penicillamine and trientene may reverse symptoms.[59]

The clinical hallmarks of cerebrotendinous xanthomatosis (CTX) include tendon xanthomas, cerebellar ataxia, dementia, cataracts, premature atherosclerosis, and pulmonary dysfunction, with increased cholestenol and bile alcohols found in serum and urine.[60] Supplementation with chenodeoxycholic acid (CDCA) inhibits abnormal bile acid synthesis by providing feedback inhibition, which is deficient in these patients. A hallmark 1984 study showed that, in 17 patients with CTX given CDCA, several had improvement of dementia and cerebellar ataxia.[61] A more recent study in 2 patients with CTX started on CDCA at 3 and 5 months showed that the neurologic deficits could be improved but not completely reversed, suggesting that there even earlier detection and treatment of CTX may lead to normal development.[62]

Niemann-Pick type C (NPC) is caused by a mutation in the *NPC1* or *NPC2* gene, and the adolescent onset forms of NPC usually result in cerebellar dysfunction, including ataxia, dysarthria, dysmetria, and dysphagia, as well as gelastic cataplexy.[63] On examination, patients with NPC have characteristic impaired vertical saccades.[64] Miglustat inhibits the synthesis of glycosphingolipids and has been approved for the treatment of NPC. Miglustat improves swallowing function and stabilizes other neurologic manifestations in the years after its administration in patients with NPC.[65] Other potential treatments for NPC include 2-hydroxypropyl-beta-cyclodextrins, which may delay Purkinje cell loss and slows disease progression in patients with NPC.[66]

Other AR ataxias that are due to nutritional deficiencies may be stabilized or improved with correct nutritional supplementation. In a patient with ataxia, dysarthria, vision loss due to retinitis pigmentosa, head tremor, and areflexia, a diagnosis of ataxia with vitamin E deficiency (AVED) must be considered. Patients with AVED have mutations in the alpha-tocopherol transfer protein (alpha-TTP) leading to reduced intrahepatocyte vitamin E incorporation into very low-density lipoproteins. Serum vitamin E levels are very low in patients with AVED, and early supplementation of vitamin E in these patients can improve cerebellar ataxia.[67] AR cerebellar ataxia type 2 is caused by a mutation in the ADCK3 gene, which results in coenzyme Q10 deficiency. Studies show that patients seem to respond to idebenone supplementation.[68]

A success in AR cerebellar ataxia treatment has been seen in patients with biotinidase deficiency identified on newborn screening, who subsequently received biotin supplementation.[69] A study following 44 patients started on biotin supplementation as infants lived normal adult lives, significantly different from the natural history of biotinidase deficiency. Interestingly, biotin supplementation seems only to slow or stop disease progression but cannot reverse symptoms. A case report described patients with novel mutations in the SLC19A3 gene who had recurrent episodes of encephalopathy and at baseline had generalized dystonia, epilepsy, and bilateral caudate and putaminal hyperintensities, and had clinical improvement during encephalopathic episodes with administration of high doses of biotin and thiamine.[70]

The most common AR cerebellar ataxia is Friedreich ataxia, accounting for ~25% of all AR cerebellar ataxias. Friedreich ataxia is caused by a homozygous GAA trinucleotide repeat in intron 1 of the FXN gene on chromosome 9q13,[71] which reduces expression of the protein product, frataxin. Several preclinical studies in rodent cell lines have shown that administration of wild-type frataxin either through bone-marrow transplants,[72] administration of antisense oligonucleotides (ASOs),[73] or injecting FXN-expressing adeno-associated virus[74] can improve some of the symptoms of Friedreich ataxia in preclinical models.

Table 4 provides a more comprehensive summary of the different AR cerebellar ataxias and their treatments.[75–84] Most evidence for the treatments of AR cerebellar ataxias rely on case reports and open-label studies, likely because of the rarity of the illnesses. However, it is still important to consider the possibility of AR cerebellar ataxias in patients with early onset ataxia with or without sensory neuropathy, because many AR ataxias can stabilize or improve if treatments are started early. The potential for gene therapy or strategies to enhance FXN expression in the treatment of Friedreich ataxia portends great hope for the treatment of AR cerebellar ataxias.

Treatment of Autosomal Dominant Cerebellar Ataxias

In patients presenting with a slowly progressive cerebellar ataxia in middle-age who may have a family history of ataxia, the diagnosis of AD ataxias should be aggressively pursued. Most AD cerebellar ataxias are categorized as SCAs, but with exceptions, such as dentatorubro-pallidoluysian atrophy and episodic ataxias. The most common SCAs involve polyglutamine expansion repeats, which lead to protein misfolding and aggregation,[85] and SCA1, 2, 3, 6, 7, and 17 belong to this group. There are no definitive disease-modifying therapies for AD cerebellar ataxias. Nonetheless, we list several relevant clinical and preclinical studies as potential therapies for AD cerebellar ataxias.

A randomized, open-label study of valproic acid in 12 patients with SCA3 showed improvement in SARA scores, with dizziness and loss of appetite as side effects,[86] with 2 patients dropping out as a result of these side effects. The possible mechanism of action is thought to be inhibition of histone deacetylases to regulate the expression of pathologic proteins. Proteins carrying polyglutamine repeats are known to activate

Table 4
Disease-modifying therapies for autosomal recessive ataxias

Ataxia Type	Treatment	Evidence	Mechanism of Action	References
Wilson disease	Copper chelators	Observational studies	Blockade of intestinal copper absorption	Aggarwal and Bhatt,[59] 2018
Niemann-Pick disease	Miglustat	A prospective randomized control study	Inhibition of glycosphingolipid synthesis	Pineda et al,[65] 2018
Niemann-Pick disease	Intrathecal 2-hydroxypropyl-β-cyclodextrins	An open-label, observational study	Unclear	Ory et al,[66] 2017
Ataxia telangiectasia	Glucocorticoids	An prospective, cohort study	Unclear, possible restoration of ATM gene expression	Menotta et al,[75] 2017; Zannolli et al,[76] 2012
Cerebrotendinous xanthomatosis	Chenodeoxycholic acid supplementation	An open-label, observational study	Replace missing bile acids; lipid metabolism deficit	Berginer et al,[61] 1984; Nie et al,[60] 2014; Pierre et al,[62] 2008
Ataxia with vitamin E deficiency	Vitamin E	An open-label, observational study	Replacement therapy	Gabsi et al,[67] 2001
Riboflavin transporter deficiency neuronopathy (*SLC52A2* gene mutation)	Riboflavin	An open-label, observational study	Supplementation to boost absorption	Foley et al,[77] 2014; Guissart et al,[78] 2016
Autosomal recessive cerebellar ataxia 2	Ubidecarenone	An open-label, observational study	Replacement therapy	Mignot et al,[68] 2013
Abetalipoproteinemia	Low-fat diet, essential fatty acid supplementation	A case series	Replacement therapy	Chardon et al,[79] 2009; Lee and Hegele,[80] 2014
Biotinidase deficiency	Biotin	A case series	Replacement therapy	Wolf,[69] 2017
SLC19A3 gene mutation	Biotin, thiamine	A case series	Replacement therapy	Debs et al,[70] 2010
CoQ10, CoQ4 deficiency	Coenzyme Q10	A case series	Replacement therapy	Caglayan et al,[81] 2019

(continued on next page)

Table 4
(continued)

Ataxia Type	Treatment	Evidence	Mechanism of Action	References
Refsum disease	Phytanic acid restriction, lipid apheresis	A case report and 2 case series	Toxic substrate reduction	Baldwin et al,[82] 2010; Gibberd et al,[83] 1979; Zolotov et al,[84] 2012
Friedreich ataxia	Frataxin-expressing adeno-associated virus	A preclinical, rodent study	Frataxin replacement	Piguet et al,[74] 2018
Friedreich ataxia	Allogenic stem cell transplantation	A preclinical, rodent study	Increasing frataxin levels	Kemp et al,[72] 2018
Friedreich ataxia	ASO targeting triplet expansion in frataxin	A preclinical, rodent study	Increasing frataxin expression	Li et al,[73] 2018

Abbreviations: CoQ4, coenzyme Q4; CoQ10, coenzyme Q10.

the mitochondrial apoptotic pathway leading to neuronal death; therefore, mitochondrial dysfunction might be one of the shared pathways for SCAs. A retrospective study demonstrated that patients with SCA who took coenzyme Q10, a cofactor in the mitochondrial respiratory chain, had better SARA scores than those who did not. In addition, a dose-dependent effect was found in SCA3 patients.[87] This study suggests that coenzyme Q10 may have disease-modifying effects for SCAs, and warrants further randomized, placebo-controlled trials.

Citalopram was initially identified in a screen of Food and Drug Administration-approved drugs to rescue neuronal dysfunction in an SCA3 *C elegans* model. Citalopram, a serotonin reuptake inhibitor, was further demonstrated to reduce ataxin-3 neuronal inclusions and astrogliosis, as well as improving motor symptoms in SCA3 mouse models.[88] These preclinical animal studies provide strong rationale for future randomized placebo-controlled trials for citalopram in SCA3. Excessive glutamate-mediated neuronal transmission leading to neuronal toxicity is a major mechanism for neurodegenerative disorders; therefore, modulating glutamatergic neuronal transmission could be disease modifying in SCAs. Toward this goal, there is an ongoing clinical trial treating patients with SCA with a glutamate modulator, troriluzole, to examine its effects on slowing disease progression.

As SCAs are monogenetic disorders, therapies specifically through ASO targeting mutated genes hold promise as disease-modifying therapies. There are several preclinical studies showing that knocking down of mutated protein expression by gene therapy can be disease-modifying therapy in animal models of SCAs. ASOs targeting *ATXN2* in an SCA2 mouse model improved motor function and Purkinje cell firing.[89] A similar study showed efficacy of ASOs in reducing ATXN1 protein in a SCA1 mouse model with improvement in motor coordination.[90] ASOs targeting ATXN3 also showed promising results in SCA3 mouse models,[91] and knockout of the entire *ATXN3* gene is well tolerated in a SCA3 mouse model,[92] providing some preclinical safety evidence. Other than ASOs, intraventricular injections of small hairpin RNA silencing mutant *ATXN3* have also been shown to improve motor symptoms in SCA3 mouse models.[93] In an SCA6 mouse model, delivery of microRNA against the toxic gene product can also improve the motor performance and halt Purkinje cell degeneration.[94]

Table 5 summarizes the potential disease-modifying treatments highlighted above, as well as other promising preclinical studies not mentioned in the text.[95–99]

Treatments for Idiopathic Neurodegenerative Ataxias

Multiple system atrophy (MSA) is a common diagnosis in patients with late onset, progressive cerebellar ataxia, and is often accompanied by parkinsonism and autonomic dysfunction. A recent genetic study found an association between a rare variant of *COQ2* and MSA in East Asian populations.[100,101] *COQ2* encodes for a protein that is essential in the synthesis of coenzyme Q10. Interestingly, reduction of coenzyme Q10 levels is observed both in the serum[93] and in the postmortem cerebellum of MSA patients.[102] A clinical trial of ubiquinol, a form of coenzyme Q10, in the treatment of MSA is currently underway.

Other potential treatments for MSA include modulation of the serotonergic system with the selective serotonergic reuptake inhibitors, which have been shown to reduce alpha-synuclein uptake in neuronal and oligodendroglial cells and thus could be disease modifying.[103] A small double-blind, placebo-controlled study of 19 patients with MSA showed that paroxetine (a serotonin reuptake inhibitor)-treated patients showed better limb agility compared with placebo-treated patients.[104] Another promising potential treatment of MSA is myeloperoxidase inhibitors, which have been shown to improve motor function in an MSA mouse model and to reduce

Table 5
Disease-modifying therapy in autosomal dominant ataxias

Treatment	Ataxia Type	Evidence	Mechanism of Action	References
Valproic acid	SCA3	A randomized, open-label, dose-escalation	Histone deacetylase inhibition	Lei et al,[86] 2016
Coenzyme Q10	SCA 1, SCA3	An observational study	Enhancing mitochondrial respiratory chain	Lo et al,[87] 2015
Troriluzole (BHV4157)	SCA1, SCA2, SCA3, SCA6, SCA7, SCA8, SCA10	An ongoing phase III, randomized, double-blind, placebo-controlled study	Modulation of glutamate neurotransmission	ClinicalTrials.gov Identifier: NCT03701399
Citalopram	SCA3	A preclinical, rodent study	Reduction of ATXN3 neuronal inclusions and astrogliosis	Teixeira-Castro et al,[88] 2015
ASO targeting ATXN1	SCA1	A preclinical, rodent study	Downregulation of ATXN1	Friedrich et al,[90] 2018
ASO targeting ATXN2	SCA2	A preclinical, rodent study	Downregulation of ATXN2	Scoles et al,[89] 2017
ASO vitreal injections	SCA7	A preclinical, rodent study	Downregulation of ATXN7	Niu et al,[95] 2018
ASO targeting ATXN3	SCA3	A preclinical, rodent study	Downregulation of ATXN3	Toonen et al,[91] 2017; Moore et al,[92] 2017
Small hairpin RNA silencing ATXN3	SCA3	A preclinical, rodent study	Downregulation of ATXN3	Nóbrega et al,[96] 2019; Nóbrega et al,[97] 2013
RNAi targeting ATXN7	SCA7	A preclinical, rodent study	Reduction of wild-type and mutant ATXN7	Ramachandran et al,[98] 2014
MicroRNA blocking IRES-driven translation CACNA1A second cistern	SCA6	A preclinical, rodent study	Selective downregulation of toxic gene product	Miyazaki et al,[94] 2016
Gluten-free diet	SCA35	A case report	Toxic substrate reduction	Lin et al,[99] 2019

Abbreviations: ASO, antisense oligonucleotide; SCA, spinocerebellar ataxia.

alpha-synuclein aggregates.[105] A phase III trial of an irreversible myeloperoxidase inhibitor, BHV-3241, is currently underway.

SUMMARY

The purpose of this paper is to describe the wide range of treatments available for cerebellar ataxia and to highlight promising therapies on the horizon. With the recent advances in gene therapy and ASO approaches, targeted therapies for ataxia hold the promise of improving quality of life for patients with ataxia and possibly even slow or reverse the disease course. Moreover, continued improvement of clinical trial design for ataxia will also advance our ability to demonstrate therapeutic efficacy.

Several challenges remain to be addressed in the currently burgeoning field of ataxia research. First, although most studies rely on SARA or ICARS scores, additional patient-oriented outcome measures need to be developed to demonstrate improvement in quality of life for patients with ataxia. Second, as we begin to understand the role of the cerebellum in cognitive and emotional processing, nonmotor rating scales, such as the cerebellar cognitive affective scale,[106] will need to be implemented to comprehensively assess the aspects of patients' lives affected by cerebellar dysfunction. Third, all clinical rating scales are limited by their ability to capture only a moment in time in the clinic and as such the development of wearable instruments are needed to more fully describe "real life" motor performance at home. Fourth, imaging and fluid biomarkers should be used as part of clinical trials for ataxia to test for target engagement and as additional evidence for disease-modifying effects.

There are a multitude of treatments for ataxia that can be offered: both symptomatic therapies that may help regardless of the cause of ataxia as well as potential disease-modifying therapies targeting specific types of ataxia. It is not only the time to dispel the myth that there is no treatment of ataxia, but in fact there is a reason to be hopeful about the current state and future of ataxia treatments.

DISCLOSURE

The authors have no relationship with a commercial company that has a direct financial interest in the subject matter or materials discussed in this article or with a company making a competing product.

SUPPLEMENTARY DATA

Supplementary data related to this article can be found online at https://doi.org/10.1016/j.ncl.2020.01.008.

REFERENCES

1. Manto M, Bower JM, Conforto AB, et al. Consensus paper: roles of the cerebellum in motor control—the diversity of ideas on cerebellar involvement in movement. Cerebellum 2012;11(2):457–87.
2. Stoodley CJ, Schmahmann JD. Functional topography of the human cerebellum. Handb Clin Neurol 2018;154:59–70.
3. Subramony SH. Degenerative ataxias: challenges in clinical research. Ann Clin Transl Neurol 2017;4(1):53–60.
4. Ruano L, Melo C, Silva MC, et al. The global epidemiology of hereditary ataxia and spastic paraplegia: a systematic review of prevalence studies. Neuroepidemiology 2014;42(3):174–83.

5. Klockgether T. Sporadic ataxia with adult onset: classification and diagnostic criteria. Lancet Neurol 2010;9(1):94–104.

6. Pandolfo M, Manto M. Cerebellar and afferent ataxias. Continuum (Minneap Minn) 2013;19(5 Movement Disorders):1312–43.

7. Fogel BL, Perlman S. An approach to the patient with late-onset cerebellar ataxia. Nat Clin Pract Neurol 2006;2(11):629–35 [quiz 1 p following 635].

8. Schmitz-Hübsch T, du Montcel ST, Baliko L, et al. Scale for the assessment and rating of ataxia: development of a new clinical scale. Neurology 2006;66(11): 1717–20.

9. Jacobi H, du Montcel ST, Bauer P, et al. Long-term disease progression in spinocerebellar ataxia types 1, 2, 3, and 6: a longitudinal cohort study. Lancet Neurol 2015;14(11):1101–8.

10. Ashizawa T, Figueroa KP, Perlman SL, et al. Clinical characteristics of patients with spinocerebellar ataxias 1, 2, 3 and 6 in the US; a prospective observational study. Orphanet J Rare Dis 2013;8:177.

11. Trouillas P, Takayanagi T, Hallett M, et al. International Cooperative Ataxia Rating Scale for pharmacological assessment of the cerebellar syndrome. The Ataxia Neuropharmacology Committee of the World Federation of Neurology. J Neurol Sci 1997;145(2):205–11.

12. Morton SM, Tseng Y-W, Zackowski KM, et al. Longitudinal tracking of gait and balance impairments in cerebellar disease. Mov Disord 2010;25(12):1944–52.

13. Strupp M, Kalla R, Claassen J, et al. A randomized trial of 4-aminopyridine in EA2 and related familial episodic ataxias. Neurology 2011;77(3):269–75.

14. Tsunemi T, Ishikawa K, Tsukui K, et al. The effect of 3,4-diaminopyridine on the patients with hereditary pure cerebellar ataxia. J Neurol Sci 2010;292(1–2):81–4.

15. Youn J, Shin H, Kim JS, et al. Preliminary study of intravenous amantadine treatment for ataxia management in patients with probable multiple system atrophy with predominant cerebellar ataxia. J Mov Disord 2012;5(1):1–4.

16. Heo J-H, Lee S-T, Chu K, et al. The efficacy of combined estrogen and buspirone treatment in olivopontocerebellar atrophy. J Neurol Sci 2008;271(1–2): 87–90.

17. Rohr A, Eichler K, Hafezi-Moghadam N. Citalopram, a selective serotonin reuptake inhibitor, improves symptoms of Friedreich's ataxia. Pharmacopsychiatry 1999;32(3):113–4.

18. Egorova PA, Zakharova OA, Vlasova OL, et al. In vivo analysis of cerebellar Purkinje cell activity in SCA2 transgenic mouse model. J Neurophysiol 2016;115(6): 2840–51.

19. Bushart DD, Chopra R, Singh V, et al. Targeting potassium channels to treat cerebellar ataxia. Ann Clin Transl Neurol 2018;5(3):297–314.

20. Ristori G, Romano S, Visconti A, et al. Riluzole in cerebellar ataxia: a randomized, double-blind, placebo-controlled pilot trial. Neurology 2010;74(10): 839–45.

21. Romano S, Coarelli G, Marcotulli C, et al. Riluzole in patients with hereditary cerebellar ataxia: a randomised, double-blind, placebo-controlled trial. Lancet Neurol 2015;14(10):985–91.

22. Zesiewicz TA, Greenstein PE, Sullivan KL, et al. A randomized trial of varenicline (Chantix) for the treatment of spinocerebellar ataxia type 3. Neurology 2012; 78(8):545–50.

23. Yabe I, Sasaki H, Yamashita I, et al. Clinical trial of acetazolamide in SCA6, with assessment using the Ataxia Rating Scale and body stabilometry. Acta Neurol Scand 2001;104(1):44–7.

24. Baloh RW, Winder A. Acetazolamide-responsive vestibulocerebellar syndrome: clinical and oculographic features. Neurology 1991;41(3):429–33.

25. Griggs RC, Moxley RT, Lafrance RA, et al. Hereditary paroxysmal ataxia: response to acetazolamide. Neurology 1978;28(12):1259–64.

26. Harno H, Hirvonen T, Kaunisto MA, et al. Acetazolamide improves neurotological abnormalities in a family with episodic ataxia type 2 (EA-2). J Neurol 2004; 251(2):232–4.

27. Martínez-Monseny AF, Bolasell M, Callejón-Póo L, et al. AZATAX: acetazolamide safety and efficacy in cerebellar syndrome in PMM2 congenital disorder of glycosylation (PMM2-CDG). Ann Neurol 2019;85(5):740–51.

28. França C, de Andrade DC, Teixeira MJ, et al. Effects of cerebellar neuromodulation in movement disorders: a systematic review. Brain Stimul 2018;11(2): 249–60.

29. Grimaldi G, Argyropoulos GP, Boehringer A, et al. Non-invasive cerebellar stimulation—a consensus paper. Cerebellum 2014;13(1):121–38.

30. Ilg W, Synofzik M, Brötz D, et al. Intensive coordinative training improves motor performance in degenerative cerebellar disease. Neurology 2009;73(22): 1823–30.

31. Kawamura K, Etoh S, Shimodozono M. Transcranial magnetic stimulation for diplopia in a patient with spinocerebellar ataxia type 6: a case report. Cerebellum Ataxias 2018;5:15.

32. Shiga Y, Tsuda T, Itoyama Y, et al. Transcranial magnetic stimulation alleviates truncal ataxia in spinocerebellar degeneration. J Neurol Neurosurg Psychiatry 2002;72(1):124–6.

33. Shimizu H, Tsuda T, Shiga Y, et al. Therapeutic efficacy of transcranial magnetic stimulation for hereditary spinocerebellar degeneration. Tohoku J Exp Med 1999;189(3):203–11.

34. Kim W-S, Jung SH, Oh MK, et al. Effect of repetitive transcranial magnetic stimulation over the cerebellum on patients with ataxia after posterior circulation stroke: a pilot study. J Rehabil Med 2014;46(5):418–23.

35. Benussi A, Koch G, Cotelli M, et al. Cerebellar transcranial direct current stimulation in patients with ataxia: a double-blind, randomized, sham-controlled study. Mov Disord 2015;30(12):1701–5.

36. Grimaldi G, Manto M. Anodal transcranial direct current stimulation (tDCS) decreases the amplitudes of long-latency stretch reflexes in cerebellar ataxia. Ann Biomed Eng 2013;41(11):2437–47.

37. Hashimoto T, Muralidharan A, Yoshida K, et al. Neuronal activity and outcomes from thalamic surgery for spinocerebellar ataxia. Ann Clin Transl Neurol 2018; 5(1):52–63.

38. dos Santos Ghilardi MG, Cury RG, dos Ângelos JS, et al. Long-term improvement of tremor and ataxia after bilateral DBS of VoP/zona incerta in FXTAS. Neurology 2015;84(18):1904–6.

39. Teixeira MJ, Cury RG, Galhardoni R, et al. Deep brain stimulation of the dentate nucleus improves cerebellar ataxia after cerebellar stroke. Neurology 2015; 85(23):2075–6.

40. Weiss D, Mielke C, Wächter T, et al. Long-term outcome of deep brain stimulation in fragile X-associated tremor/ataxia syndrome. Parkinsonism Relat Disord 2015;21(3):310–3.

41. Grimaldi G, Oulad Ben Taib N, Manto M, et al. Marked reduction of cerebellar deficits in upper limbs following transcranial cerebello-cerebral DC stimulation:

tremor reduction and re-programming of the timing of antagonist commands. Front Syst Neurosci 2014;8:9.

42. Benussi A, Dell'Era V, Cantoni V, et al. Cerebello-spinal tDCS in ataxia: a randomized, double-blind, sham-controlled, crossover trial. Neurology 2018; 91(12):e1090–101.

43. Miyai I, Ito M, Hattori N, et al. Cerebellar ataxia rehabilitation trial in degenerative cerebellar diseases. Neurorehabil Neural Repair 2012;26(5):515–22.

44. Rodríguez-Díaz JC, Velázquez-Pérez L, Rodríguez Labrada R, et al. Neurorehabilitation therapy in spinocerebellar ataxia type 2: a 24-week, rater-blinded, randomized, controlled trial. Mov Disord 2018;33(9):1481–7.

45. Velázquez-Pérez L, Rodríguez-Diaz JC, Rodríguez-Labrada R, et al. Neurorehabilitation improves the motor features in prodromal SCA2: a randomized, controlled trial. Mov Disord 2019;34(7):1060–8.

46. Chang Y-J, Chou C-C, Huang W-T, et al. Cycling regimen induces spinal circuitry plasticity and improves leg muscle coordination in individuals with spinocerebellar ataxia. Arch Phys Med Rehabil 2015;96(6):1006–13.

47. Lin C-Y, Kuo S-H. The role of the cerebellum in rock climbing. J Neurol Sci 2017; 383:158–60.

48. Perry SE, Sevitz JS, Curtis JA, et al. Skill training resulted in improved swallowing in a person with multiple system atrophy: an endoscopy study. Mov Disord Clin Pract 2018;5(4):451–2.

49. Mitoma H, Manto M, Hampe CS. Time is cerebellum. Cerebellum 2018;17(4): 387–91.

50. de Alarcon PA, Matthay KK, London WB, et al. Intravenous immunoglobulin with prednisone and risk-adapted chemotherapy for children with opsoclonus myoclonus ataxia syndrome associated with neuroblastoma (ANBL00P3): a randomised, open-label, phase 3 trial. Lancet Child Adolesc Health 2018;2(1):25–34.

51. Nanri K, Okuma M, Sato S, et al. Prevalence of autoantibodies and the efficacy of immunotherapy for autoimmune cerebellar ataxia. Intern Med 2016;55(5): 449–54.

52. Chataway J, Hardman E. Thiamine in Wernicke's syndrome—how much and how long? Postgrad Med J 1995;71(834):249.

53. Sinha S, Kataria A, Kolla BP, et al. Wernicke encephalopathy—clinical pearls. Mayo Clin Proc 2019;94(6):1065–72.

54. Kuo S-H, Debnam JM, Fuller GN, et al. Wernicke's encephalopathy: an underrecognized and reversible cause of confusional state in cancer patients. Oncology 2009;76(1):10–8.

55. Stabler SP. Clinical practice. Vitamin B12 deficiency. N Engl J Med 2013;368(2): 149–60.

56. Chakrabarty B, Dubey R, Gulati S, et al. Isolated cerebellar involvement in vitamin B12 deficiency: a case report. J Child Neurol 2014;29(11):NP161–3.

57. Mitoma H, Hadjivassiliou M, Honnorat J. Guidelines for treatment of immune-mediated cerebellar ataxias. Cerebellum Ataxias 2015;2:14.

58. Synofzik M, Puccio H, Mochel F, et al. Autosomal recessive cerebellar ataxias: paving the way toward targeted molecular therapies. Neuron 2019;101(4): 560–83.

59. Aggarwal A, Bhatt M. Advances in treatment of Wilson disease. Tremor Other Hyperkinet Mov (N Y) 2018;8:525.

60. Nie S, Chen G, Cao X, et al. Cerebrotendinous xanthomatosis: a comprehensive review of pathogenesis, clinical manifestations, diagnosis, and management. Orphanet J Rare Dis 2014;9:179.

61. Berginer VM, Salen G, Shefer S. Long-term treatment of cerebrotendinous xanthomatosis with chenodeoxycholic acid. N Engl J Med 1984;311(26):1649–52.
62. Pierre G, Setchell K, Blyth J, et al. Prospective treatment of cerebrotendinous xanthomatosis with cholic acid therapy. J Inherit Metab Dis 2008;31(Suppl 2): S241–5.
63. Pedroso JL, Fusão EF, Ladeia-Frota C, et al. Teaching video neuroimages: gelastic cataplexy as the first neurologic manifestation of Niemann-Pick disease type C. Neurology 2012;79(22):e189.
64. Gupta DK, Blanco-Palmero VA, Chung WK, et al. Abnormal vertical eye movements as a clue for diagnosis of Niemann-Pick type C. Tremor Other Hyperkinet Mov (N Y) 2018;8:560.
65. Pineda M, Walterfang M, Patterson MC. Miglustat in Niemann-Pick disease type C patients: a review. Orphanet J Rare Dis 2018;13(1):140.
66. Ory DS, Ottinger EA, Farhat NY, et al. Intrathecal 2-hydroxypropyl-β-cyclodextrin decreases neurological disease progression in Niemann-Pick disease, type C1: a non-randomised, open-label, phase 1-2 trial. Lancet 2017;390(10104): 1758–68.
67. Gabsi S, Gouider-Khouja N, Belal S, et al. Effect of vitamin E supplementation in patients with ataxia with vitamin E deficiency. Eur J Neurol 2001;8(5):477–81.
68. Mignot C, Apartis E, Durr A, et al. Phenotypic variability in ARCA2 and identification of a core ataxic phenotype with slow progression. Orphanet J Rare Dis 2013;8:173.
69. Wolf B. Successful outcomes of older adolescents and adults with profound biotinidase deficiency identified by newborn screening. Genet Med 2017;19(4): 396–402.
70. Debs R, Depienne C, Rastetter A, et al. Biotin-responsive basal ganglia disease in ethnic Europeans with novel SLC19A3 mutations. Arch Neurol 2010;67(1): 126–30.
71. Campuzano V, Montermini L, Moltò MD, et al. Friedreich's ataxia: autosomal recessive disease caused by an intronic GAA triplet repeat expansion. Science 1996;271(5254):1423–7.
72. Kemp KC, Hares K, Redondo J, et al. Bone marrow transplantation stimulates neural repair in Friedreich's ataxia mice. Ann Neurol 2018;83(4):779–93.
73. Li L, Shen X, Liu Z, et al. Activation of frataxin protein expression by antisense oligonucleotides targeting the mutant expanded repeat. Nucleic Acid Ther 2018;28(1):23–33.
74. Piguet F, de Montigny C, Vaucamps N, et al. Rapid and complete reversal of sensory ataxia by gene therapy in a novel model of Friedreich ataxia. Mol Ther 2018;26(8):1940–52.
75. Menotta M, Biagiotti S, Spapperi C, et al. ATM splicing variants as biomarkers for low dose dexamethasone treatment of A-T. Orphanet J Rare Dis 2017; 12(1):126.
76. Zannolli R, Buoni S, Betti G, et al. A randomized trial of oral betamethasone to reduce ataxia symptoms in ataxia telangiectasia. Mov Disord 2012;27(10): 1312–6.
77. Foley AR, Menezes MP, Pandraud A, et al. Treatable childhood neuronopathy caused by mutations in riboflavin transporter RFVT2. Brain 2014;137(Pt 1): 44–56.
78. Guissart C, Drouot N, Oncel I, et al. Genes for spinocerebellar ataxia with blindness and deafness (SCABD/SCAR3, MIM# 271250 and SCABD2). Eur J Hum Genet 2016;24(8):1154–9.

79. Chardon L, Sassolas A, Dingeon B, et al. Identification of two novel mutations and long-term follow-up in abetalipoproteinemia: a report of four cases. Eur J Pediatr 2009;168(8):983–9.

80. Lee J, Hegele RA. Abetalipoproteinemia and homozygous hypobetalipoproteinemia: a framework for diagnosis and management. J Inherit Metab Dis 2014; 37(3):333–9.

81. Caglayan AO, Gumus H, Sandford E, et al. COQ4 mutation leads to childhood-onset ataxia improved by CoQ10 administration. Cerebellum 2019;18(3):665–9.

82. Baldwin EJ, Gibberd FB, Harley C, et al. The effectiveness of long-term dietary therapy in the treatment of adult Refsum disease. J Neurol Neurosurg Psychiatry 2010;81(9):954–7.

83. Gibberd FB, Billimoria JD, Page NG, et al. Heredopathia atactica polyneuritiformis (Refsum's disease) treated by diet and plasma-exchange. Lancet 1979; 1(8116):575–8.

84. Zolotov D, Wagner S, Kalb K, et al. Long-term strategies for the treatment of Refsum's disease using therapeutic apheresis. J Clin Apher 2012;27(2):99–105.

85. Sullivan R, Yau WY, O'Connor E, et al. Spinocerebellar ataxia: an update. J Neurol 2019;266(2):533–44.

86. Lei L-F, Yang G-P, Wang J-L, et al. Safety and efficacy of valproic acid treatment in SCA3/MJD patients. Parkinsonism Relat Disord 2016;26:55–61.

87. Lo RY, Figueroa KP, Pulst SM, et al. Coenzyme Q10 and spinocerebellar ataxias. Mov Disord 2015;30(2):214–20.

88. Teixeira-Castro A, Jalles A, Esteves S, et al. Serotonergic signalling suppresses ataxin 3 aggregation and neurotoxicity in animal models of Machado-Joseph disease. Brain 2015;138(Pt 11):3221–37.

89. Scoles DR, Meera P, Schneider MD, et al. Antisense oligonucleotide therapy for spinocerebellar ataxia type 2. Nature 2017;544(7650):362–6.

90. Friedrich J, Kordasiewicz HB, O'Callaghan B, et al. Antisense oligonucleotide-mediated ataxin-1 reduction prolongs survival in SCA1 mice and reveals disease-associated transcriptome profiles. JCI Insight 2018;3(21) [pii:123193].

91. Toonen LJA, Rigo F, van Attikum H, et al. Antisense oligonucleotide-mediated removal of the polyglutamine repeat in spinocerebellar ataxia type 3 mice. Mol Ther Nucleic Acids 2017;8:232–42.

92. Moore LR, Rajpal G, Dillingham IT, et al. Evaluation of antisense oligonucleotides targeting ATXN3 in SCA3 mouse models. Mol Ther Nucleic Acids 2017; 7:200–10.

93. Mitsui J, Matsukawa T, Yasuda T, et al. Plasma coenzyme Q10 levels in patients with multiple system atrophy. JAMA Neurol 2016;73(8):977–80.

94. Miyazaki Y, Du X, Muramatsu S-I, et al. An miRNA-mediated therapy for SCA6 blocks IRES-driven translation of the CACNA1A second cistron. Sci Transl Med 2016;8(347):347ra94.

95. Niu C, Prakash TP, Kim A, et al. Antisense oligonucleotides targeting mutant Ataxin-7 restore visual function in a mouse model of spinocerebellar ataxia type 7. Sci Transl Med 2018;10(465) [pii:eaap8677].

96. Nóbrega C, Codêsso JM, Mendonça L, et al. RNA interference therapy for Machado-Joseph disease: long-term safety profile of lentiviral vectors encoding short hairpin RNAs targeting mutant Ataxin-3. Hum Gene Ther 2019;30(7): 841–54.

97. Nóbrega C, Nascimento-Ferreira I, Onofre I, et al. Silencing mutant ataxin-3 rescues motor deficits and neuropathology in Machado-Joseph disease transgenic mice. PLoS One 2013;8(1):e52396.

98. Ramachandran PS, Boudreau RL, Schaefer KA, et al. Nonallele specific silencing of ataxin-7 improves disease phenotypes in a mouse model of SCA7. Mol Ther 2014;22(9):1635–42.
99. Lin C-C, Gan S-R, Gupta D, et al. Hispanic spinocerebellar ataxia type 35 (SCA35) with a novel frameshift mutation. Cerebellum 2019;18(2):291–4.
100. Multiple-System Atrophy Research Collaboration. Mutations in COQ2 in familial and sporadic multiple-system atrophy. N Engl J Med 2013;369(3):233–44.
101. Kuo S-H, Quinzii CM. Coenzyme Q10 as a peripheral biomarker for multiple system atrophy. JAMA Neurol 2016;73(8):917–9.
102. Barca E, Kleiner G, Tang G, et al. Decreased coenzyme Q10 levels in multiple system atrophy cerebellum. J Neuropathol Exp Neurol 2016;75(7):663–72.
103. Konno M, Hasegawa T, Baba T, et al. Suppression of dynamin GTPase decreases α-synuclein uptake by neuronal and oligodendroglial cells: a potent therapeutic target for synucleinopathy. Mol Neurodegener 2012;7:38.
104. Friess E, Kuempfel T, Modell S, et al. Paroxetine treatment improves motor symptoms in patients with multiple system atrophy. Parkinsonism Relat Disord 2006;12(7):432–7.
105. Stefanova N, Georgievska B, Eriksson H, et al. Myeloperoxidase inhibition ameliorates multiple system atrophy-like degeneration in a transgenic mouse model. Neurotox Res 2012;21(4):393–404.
106. Hoche F, Guell X, Vangel MG, et al. The cerebellar cognitive affective/Schmahmann syndrome scale. Brain 2018;141(1):248–70.
107. Tercero-Pérez K, Cortés H, Torres-Ramos Y, et al. Effects of Physical Rehabilitation in Patients with Spinocerebellar Ataxia Type 7. Cerebellum Lond Engl 2019; 18:397–405.

Treatment of Functional Movement Disorders

Kathrin LaFaver, MD

KEYWORDS

- Psychogenic movement disorder • Conversion disorder • Multidisciplinary treatment
- Cognitive behavior therapy

KEY POINTS

- Functional movement disorders (FMD) are common conditions seen in neurologic practice, presenting with tremor, weakness, dystonia, jerking movements, and abnormal gait and speech, often combining several phenomenologies.
- The diagnosis of FMD relies on history and positive findings on neurologic examination and is no longer considered a diagnosis of exclusion.
- Treatment of FMD begins with an explanation of the diagnosis, often aided by demonstration of functional exam findings, exploration of physical and psychological trigger factors and emphasizing the potential for reversibility of symptoms.
- There is increasing evidence for benefits from physical, occupational, and speech therapy, as well as psychotherapeutic interventions, and treatment should be tailored to patients' symptoms and comorbidities.

INTRODUCTION

Functional movement disorders (FMD) are commonly seen in neurology clinics and are a major source of disability.[1] Despite the wide recognition of this problem,[2,3] there remains controversy over which specialists should oversee and manage the care of patients with FMD.[4] Over the last decade, important progress has been made in defining neurobiological factors that are shaping the understanding of FMD as a brain circuit disorder at the intersection of neurology and psychiatry.[5–9] Those insights are helping to inform best practices in diagnosis and treatment of patients, with emerging evidence for benefits from physical therapy, cognitive behavior therapy (CBT), and multidisciplinary treatment approaches.[5,10] An important gap in achieving best treatment outcomes for patients remains the paucity of dedicated FMD treatment centers in the United States and elsewhere and the lack of specialized training in FMD for many health care professionals. This article discusses current terminology, changes in diagnostic criteria, prognosis, and evidence-based and emerging treatments in FMD.

Department of Neurology, Northwestern University Feinberg School of Medicine, Abbott Hall, Room 1112, 710 North Lake Shore Drive, Chicago, IL 60611, USA
E-mail address: Kathrin.LaFaver@northwestern.edu
Twitter: @LaFaverMD (K.L.)

Neurol Clin 38 (2020) 469–480
https://doi.org/10.1016/j.ncl.2020.01.011   **neurologic.theclinics.com**
0733-8619/20/© 2020 Elsevier Inc. All rights reserved.

TERMINOLOGY

Nomenclature remains inconsistent, in part because practitioners from multiple disciplines approach FMD from different angles. The term conversion disorder remains prevalent in the psychiatric literature and conveys the idea of an unresolved psychological conflict expressed through physical symptoms.[11] In the latest edition of the Diagnostic and Statistical Manual of Mental Disorders (DSM), conversion disorder is now used synonymous with functional neurologic symptom disorder.[12,13] Overall, there has been a shift in the literature from psychogenic movement disorders toward FMD, underlying a greater emphasis on a biopsychosocial illness model with multiple factors contributing to symptom genesis.[14,15] It is sometimes stressed that patients perceive their symptoms as dysfunctional rather than functional but prefer this term as less stigmatizing among other options.[16] The historically used term hysteria has been abandoned,[17] and the use of medically unexplained symptoms is discouraged because of its vague nature and possible overlap with symptoms caused by unrecognized neurologic illness.

DIAGNOSTIC CRITERIA

Over the past decade, there has been an emphasis away from considering FMD a diagnosis of exclusion toward phenotype-specific, positive diagnostic criteria.[18,19] Although still considered important as predisposing and precipitating factors in FMD, psychological stress is no longer required for the diagnosis in the latest edition of the DSM, DSM-5.[12] The neurologic examination is designed to identify internal inconsistencies and incongruence of findings with so-called organic neurologic disorders. For functional tremor, variability in tremor frequency, entrainment to different external stimuli, and interruption of tremor to ballistic movements can be found.[20,21] Inability to move a limb on command but normal automatic movements when attention is shifted is an example of inconsistency in limb weakness. Electrophysiologic studies to support a diagnosis of FMD are especially helpful for functional tremor and myoclonus.[22,23] A detailed review of phenomenologic diagnostic criteria is outside of the scope of this article. Importantly, the rate of misdiagnosis for FMD has been found to be around 4%, similar to those of other neurologic conditions.[24] Increased recognition and education on functional neurological disorder (FND) during neurology training programs will further aid in providing timely and accurate diagnosis for patients.[25] Neurologists should be aware of the possible presence of FMD in the setting of other neurologic disorders, in some cases even as possible precursors for neurodegenerative disorders such as Parkinson disease.[26,27]

THE BIOPSYCHOSOCIAL MODEL

Although the pathophysiology of FND remains incompletely understood, genetic predisposition and biological, environmental, and psychological factors are thought to be contributing factors toward symptom genesis (biopsychosocial model).[7,28] Sigmund Freud's concept of hysteria, the repression of painful experiences and conversion into physical symptoms,[17] has been substituted with a complex model of predisposing vulnerabilities and precipitating and maintaining factors.[29,30] Neuroimaging studies have identified difference in sensorimotor and limbic pathways in FMD during resting state and task performance, and may provide biomarkers to aid in diagnosis and disease monitoring.[6,31,32] A recent study by Espay and colleagues[33] in patients with functional tremor found increased activation at baseline and decreased activation after a 12-week course of CBT in the anterior cingulate/paracingulate during emotional task processing. Diez and colleagues[34] found increased functional connectivity from the right amygdala to the left anterior insula, periaqueductal gray, and hypothalamus in patients with FND compared with controls, which correlated with clinical improvement at 6 months.

PROGNOSIS

There are few long-term studies on the natural history of FMD. Available studies have pointed toward an unfavorable prognosis, with many patients having persistent symptoms after years of follow-up.[35,36] Good physical health, positive social life, patients' perception of effective treatment by the physician, elimination of stressors, and treatment with a specific medication were found to be favorable factors in a single-center study of FMD with 3-year follow-up.[37] In a recent study of functional limb weakness with 14-year follow-up, ongoing symptoms were shown in most patients and a greater than expected mortality was found.[38] Better recognition of FMD with timely diagnosis, reduced stigma, and improved access to treatment may lead to improved outcomes in the future.

TREATMENT

The treatment process begins with diagnostic debriefing of patients. Providing a diagnosis of FMD should be based on positive, unambiguous signs that can be shown to the patient and normalized as frequently encountered reactions to physical and psychological stress, with a potential for reversibility.[39–41] Gaining an appropriate understanding and acceptance of the diagnosis of FMD is a prerequisite toward engaging in therapy, and treatment is rarely successful if initiated before completion of the diagnostic work-up. The patient's motivation for therapy and readiness to change should be assessed[42] and potential treatment barriers noted, including inopportune timing and lack of financial or psychosocial support. Treatment goals and expectations should be established in partnership with the patient, and movement-specific as well as functional goals addressed.

PHYSICAL THERAPY

Physical therapy (PT) can play an important role in the treatment of FMD either by itself or in combination with other treatment modalities. Physical therapists, along with physiatrists, are in a unique position to gain patients' trust and confidence, because they are experts in dysfunction of the musculoskeletal system and can also address secondary injuries in FMD related to deconditioning and abnormal movement mechanics. The main principle in PT for FMD is motor retraining, allowing patients to regain voluntary control over their movements. Several smaller prospective and retrospective studies have shown evidence for benefit from PT,[43–45] and there is an ongoing large randomized controlled trial in the United Kingdom with results expected in 2021 (www.physio4fmd.org). Importantly, PT needs to be delivered within a shared framework of FMD as a disorder with fluctuating and potentially reversible deficits, and rehabilitation techniques adapted for this patient population. In a feasibility study by Nielsen and colleagues,[46] 60 patients with FMD were randomized to receive either a 5-day protocolized PT intervention or usual care, which included a median of 5 PT sessions in the community. Although 72% of patients in the FMD-PT group reported significant improvement at 6-month follow-up, only 18% in the community-PT group rated their symptoms as improved. Recommended interventions include limited hands-on treatment, facilitating rather than supporting movements, encouraging early weight bearing, goal-directed rehabilitation focusing on function and automatic movement, minimized reinforcement of maladaptive movement patterns and postures, and avoidance of adaptive equipment and mobility aids.[47] In a UK survey, most physical therapists expressed interest in treating patients with FMD but rated their knowledge about the disorder as low.[48] This situation is likely similar in the United States, where treatment of functional neurologic disorders is not part of the core curricula for physical and occupational therapists. Remaining questions include the optimal frequency, intensity, and duration of PT. In a recent US-based retrospective FMD cohort study, the number of weekly PT sessions attended was significantly positively correlated with clinical improvement,[49] whereas a previous retrospective study with outpatient physical and occupational therapy (OT) reported good outcomes in 74% with a standardized 5-day treatment duration.[50]

OCCUPATIONAL THERAPY

Occupational therapists are trained to help patients to perform activities of daily living, work, and leisure. With a focus on physical, mental, and social determinants of health, OT is well positioned to help patients with FMD in optimizing functional outcomes. Similar to PT, therapy principles in OT need to be adapted to meet FMD treatment goals.[51] Rather than adjusting and compensating for motor deficits, the goal is relearning of normal movement patterns and suppression of unwanted movements. Although no randomized controlled treatment trials with OT as a single intervention have been performed, several multidisciplinary treatment programs included OT as one of the interventions offered, and these are discussed later. In a study with 10 patients with functional tremor, retraining of tremor to tactile and auditory external cueing and visual feedback resulted in significant tremor improvement for up to 6 months in 60%.[52] Typically used as part of the neurologic examination in functional tremor, the therapeutic use of entrainment strategies should be tested in larger studies. Further research on other specific interventions, including mirror therapy, constraint-induced movement therapy,[53] and the use of virtual reality in FMD rehabilitation, is needed.[54]

SPEECH THERAPY

Functional speech and voice disorders are frequently present in FMD. Characteristics of functional speech disorders include dysphonia, stuttering, prosodic abnormalities, articulation abnormalities, and foreign accent syndrome.[55,56] Speech therapy can be beneficial in restoring normal speech patterns, although treatment outcomes have been noted to be variable and generally not favorable if the diagnosis of a functional speech disorder is not accepted.[57,58] Speech therapists can also help with restoring normal breathing and swallowing patterns.

MULTIDISCIPLINARY TREATMENT

Multidisciplinary treatment, tailored to the patient's individual symptoms and medical and psychiatric comorbidities, is a common treatment approach in clinical practice. Recent reports from specialized FMD centers highlight current treatment practice, although clinical studies are needed to guide development of evidence-based treatment recommendations and determine the best setting, frequency, intensity, and length of interventions.[59–61] Common characteristics of FMD specialist clinics include (1) multidisciplinary patient assessment; (2) dedicated patient education about the diagnosis; and (3) multidisciplinary treatments with a combination of

PT, OT, speech therapy, and psychotherapy interventions. Differences in treatment duration, frequency, therapy setting, length of follow-up, and reported outcomes do not allow for a direct comparison between treatment programs. For patients with significant impairment in daily activities, inpatient rehabilitation may offer benefits in providing a treatment environment with special expertise by all team members, a separation from the patient's usual environment with distancing from possible maintaining factors, and close monitoring for patients with higher psychiatric care needs. In a study by Jordbru and colleagues,[62] 60 patients with a functional gait disorder were randomized to immediate or delayed 3-week inpatient treatment with PT offered in a cognitive behavioral framework, showing improved ability to walk and quality of life maintained at 1 year follow-up. In a prospective study of 66 patients admitted for a 4-week treatment program in a neuropsychiatric inpatient setting, two-thirds of patients rated better or much better at discharge and 1-year follow-up, although a high percentage of patients was lost to follow-up.[63] Other inpatient programs reported in the literature varied in length of stay from 1 week to an average of 3 months, and differ in patient baseline characteristics and length of follow-up. Retrospectively reported outcomes for several programs show that improvements in motor symptoms and quality of life are possible even for patients with long-standing symptoms, although reintegration in work for previously disabled patients is not commonly seen.[64–66]

PSYCHOLOGICAL TREATMENT

In the past, psychotherapy has been considered the mainstay for treatment of FND, with the largest evidence for benefit of adapted CBT in psychogenic nonepileptic seizures (PNES). CBT is intended to change cognitive distortions to improve emotions and behaviors, and is commonly used in the treatment of depression, anxiety, and eating disorders. In a study by LaFrance and colleagues,[67] 38 patients with PNES were randomized to medication treatment with sertraline only, CBT-informed psychotherapy (CBT-ip) only, CBT-ip with sertraline, or treatment as usual. Significant improvements in seizure frequency and global functioning were found in the CBT-ip groups with and without sertraline.[67] The Cognitive Behavioral Therapy for Dissociative (Non-Epileptic) Seizures (CODES) trial is the largest randomized controlled study in patients with PNES to date and stratified 298 patients to either specifically tailored CBT plus standardized medical care or standardized medical care alone, with results expected to be reported in 2020 (www.codestrial.org).[68] A randomized controlled study of a guided self-help intervention using a CBT-based manual showed moderately improved outcomes at 3 and 6 months in a mixed group of patients with FND compared with usual care.[69] A brief psychotherapeutic intervention for a mixed group of patients with FND offered as part of interdisciplinary care with a neurologist showed significantly improved physical and psychological symptoms and a reduction in new hospital stays compared with standard care.[70] In FMD, CBT delivered over 12 weekly treatment sessions was found to markedly reduce functional tremor in 73% of patients, although the lack of a control group and long-term follow-up were limiting factors.[33]

In addition to CBT, psychodynamic therapy has been studied in FND, focusing on interpersonal relationships and emotional processing. A trial of brief augmented psychodynamic interpersonal therapy in a mixed group of FND showed significant benefits in emotional processing and health-related quality of life.[71] Although a retrospective case series of 30 patients with FMD showed symptomatic improvement in 60% of patients treated with psychodynamic therapy, a study of 15 patients with FMD using a crossover design of psychodynamic psychotherapy versus neurologic observation and support showed no changes in motor or mood symptoms at 3 and 6 months.[72,73] Other treatments currently under exploration in FND include acceptance and commitment therapy and mindfulness interventions. Of note, a recent prospective study with 193 newly diagnosed patients with FND in the Netherlands under naturalistic treatment settings showed no independent significant impact of the use of psychotherapy on favorable outcomes at 12 months, and high levels of somatization were associated with worse treatment outcomes.[74] Taken together, the current data on psychotherapy in FMD suggests benefit from relative short interventions, but that it may not be needed for all patients if substituted with psychologically informed rehabilitation-based interventions.

COMPLEMENTARY AND INTEGRATIVE MEDICINE

Relaxation training, including mindfulness meditation, guided imagery, diaphragmatic breathing, and progressive muscle relaxation, may be of benefit in FMD but has not been systematically studied. There is insufficient evidence to date to support a role of acupuncture in the treatment of FMD and other FND.[75] Hypnosis has historically been used in FMD and induces a trancelike state with high suggestibility, which is used therapeutically to induce behavioral modifications. A randomized controlled trial of manualized hypnosis compared with wait-list control showed significant improvement in behavioral symptoms and motor disability at 6-month follow-up, although a second study by the same author comparing the addition of manualized hypnosis with a multidisciplinary treatment program showed no added benefit of the hypnosis intervention.[76,77]

PHARMACOLOGIC TREATMENT

The role of pharmacologic treatment in FMD should be individualized depending on comorbidities, including depression, anxiety, and chronic pain. Treatment with antidepressants alone has not been shown to improve motor function in FMD, although no randomized controlled or adequately powered studies have been conducted.[78] Patients previously started on medications not indicated for FMD, such as carbidopa/levodopa or antiepileptic agents, should be weaned off. It is often helpful to wait with tapering of medications until the patient is engaged in other treatment modalities and learns strategies to deal with worsening or reemerging symptoms. For severe FMD without benefit from other treatments, sedation with propofol to show the reversibility of symptoms such as fixed dystonia may have a role, usually combined with psychoeducation and multidisciplinary treatment.[79]

BOTULINUM TOXIN

A recent double-blinded randomized controlled study compared injections with botulinum neurotoxin versus placebo in jerky and tremulous FMD and found no difference in symptom improvement between the treatment groups.[80] The high percentage of patients showing symptom improvement after an open-label phase regardless of initial treatment allocation may support further research in placebo therapies in FMD.

OTHER TREATMENTS

There has been a long-standing interest in the use of transcranial magnetic stimulation (TMS) as a noninvasive method to test cortical excitability and connectivity. Repetitive TMS (rTMS) can induce neuromodulatory effects with long-term potentiation or depression. A recent study of TMS over the motor cortex contralateral to symptoms versus the spinal roots in the control group in 33 patients with FMD showed symptomatic benefit in both groups, suggesting a behavioral or placebo response.[81] A randomized controlled study of rTMS versus sham stimulation in 33 patients with functional tremor showed sustained benefits in the treatment groups up to 12 months, although addition of hypnosis in an open-label phase of the study may have been a confounding factor.[82] Further research in this area is of interest to test pathways involved in symptom genesis and identify new treatment targets.

Transcutaneous electrical nerve stimulation showed benefit in a single center study of 19 patients with FMD, but lacked a control or sham stimulation group.[83] The use of placebo treatment may hold promise in FMD, but is associated with ethical challenges.[84,85]

TREATMENT OBSTACLES

It is important to acknowledge that, even with the best efforts, not all patients are able to improve their symptoms. Possible treatment obstacles include ambiguity about the diagnosis, and barriers toward full engagement in therapy, such as pending litigation or lack of psychosocial support. A recent study examined the impact of motivational interviewing (MI) on adherence to psychotherapy for PNES and found a 65% adherence rate in the intervention group versus 31% in the control group, as well as a significant improvement in PNES frequency in the MI group.[86] The use of MI and other strategies to improve patient engagement in treatment is an important area of future research. Furthermore, efforts to adequately train health care professionals of multiple disciplines in treatment of FMD will be an important step in improving access to care and patient outcomes.

SUMMARY

FMD is a common neuropsychiatric condition that can be difficult to diagnose and treat. Over the past decade, important progress has been made toward better understanding of neurobiological factors involved in FMD and defining effective treatment interventions. There remains a need for randomized controlled studies to compare different treatment modalities and measure long-term treatment outcomes. Concerted efforts to develop standardized FND outcome measures are an important step in developing future clinical trials.[87] Further work is also needed to optimize factors associated with positive engagement in therapy and educate health care professionals in multiple disciplines on FMD treatment to improve access to care.

DISCLOSURE

K. LaFaver has received speaker's honoraria from the American Academy of Neurology and the International Parkinson and Movement Disorder Society. Also, he received grant funding from the Ayers Foundation.

REFERENCES

1. Carson A, Lehn A. Epidemiology. Handb Clin Neurol 2016;139:147–60.
2. Hallett M. Psychogenic movement disorders: a crisis for neurology. Curr Neurol Neurosci Rep 2006;6(4):269–71.
3. Hallett M. Functional movement disorders: Is the crisis resolved? Mov Disord 2019;34(7):971–4.
4. Perez DL, Haller AL, Espay AJ. Should neurologists diagnose and manage functional neurologic disorders? It is complicated. Neurol Clin Pract 2019;9(2):165–7.

5. Espay AJ, Aybek S, Carson A, et al. Current concepts in diagnosis and treatment of functional neurological disorders. JAMA Neurol 2018;75(9):1132–41.
6. Begue I, Adams C, Stone J, et al. Structural alterations in functional neurological disorder and related conditions: a software and hardware problem? Neuroimage Clin 2019;22:101798.
7. Pick S, Goldstein LH, Perez DL, et al. Emotional processing in functional neurological disorder: a review, biopsychosocial model and research agenda. J Neurol Neurosurg Psychiatry 2019;90(6):704–11.
8. Perez DL, Dworetzky BA, Dickerson BC, et al. An integrative neurocircuit perspective on psychogenic nonepileptic seizures and functional movement disorders: neural functional unawareness. Clin EEG Neurosci 2015;46(1):4–15.
9. Baizabal-Carvallo JF, Hallett M, Jankovic J. Pathogenesis and pathophysiology of functional (psychogenic) movement disorders. Neurobiol Dis 2019;127:32–44.
10. Adams C, Anderson J, Madva EN, et al. You've made the diagnosis of functional neurological disorder: now what? Pract Neurol 2018;18(4):323–30.
11. Cretton A, Brown RJ, LaFrance WC Jr, et al. What does neuroscience tell us about the conversion model of functional neurological disorders? J Neuropsychiatry Clin Neurosci 2020;32(1):24–32.
12. American Psychiatric Association. Diagnostic and Statistical Manual of Mental Disorders. 5th edition. Washington, DC: American Psychiatric Association; 2013.
13. Demartini B, D'Agostino A, Gambini O. From conversion disorder (DSM-IV-TR) to functional neurological symptom disorder (DSM-5): When a label changes the perspective for the neurologist, the psychiatrist and the patient. J Neurol Sci 2016;360:55–6.
14. Edwards MJ, Stone J, Lang AE. From psychogenic movement disorder to functional movement disorder: it's time to change the name. Mov Disord 2014; 29(7):849–52.
15. Fahn S, Olanow CW. Reply to: psychogenic movement disorders: what's in a name? Mov Disord 2014;29(13):1699–701.
16. Stone J, Wojcik W, Durrance D, et al. What should we say to patients with symptoms unexplained by disease? The "number needed to offend". BMJ 2002; 325(7378):1449–50.
17. Kanaan RAA. Freud's hysteria and its legacy. Handb Clin Neurol 2016;139:37–44.
18. Espay AJ, Lang AE. Phenotype-specific diagnosis of functional (psychogenic) movement disorders. Curr Neurol Neurosci Rep 2015;15(6):32.
19. Gasca-Salas C, Lang A. Neurologic diagnostic criteria for functional neurologic disorders. Handb Clin Neurol 2016;139:1930212.
20. Zeuner KE, Shoge RO, Goldstein SR, et al. Accelerometry to distinguish psychogenic from essential or parkinsonian tremor. Neurology 2003;61(4):548–50.
21. Kumru H, Valls-Sole J, Valldeoriola F, et al. Transient arrest of psychogenic tremor induced by contralateral ballistic movements. Neurosci Lett 2004;370(2–3): 135–9.
22. Hallett M. Physiology of psychogenic movement disorders. J Clin Neurosci 2010; 17(8):959–65.
23. Schwingenschuh P, Saifee TA, Katschnig-Winter P, et al. Validation of "laboratory-supported" criteria for functional (psychogenic) tremor. Mov Disord 2016;31(4): 555–62.
24. Stone J, Smyth R, Carson A, et al. Systematic review of misdiagnosis of conversion symptoms and "hysteria. BMJ 2005;331(7523):989.
25. Perez DL, Hunt A, Sharma N, et al. Cautionary notes on diagnosing functional neurologic disorder as a neurologist-in-training. Neurol Clin Pract 2019.

26. Wissel BD, Dwivedi AK, Merola A, et al. Functional neurological disorders in Parkinson disease. J Neurol Neurosurg Psychiatry 2018;89(6):566–71.
27. Stone J, Carson A, Duncan R, et al. Which neurological diseases are most likely to be associated with "symptoms unexplained by organic disease. J Neurol 2012; 259(1):33–8.
28. Reuber M. The etiology of psychogenic non-epileptic seizures: toward a biopsychosocial model. Neurol Clin 2009;27(4):909–24.
29. Stone J, Carson A. Functional and dissociative (psychogenic) neurological symptoms. In: Daroff R, Fenichel G, Jankovic J, et al, editors. Bradley's neurology in clinical practice. Philadelphia: Elsevier; 2012. p. 2147–62.
30. McKee K, Glass S, Adams C, et al. The inpatient assessment and management of motor functional neurological disorders: an interdisciplinary perspective. Psychosomatics 2018;59(4):358–68.
31. Roelofs JJ, Teodoro T, Edwards MJ. Neuroimaging in Functional Movement Disorders. Curr Neurol Neurosci Rep 2019;19(3):12.
32. Maurer CW, LaFaver K, Ameli R, et al. Impaired self-agency in functional movement disorders: A resting-state fMRI study. Neurology 2016;87(6):564–70.
33. Espay AJ, Ries S, Maloney T, et al. Clinical and neural responses to cognitive behavioral therapy for functional tremor. Neurology 2019;93(19):e1787–98.
34. Diez I, Ortiz-Teran L, Williams B, et al. Corticolimbic fast-tracking: enhanced multimodal integration in functional neurological disorder. J Neurol Neurosurg Psychiatry 2019;90(8):929–38.
35. McKeon A, Ahlskog JE, Bower JH, et al. Psychogenic tremor: long-term prognosis in patients with electrophysiologically confirmed disease. Mov Disord 2009;24(1):72–6.
36. Gelauff J, Stone J, Edwards M, et al. The prognosis of functional (psychogenic) motor symptoms: a systematic review. J Neurol Neurosurg Psychiatry 2014;85(2): 220–6.
37. Thomas M, Vuong KD, Jankovic J. Long-term prognosis of patients with psychogenic movement disorders. Parkinsonism Relat Disord 2006;12(6):382–7.
38. Gelauff JM, Carson A, Ludwig L, et al. The prognosis of functional limb weakness: a 14-year case-control study. Brain 2019;142(7):2137–48.
39. Stone J, Edwards M. Trick or treat? Showing patients with functional (psychogenic) motor symptoms their physical signs. Neurology 2012;79(3):282–4.
40. Stone J, Carson A, Hallett M. Explanation as treatment for functional neurologic disorders. Handb Clin Neurol 2017;139:543–53.
41. Carson A, Lehn A, Ludwig L, et al. Explaining functional disorders in the neurology clinic: a photo story. Pract Neurol 2016;16(1):56–61.
42. Heider J, Kock K, Sehlbrede M, et al. Readiness to change as a moderator of therapy outcome in patients with somatoform disorders. Psychother Res 2018; 28(5):722–33.
43. Nielsen G, Ricciardi L, Demartini B, et al. Outcomes of a 5-day physiotherapy programme for functional (psychogenic) motor disorders. J Neurol 2015;262(3): 674–81.
44. Nielsen G, Stone J, Edwards MJ. Physiotherapy for functional (psychogenic) motor symptoms: a systematic review. J Psychosom Res 2013;75(2):93–102.
45. Dallocchio C, Arbasino C, Klersy C, et al. The effects of physical activity on psychogenic movement disorders. Mov Disord 2010;25(4):421–5.
46. Nielsen G, Buszewicz M, Stevenson F, et al. Randomised feasibility study of physiotherapy for patients with functional motor symptoms. J Neurol Neurosurg Psychiatry 2017;88(6):484–90.

47. Nielsen G, Stone J, Matthews A, et al. Physiotherapy for functional motor disorders: a consensus recommendation. J Neurol Neurosurg Psychiatry 2015; 86(10):1113–9.

48. Edwards MJ, Stone J, Nielsen G. Physiotherapists and patients with functional (psychogenic) motor symptoms: a survey of attitudes and interest. J Neurol Neurosurg Psychiatry 2012;83(6):655–8.

49. Maggio JB, Ospina JP, Callahan J, et al. Outpatient physical therapy for functional neurological disorder: a preliminary feasibility and naturalistic outcome study in a U.S. cohort. J Neuropsychiatry Clin Neurosci 2020;32(1):85–9.

50. Czarnecki K, Thompson JM, Seime R, et al. Functional movement disorders: successful treatment with a physical therapy rehabilitation protocol. Parkinsonism Relat Disord 2012;18(3):247–51.

51. Gardiner P, MacGregor L, Carson A, et al. Occupational therapy for functional neurological disorders: a scoping review and agenda for research. CNS Spectr 2018;23(3):205–12.

52. Espay AJ, Edwards MJ, Oggioni GD, et al. Tremor retrainment as therapeutic strategy in psychogenic (functional) tremor. Parkinsonism Relat Disord 2014; 20(6):647–50.

53. Taub E, Uswatte G, Mark VW. The functional significance of cortical reorganization and the parallel development of CI therapy. Front Hum Neurosci 2014;8:396.

54. Bullock K, Won AS, Bailenson J, et al. Virtual reality-delivered mirror visual feedback and exposure therapy for FND: a midpoint report of a randomized controlled feasibility study. J Neuropsychiatry Clin Neurosci 2020;32(1):90–4.

55. Chung DS, Wettroth C, Hallett M, et al. Functional speech and voice disorders: case series and literature review. Mov Disord Clin Pract 2018;5(3):312–6.

56. Baizabal-Carvallo JF, Jankovic J. Speech and voice disorders in patients with psychogenic movement disorders. J Neurol 2015;262(11):2420–4.

57. Duffy JR. Functional speech disorders: clinical manifestations, diagnosis, and management. Handb Clin Neurol 2016;139:379–88.

58. Reiter R, Rommel D, Brosch S. Long term outcome of psychogenic voice disorders. Auris Nasus Larynx 2013;40(5):470–5.

59. Glass SP, Matin N, Williams B, et al. Neuropsychiatric factors linked to adherence and short-term outcome in a U.S. functional neurological disorders clinic: a retrospective cohort study. J Neuropsychiatry Clin Neurosci 2018;30(2):152–9.

60. Jacob AE, Smith CA, Jablonski ME, et al. Multidisciplinary clinic for functional movement disorders (FMD): 1-year experience from a single centre. J Neurol Neurosurg Psychiatry 2018;89(9):1011–2.

61. Aybek S, Lidstone SC, Nielsen G, et al. What is the role of a specialist assessment clinic for FND? lessons from three national referral centers. J Neuropsychiatry Clin Neurosci 2020;32(1):79–84.

62. Jordbru AA, Smedstad LM, Klungsoyr O, et al. Psychogenic gait disorder: a randomized controlled trial of physical rehabilitation with one-year follow-up. J Rehabil Med 2014;46(2):181–7.

63. Demartini B, Batla A, Petrochilos P, et al. Multidisciplinary treatment for functional neurological symptoms: a prospective study. J Neurol 2014;261(12):2370–7.

64. Saifee TA, Kassavetis P, Parees I, et al. Inpatient treatment of functional motor symptoms: a long-term follow-up study. J Neurol 2012;259(9):1958–63.

65. McCormack R, Moriarty J, Mellers JD, et al. Specialist inpatient treatment for severe motor conversion disorder: a retrospective comparative study. J Neurol Neurosurg Psychiatry 2014;85(8):895–900.

66. Jacob AE, Kaelin DL, Roach AR, et al. Motor retraining (MoRe) for functional movement disorders: outcomes from a 1-week multidisciplinary rehabilitation program. PM R 2018;10(11):1164–72.

67. LaFrance WC Jr, Baird GL, Barry JJ, et al. Multicenter pilot treatment trial for psychogenic nonepileptic seizures: a randomized clinical trial. JAMA Psychiatry 2014;71(9):997–1005.

68. Goldstein LH, Mellers JD, Landau S, et al. COgnitive behavioural therapy vs standardised medical care for adults with Dissociative non-Epileptic Seizures (CODES): a multicentre randomised controlled trial protocol. BMC Neurol 2015; 15:98.

69. Sharpe M, Walker J, Williams C, et al. Guided self-help for functional (psychogenic) symptoms: a randomized controlled efficacy trial. Neurology 2011;77(6): 564–72.

70. Hubschmid M, Aybek S, Maccaferri GE, et al. Efficacy of brief interdisciplinary psychotherapeutic intervention for motor conversion disorder and nonepileptic attacks. Gen Hosp Psychiatry 2015;37(5):448–55.

71. Williams IA, Howlett S, Levita L, et al. Changes in emotion processing following brief augmented psychodynamic interpersonal therapy for functional neurological symptoms. Behav Cogn Psychother 2018;46(3):350–66.

72. Sharma VD, Jones R, Factor SA. Psychodynamic psychotherapy for functional (psychogenic) movement disorders. J Mov Disord 2017;10(1):40–4.

73. Kompoliti K, Wilson B, Stebbins G, et al. Immediate vs. delayed treatment of psychogenic movement disorders with short term psychodynamic psychotherapy: randomized clinical trial. Parkinsonism Relat Disord 2014;20(1):60–3.

74. Vermeulen M, de Haan RJ. Favourable outcome without psychotherapy in patients with functional neurologic disorder. J Clin Neurosci 2020;71:141–3.

75. Kawakita K, Okada K. Acupuncture therapy: mechanism of action, efficacy, and safety: a potential intervention for psychogenic disorders? Biopsychosoc Med 2014;8(1):4.

76. Moene FC, Spinhoven P, Hoogduin KA, et al. A randomized controlled clinical trial of a hypnosis-based treatment for patients with conversion disorder, motor type. Int J Clin Exp Hypn 2003;51(1):29–50.

77. Moene FC, Spinhoven P, Hoogduin KA, et al. A randomised controlled clinical trial on the additional effect of hypnosis in a comprehensive treatment programme for in-patients with conversion disorder of the motor type. Psychother Psychosom 2002;71(2):66–76.

78. Voon V, Lang AE. Antidepressant treatment outcomes of psychogenic movement disorder. J Clin Psychiatry 2005;66(12):1529–34.

79. Stone J, Hoeritzauer I, Brown K, et al. Therapeutic sedation for functional (psychogenic) neurological symptoms. J Psychosom Res 2014;76(2):165–8.

80. Dreissen YEM, Dijk JM, Gelauff JM, et al. Botulinum neurotoxin treatment in jerky and tremulous functional movement disorders: a double-blind, randomised placebo-controlled trial with an open-label extension. J Neurol Neurosurg Psychiatry 2019;90(11):1244–50.

81. Garcin B, Mesrati F, Hubsch C, et al. Impact of transcranial magnetic stimulation on functional movement disorders: cortical modulation or a behavioral effect? Front Neurol 2017;8:338.

82. Taib S, Ory-Magne F, Brefel-Courbon C, et al. Repetitive transcranial magnetic stimulation for functional tremor: A randomized, double-blind, controlled study. Mov Disord 2019;34(8):1210–9.

83. Ferrara J, Stamey W, Strutt AM, et al. Transcutaneous electrical stimulation (TENS) for psychogenic movement disorders. J Neuropsychiatry Clin Neurosci 2011;23(2):141–8.

84. Burke MJ, Kaptchuk TJ, Pascual-Leone A. Challenges of differential placebo effects in contemporary medicine: The example of brain stimulation. Ann Neurol 2019;85(1):12–20.

85. Rommelfanger KS. The role of placebo in the diagnosis and treatment of functional neurologic disorders. Handb Clin Neurol 2016;139:607–17.

86. Tolchin B, Baslet G, Suzuki J, et al. Randomized controlled trial of motivational interviewing for psychogenic nonepileptic seizures. Epilepsia 2019;60(5):986–95.

87. Nicholson TR, Carson A, Edwards MJ, et al. Outcome measures for functional neurological disorder: a review of the theoretical complexities. J Neuropsychiatry Clin Neurosci 2020;32(1):33–42.

Printed and bound by CPI Group (UK) Ltd, Croydon, CR0 4YY

03/10/2024

01040402-0008